Sources in the History of Medicine

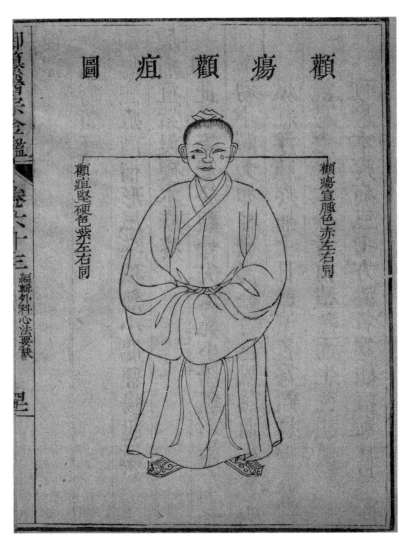

In 1869, the Emperor of China, Tung-ji, presented the U.S. government with 933 volumes of material on the subjects of Chinese herbal medicine and ancient agricultural practices, including the *Yizong Jin-jian,* or *Complete Survey of Medical Knowledge.* This presentation marked the beginning of the Asian Collection in the Library of Congress.

Sources in the History of Medicine

The Impact of Disease and Trauma

EDITED BY
ROBIN L. ANDERSON

Arkansas State University

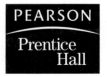

Upper Saddle River, New Jersey 07458

Library of Congress Cataloging-in-Publication Data

Sources in the history of medicine : the impact of disease and trauma / edited by Robin L. Anderson.
   p. ; cm.
  Includes bibliographical references.
  ISBN 0-13-191348-4
  1. Medicine—History.   2. Disease—History.   3. Diseases and history.
  [DNLM: 1. History of Medicine.   2. Communicable Diseases—history. WZ 40 S724 2007]
I. Anderson, Robin L. (Robin Leslie)
  R133.S67 2007
  610.9—dc22

                                2005034127

Editorial Director: Charlyce Jones-Owen
Executive Editor: Charles Cavaliere
Editorial Assistant: Maria Guarascio
Production Liaison: Joanne Hakim
Executive Marketing Manager: Heather Shelstad
Marketing Manager: Emily Cleary
Marketing Assistant: Jennifer Lang
Manufacturing Buyer: Benjamin Smith
Cover Art Director: Jayne Conte
Cover Design: Bruce Kenselaar
Cover Illustration/Photo: Courtesy of the Library of Congress. From Johannes de Ketham's 1495 *Fasciculus Medicinae*, the first printed European general medical text to include illustrations, showing a seated teacher surrounded by Arabic, Jewish, and Greek medical texts. The three patients on the bottom are waiting to have their urine examined.
Director, Image Resource Center: Melinda Reo
Manager, Rights and Permissions: Zina Arabia
Manager, Visual Research: Beth Brenzel
Manager, Cover Visual Research & Permissions: Karen Sanatar
Image Permission Coordinator: Jennifer Puma
Photo Researcher: Rachel Lucas
Composition/Full-Service Project Management: Kelly Ricci, TechBooks/GTS
Printer/Binder: RR Donnelley & Sons Company

Credits and acknowledgments borrowed from other sources and reproduced, with permission, in this textbook appear on page 347.

Pearson Education LTD., London
Pearson Education Singapore, Pte. Ltd
Pearson Education, Canada, Ltd
Pearson Education—Japan
Pearson Education Australia PTY, Limited

Pearson Education North Asia Ltd
Pearson Educación de Mexico, S.A. de C.V.
Pearson Education Malaysia, Pte. Ltd
Pearson Education, Upper Saddle River, New Jersey

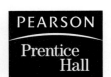

10 9 8 7 6 5 4 3 2 1
ISBN: 0-13-191348-4

Graças a Deus
Thanks be to God

Contents

Chapter Three
CHINA AND INDIA IN ANTIQUITY

Chapter Four
GREECE

Chapter Five
ROME AND BYZANTIUM

Chapter Six
EUROPE, 500–1500   **107**

Chapter Seven
MEDICINE IN THE MUSLIM WORLD AND THE   **130**
AMERICAS, 700–1500

Chapter Eleven
THE NINETEENTH CENTURY: CHANGE AND UPHEAVAL   230

Chapter Twelve
THE TWENTIETH CENTURY: ADVANCES AND CHALLENGES   262

Preface

This reader is not so much about the history of medicine per se as it is a series of glimpses into medical practices and the effects that disease and trauma have had on people throughout history. Although a few readings deal with some of the great discoveries of medical science, the focus is on people—ordinary folks—and how they have dealt with illness, with battlefield injuries and work-related accidents, with childbirth, and with the individuals who provided care and cures for such problems.

What emerges from these readings is a picture of human response to adversity, beginning with the earliest humans and ending with the challenges facing everyone in the twenty-first century. The broad diversity of such responses is due to differences in culture, religion, and worldview, just as much as it is the result of the evolution of the medical arts. People in different cultures at different points in time have reacted to illnesses and injuries in many ways. Yet, some unifying threads can also be found throughout history: the desire to alleviate pain and suffering, the attempts to protect oneself and others from what we now know as infectious diseases, the determination to prolong life. No matter what culture, no matter what century, human beings have had such common goals, and they have looked to their shamans, their physicians, their midwives, and most often themselves to provide assistance in reaching these goals. Methods and means vary enormously during the human experience, but the goals remain relatively unchanged.

This reader covers a wide variety of problems and issues. Predictably, some of the selections are on surgery; on diseases such as smallpox, tuberculosis, and influenza; and on obstetrics and child care. In addition, however, I have included pieces about alcoholism, famine, sports, dentistry, and insanity. The list of health problems that have faced humankind is lengthy, and I have made an effort to include as many as possible. Several selections are designed to give the reader a broader knowledge of non-Western health-care traditions such as the Chinese, Indian, and Muslim. Finally, in the chapters on twentieth- and twenty-first-century medicine, selections were chosen to give the reader a feel for some of the problems facing human populations today, including a broad spectrum of topics from AIDS, to ethical decisions in health care, to the specter of bioterrorism.

Many other topics and issues were not included because of space constraints. If, having read these selections, the reader becomes curious about the human response to disease and trauma and wants to research further, my purpose will have been achieved.

In the interests of readability, all footnotes, citations, abstracts, and bibliographic references have been removed from the readings. Many of the selections have also been edited for length. Should the reader require the deleted information, full citations to the original materials have been included. All dating in this reader conforms to the B.C.E.-C.E. format, designating, respectively, "before the common era" and "the common era."

Acknowledgments

The work on this reader has been a labor of love, with emphasis on both the words *labor* and *love.* It could not have been accomplished without the help of a number of individuals. In particular, I would like to thank Charles Cavaliere of Prentice Hall for having faith in the project and helping to bring it to fruition; Moira Allen for her editorial expertise; Kathleen Riley-King for her fantastic editing job; Wendy Anderson for her hours of typing, copying, and submitting requests for articles; and especially Margarett Daniels, the head of Inter-Library Loan at Arkansas State University, for her tremendous assistance in locating literally several thousand articles considered for inclusion in the reader. To the individuals who reviewed the manuscript—James Whorton, University of Washington; Karol Weaver, Susquehanna University; and Paul Farber, Oregon State University—I also owe many thanks. Finally, I owe a huge debt of gratitude to my History of Medicine class who reviewed and critiqued the manuscript in great detail. Thank you one and all; without your help, this reader could not have been written.

Robin L. Anderson

Sources in the History
of Medicine

Chapter One

Paleopathology and Primitive Medicine

INTRODUCTION

As long as hominids have walked the earth, they have been faced with the threats of accidents and disease, both of which often lead to death. In fact, one theory is that religion developed to explain what was happening to a sick or wounded group member. **Paleopathology,** as the name suggests, is the study of physical evidence of disease and trauma in search of a clear picture of early human afflictions. The paleopathologist must, however, resist the temptation to read too much into the physical evidence. Rarely can motives be extrapolated from the evidence; thus, for example, we cannot assume that early humans drank willow-bark tea to cure a headache. Even though this tea contains the same chemical that is in aspirin, our ancestors may have simply drunk it because it tasted good.

The principal constraint in paleopathology has always been the nature of the evidence: skeletal remains, fossilized feces **(coprolites),** and a relatively few mummified bodies. Whereas recognizing arthritis (probably humanity's oldest affliction), broken bones, and dental damage is relatively easy, determining the nature and impact of diseases such as cancer that primarily affect only soft tissue has been nearly impossible. Tuberculosis is one disease which causes damage in both soft tissue and bony structure, but both pathologies are not always present in the same body.

Nevertheless, modern technology and forensic methods are rapidly expanding our knowledge base about health problems in early humans. Noninvasive methods such as computed tomography (CT) and magnetic resonance imaging (MRI) have allowed us to learn a great deal about mummified cadavers without having to destroy them by opening them. Innovative laboratory testing methods have permitted new hypotheses to be developed about nutrition and growth—for example, by looking at dental enamel erosion patterns and bone densities. Likewise, DNA testing has opened whole new worlds of information. As modern science addresses such questions, dry bones will yield an enormous amount of new information.

However, we are limited in what we can learn by using such methods. We are discovering many new facts about the health problems found among *Homo neanderthalensis*, Cro-Magnon man, and others; but to what extent can we extrapolate their reactions to disease and trauma from such evidence? In the past, researchers often looked at the few extant Stone Age cultures remaining in the modern world and suggested that their reactions would have been similar to their predecessors'. Such leaps of intuition are dangerous at best and often misleading. Contemporary forensic anthropologists must recognize the limitations of the evidence and admit that the cultural response to disease and trauma in the earliest human groups is not yet clearly definable. We are learning a great deal about early humans' afflictions and their diet, living conditions, and social groupings, but as yet we can only guess at the ways in which they responded to the health problems they faced.

TIME LINE

4 million B.P.–8000 B.C.E.*	**Paleolithic Humans**
4 million–2 million B.P.	Australopithecines
2.6 million–1.5 million B.P.	*Homo habilis* (first toolmakers)
2.6 million B.P.	First known stone tool
2 million–200,000 B.P.	*Homo erectus*
500,000 B.P.	First systematic use of fire
200,000 B.P.–8000 B.C.E.	Paleolithic *Homo sapiens*
200,000–30,000 B.P.	*Homo sapiens neanderthalensis*
130,000 B.P.–8000 B.C.E.	*Homo sapiens sapiens*
50,000 B.P.	*H. sapiens sapiens* move into Australia
30,000 B.P.	*H. sapiens neanderthalensis* disappear
30,000 B.P.–8000 B.C.E.	Cro-Magnon man
18,000 B.C.E.	*H. sapiens sapiens* move into Americas
10,000 B.C.E.	First permanent *H. sapiens sapiens* settlements; humans learn to use fire to cast copper and harden pottery
8000–4000 B.C.E.	**Neolithic Humans**
8000	Middle East
7000–5000	Mesoamerica, India
6500	Balkans
6000	Northern China, Egypt
5000	Southeast Asia, southern China
4000	France
3300–500 B.C.E.	**Humanity in the Age of Metals**
3300–1200	Bronze Age
1200–500	Iron Age

*Dates prior to 20,000 B.C.E. ("before the common era") are designated B.P. ("before the present").

Can Paleopathology Provide Evidence for "Compassion"?

K. A. DETTWYLER

Although archaeologists can discover a great deal about ancient humans and their general state of health and nutrition, physical evidence has some limitations. For instance, discerning what was eaten is relatively easy, but reconstructing food distribution patterns is another matter altogether. Likewise, whether abstract information such as ethics and morals can be extrapolated from physical remains is highly debatable. In this reading, the author challenges a romanticized interpretation of such evidence that suggests proof of a sense of compassion existed within Paleolithic groups.

. . . Accepting the necessity of using one's imagination in reconstructing prehistoric behavior, anthropologists have, nevertheless, generally refrained from speculating about the motives that might have prompted such behavior, beyond the obvious ones of human requirements for food, shelter, and safety. They seldom attempt to recreate what past populations thought or felt about what they were doing, and even less often do they offer value judgments about the appropriateness or moral rightness of past behavior.

However, in certain situations, the normally self-imposed constraints on archeological interpretation have been disregarded, and otherwise careful scholars have overstepped the boundaries of reasonable inference. . . . In a number of cases, the recovery from archeological sites of the skeletal remains of individuals with physical impairments has prompted archeologists to claim that the survival of these individuals provides evidence for compassion and moral decency among prehistoric peoples, who would have had to provide food, medical care (however rudimentary), and perhaps transportation for these "handicapped" individuals. . . .

Why should the discovery of individuals with "severe" physical impairments, as reflected in skeletal and fossil evidence, invite speculation about the thought patterns of prehistoric populations and judgments about the moral rightness of past behavior? . . . [T]hese interpretations are based in part on notions of "noble (prehistoric) savages," which are often explicitly advanced to counter the "older stereotypes often found in the popular image of early prehistoric populations.". . . [T]hese interpretations have equally strong roots in modern (albeit unconscious) prejudice against the disabled, by assuming that disabled individuals could not contribute to society and that they survived only because of the "compassion" of nondisabled members of the population. . . .

. . . Shanidar I, discovered by Ralph Solecki, is commonly cited as offering the first evidence for compassion in the human evolutionary record. Dating to the Middle Paleolithic, Shanidar I was an adult male Neanderthal (*Homo sapiens neanderthalensis*), who died at an age between 30 and 45 years. Initially studied by T. Dale Stewart, the Shanidar material was recently reevaluated by Erik Trinkaus. According to Trinkaus, Shanidar I

Reprinted by permission of K. A. Dettwyler, Ph.D., Department of Anthropology, Texas A&M University, from K. A. Dettwyler, "Can Paleopathology Provide Evidence for 'Compassion'?" *American Journal of Physical Anthropology* 84 (1991): 375–84.

"suffered multiple fractures involving the cranium, right humerus, and right fifth metatarsal; and the right knee, ankle, and first tarsometatarsal joint show degenerative joint disease that was probably trauma related."

What did these injuries mean in terms of functional capacity? According to Solecki, "Shanidar I was crippled, with a useless right arm." According to Trinkaus, these injuries meant "paralysis (of the right arm) with hypotrophy/atrophy . . ." and "probably . . . blindness in the left eye."

Solecki concludes that Shanidar I "was at a distinct disadvantage in an environment where even men in the best of condition had a hard time. He could barely forage and fend for himself. . . ." According to Trinkaus, Shanidar I was "one of the most severely traumatized Pleistocene hominids for whom we have evidence" and he was "partially incapacitated by (his) injuries.

In discussing how Shanidar I was treated by the fellow members of the population, Solecki says: ". . . although he was born into a savage and brutal environment, Shanidar I man provides proof that his people were not lacking in compassion. . . . We must assume that he was accepted and supported by his people up to the day he died." He concludes: "the very fact that their lame and wounded (Shanidar Neanderthals I and II) had been cared for in the cave is excellent testimony for communal living and cooperation."

Shanidar I is famous throughout the anthropological literature. . . . [He] was further immortalized by Jean Auel in her book *The Clan of the Cave Bear* where he appears as the character Creb. . . .

. . . The second example comes from the work of David Frayer and his colleagues at the late Upper Paleolithic cave site of Riparo del Romito in Calabria, southern Italy. . . . From the combination of specific skeletal abnormalities, Romito 2 has been diagnosed as having acromesomelic dysplasia, a condition caused by homozygosity for an autosomal recessive allele. This condition is characterized by severe growth deficiency, resulting in dwarfism and marked bowing of the forearm bones, with consequent restricted extension of the elbow. Romito 2's stature is estimated to have been only between 1.0 and 1.3 m. In addition to being short, "the individual could not have extended his elbow fully, but rather was capable of only a 130° extension." . . .

In evaluating Romito 2's level of productivity, Frayer et al. conclude: "this problem must have been a serious handicap in the Palaeolithic, given the demands of subsistence in a rigorous environment and of a nomadic life." . . .

Romito 2 was buried in circumstances suggesting that he was a high-status individual. . . . Gould comments: "other Paleolithic skeletons show evidence of disability after injury or of decrepitude in old age. But the Romito dwarf offers our oldest evidence for the nurturing and protection—presumably at some expense to the group—of a handicapped individual who was profoundly different from his peers and physically disadvantaged from birth. . . . If we consider care of the handicapped (particularly at some cost to caretakers) as a key attribute of humanity, then the Romito people surely practiced compassion at this level."

. . . The third example comes from the Early Archaic site of Windover in Florida, excavated by D. N. Dickel, G. H. Doran, and colleagues from Florida State University. From a cemetery dating to approximately 7,500 BP, they have recovered the remains of a teenage boy with numerous skeletal lesions. . . .

Most of this individual's lesions are attributed either directly or indirectly to spina bifida. **Spina bifida** is a congenital condition in which the neural arches of the spine fail to form properly or to fuse, allowing the spinal cord to protrude beyond the bony protection of the vertebra. . . . [S]ensory deprivation caused by the spina bifida led to lesions and infections in the right tibia and fibula, estimated to have been of at least 2 years' duration at the time of death. . . .

. . . [T]he fact that he was "maintained" at some expense to the community implies that the community could *afford* to provide food for an unproductive member of the group. Doran believes that the boy's survival supports an interpretation that the population lived in a relatively rich environment. . . .

Assumptions Underlying Inferences of "Compassion"

. . . [T]he statements of anthropologists have been used to justify claims in the popular media that the survival of disabled individuals in the past provides evidence for the existence of "compassion" and "moral decency" in these populations.

I maintain that, far from being reasonable interpretations of the skeletal/fossil record, these conclusions clearly overstep the limits of inference from skeletal pathology and contribute to further misunderstandings about the cultural nature of "handicaps." I examine now some of the implicit assumptions that underlie these (and similar) interpretations. . . .

Assumption 1: The vast majority of a population's members are productive and self-sufficient most of the time. . . . In reality, every population has members who are, for varying lengths of time, nonproductive and nonself-supporting. Infants and children are the most obvious group. . . . [I]t is reasonable to assume from ethnographic analogy that older members of the population provide the majority of food, shelter, protection, and other amenities for infants and children for a number of years.

. . . In most populations today, as well as in the past, women in the final stages of pregnancy and in the immediate postpartum period are unlikely to be able to provide all of their own food. . . . Illness and injuries probably incapacitate most members of a population occasionally, if temporarily, and, for those who survive to old age, arthritis and tooth loss suggest at least a diminution of self-sufficiency.

. . . [B]ecause of the helpless state of human newborns and the extended period of human infant dependence, and because humans are subject to a variety of illnesses and injuries, all successful human groups have extensive experience in taking care of nonproductive members.

Assumption 2: Individuals who do not show skeletal/fossil evidence of impairments were not disabled. . . . Evidence for the survival of disabled individuals is sparse in the fossil record, which is one reason why discoveries such as the Romito dwarf and the Windover spina bifida boy attract such attention. However, such individuals may have been less rare than the skeletal evidence suggests, since many impairments do not have skeletal manifestations. Many cases of deafness, blindness (or even mere nearsightedness), mental retardation, and mental illness have no physical manifestations, or only soft-tissue manifestations (for example, river blindness). We have no basis for concluding that disabled individuals or disabling conditions were either more frequent or less frequent in the past than they are today.

Assumption 3: A person with a physical impairment is, necessarily, nonproductive. . . . [W]hat we . . . know suggests that, as with children, disabled people in most societies participate as much as they can in those activities that they are capable of performing. Every society, regardless of its subsistence base, has necessary jobs that can be done by people with disabilities. For example, studies of the !Kung San of the Kalahari and other foragers show us that, even in these groups, not everyone forages or hunts every day for their own food. Food is gathered by adult women for themselves, their spouses, and their children. Food is hunted by adult men and shared among all the members of the group. Activities such as the collection of firewood, the hauling of water, and the gathering of plant foods, food processing . . . and many aspects of child care can be carried out by disabled people with limited mobility. . . .

Disabled members of a society may contribute to it differently from nondisabled members, but they do contribute. Whether or not their disability becomes a "handicap" depends on the reaction of other members of the group, not on the disability itself. . . .

The ethnographic record tells us that societies sometimes take extreme positions with respect to people who are different, including twins or triplets, albinos, people with cleft lip or palate or polydactyly, or people who are mentally ill. In some groups, individuals with abnormalities are feared or hated, and they may even be killed at birth. . . . In other groups, such individuals are revered. . . .

Assumption 4: "Survival" of disabled individuals is indicative of "compassion." . . . There is a wide gap between "survival" and being treated nicely. For all we know, these individuals were ridiculed, teased, taunted, beaten, treated as slaves, physically and emotionally abused, constantly reminded of their differences and shortcomings, and threatened with bodily harm or abandonment. If they were viewed as a "burden" to the group, they may have been reminded of this daily. . . .

. . . We can observe how disabled people are treated today, cross-culturally, and we can study whether cultural attitudes result in a handicap, but we cannot know with any certainty how disabled individuals were treated from archeological remains. As with compassion, cruelty and indifference leave few traces in the archeological record.

. . . Unfortunately, the ethnographic record, including that of our own society, supports the more dismal view of human nature more often than it supports a view of society as compassionate. The archeological record, however, cannot tell us whether disabled individuals were treated with compassion, or with tolerance, or with cruelty.

Assumption 5: Providing for, caring for, and facilitating the survival of a disabled individual is always the "compassionate" thing to do. . . . If keeping disabled individuals alive is evidence of compassion, kindness, and moral decency, then the alternative, that is, not putting forth any effort to keep disabled individuals alive, is, by default, the noncompassionate choice, and evinces a lack of "moral decency." I suggest that this dichotomy between survival/compassion and nonsurvival/noncompassion is not at all clear-cut.

The question of which is the compassionate choice—to expend effort to keep nonnormal individuals alive or to kill them (or, the genteel version, "allow them to die")—is far from being answered, even in the United States. . . . In many societies, infants who are obviously impaired or deformed at birth may either be killed outright or "allowed to die" through the deliberate withholding of food, water, medical care, or all three. . . .

To claim that facilitating the survival of a disabled person necessarily indicates compassion and moral decency . . . suggests a certainty about the moral issues in these situations, which, as

"objective" scientists, we are not justified in claiming. These complex questions of medical ethics and quality of life have not been answered in U.S. society. Speculation about the moral qualities of people who lived thousands of years ago, based on paleopathological analyses of archeological remains, is particularly inappropriate.

Discussion and Conclusions

. . . In the case of Shanidar I, his lack of a right arm and blindness in one eye may have meant that he could not be an effective hunter. He nevertheless might have gotten along quite well by collecting plants, processing food, cooking, and performing other mundane, secular functions. It is not necessary to postulate a shamanistic role for him. If his "useless right arm" was congenital, he would never have known anything different, and, if his blindness occurred after adulthood, it might also have been relatively easy for him to adapt.

For Romito 2, his shortness may have been an advantage in some way we cannot perceive. . . . It is also possible that the rest of the group went off and left Romito 2 behind every time they moved, and he had to follow along by himself, hoping that he could find the group again that night. Or, perhaps he was considered a sign from the gods and was treated very well. . . .

Likewise, the Windover boy may have been able to move around somewhat independently. . . . Perhaps [he] had some sort of crutch or cane, or the group devised a carrying device to pull him around, like a travois. Perhaps he stayed in a semi-permanent camp with a few people—the young, the old, the sick, the newly delivered mothers. Perhaps he was the youngest child in a large family, and his numerous older siblings helped care for him, or perhaps his mother resented him every day of his life and no one talked to him or played with him. Perhaps he was the son of a respected leader, who made other members of the population care for him against their will. Perhaps they were glad when he died. Again, we cannot evaluate these possibilities, because the archeological record does not provide answers to the questions of how individuals were treated or what other people thought of them.

Why have anthropologists and popular writers . . . been so quick to accept this particular perspective on paleopathological and archeological data and to treat it with so little critical thought? Is it because they think that most people still operate under what Dickel and Doran call "older stereotypes often found in the popular image of early prehistoric populations," which consider prehistoric life to have been nasty, brutish, and short? Are they merely trying to project a new image of a "noble (prehistoric) savage" to counteract the older image? That may be their intent. Or, perhaps unconsciously, they have adopted another stereotype, one common in modern Western society, which assumes that disabled people cannot contribute to society and survive only because of the compassion of nondisabled members of the population. This view of disabled people, which is pervasive in the United States, often represents a significant social handicap that individuals must struggle to overcome.

Were disabled individuals rare in prehistoric populations? Were they able to contribute to their own subsistence or to the group's survival? Were they treated nicely? By helping them to survive,

did other members of the population act "compassionately"? I suggest that these questions cannot be answered in archeological contexts, certainly not in the absence of ethnographic information about these same questions in modern contexts. Those who interpret the fossil and archeological record, in their attempts to reconstruct past behavior, need to *think* about the assumptions underlying their interpretations and the implications of their statements. I urge them to be more cautious in their recreations of what life was like for disabled individuals in the past—how they were treated, how other people felt about them, and particularly whether their survival tells us anything about the moral standards of the population.

The paleopathological analysis of skeletal remains can tell us about physical impairment, from which we may be able to infer the extent of an individual's disability. Whether or not an individual was "handicapped" by his disability cannot be determined from archeological evidence alone. To Gould's question, "what, then, can we learn of compassion from a study of bones and artifacts?" the answer must be, "practically nothing."

▲

Cranial Surgery in Ancient Peru

STEPHANIE RIFKINSON-MANN, M.D.

*One of the oldest surgical procedures known involves **trephining,** creating a hole in the skull, usually with stone or metal implements. Although the reasons for performing this procedure are still not well understood, the results are definitely impressive. Long before the use of modern anesthetics and antisepsis, the majority of these patients survived the procedure, as corroborated by healed bone around the edges of the wounds. Although evidence of trephining has been found throughout the world, most cases come from the Peruvian Andes, where it was performed more than twenty-three hundred years ago. Early humans were capable of successfully performing cranial surgery long before the advent of the modern specialty of neurosurgery.*

▲

Reprinted by permission of Lippincott Williams & Wilkins, from Stephanie Rifkinson-Mann, "Cranial Surgery in Ancient Peru," *Neurosurgery* 23, no. 4 (1988): 411–14.

As Ernest Sachs noted, "It is rather extraordinary that neurosurgery, one of the most recent specialties, should have had its beginnings in the neolithic period, long before any written records existed." The oldest known operation is trephining, which was carried out by many cultures in several parts of the world. The practice of trephination among the ancient Incas is of special interest to neurosurgeons because 2000 trephined Peruvian skulls in museums are the best evidence that cranial surgery was performed over 2300 years ago. The oldest American trephined skulls, dating back to 500 BC, were found in Peru near the imperial city of Cuzco and were studied by Paul Broca and others.

Studies have analyzed cranial bone grossly and microscopically. Incisional borders have been examined and bone thicknesses compared. The degree of skull maturation has been determined by the condition of teeth and of cranial sutures to give data on patient populations. Signs of trauma, **osteitis,** osteoma, and bone repair have been recorded. Healing after surgery has been seen at the margin of the trephination and is based on a closing **diploë,** smooth incisional borders, and the presence of osteophytes. Signs of bone repair have been interpreted to mean that these operations were done on live patients who survived years after the procedure. Survival rates were calculated by studying the number of healed openings in trephined skulls. Over 70% show evidence of healing. Some investigators ascribe the substantial survival rate to the sturdiness of the people, writing that their "resistance . . . was simply amazing, some of them having survived five successive trephinings and a dozen or more skull injuries which in others might have been fatal."

Of the 2000 Peruvian skulls in museums, 250 specimens with trephinations were studied extensively. Of these skulls, 171 (68%) were from male and 42 (17%) were from female patients; 37 (15%) were of undetermined sex. Gilbert Horrax noted that signs of trauma in so many male skulls suggested that surgery was undertaken for the wounds of soldiers hurt in hand-to-hand combat. Wilder Penfield suggested that trephination was performed for **subdural hematomas.** Sir Victor Horsley thought that the procedure was carried out for depressed fractures and that they cured focal epilepsies caused by these injuries. Most of the trephinations were performed on the left side, perhaps because trauma inflicted by a right-handed adversary would fall on that side.

The possible military importance of trephination has been suggested by the frequency with which trephined skulls have been found in the burial grounds of Incan fortresses as opposed to the relative paucity of such skulls in the coastal areas known to be inhabited by pacific communities. It has been estimated that 28% to 46% of the trephinations were performed to treat traumatic injuries; however, several investigators have concluded that such estimates are too high. Margins of fractures or other perforations may have been removed at the time of operation, thereby eliminating obvious signs of trauma for which the operation may have been performed, or complete cicatrization of bony margins may have occurred.

Many trephined skulls show no gross abnormality. There is no evidence that pre-Columbian Peruvian trephination was performed to obtain bony amulets to be used as charms. Operations may have been performed to cure cerebral disease. One cause of illness was thought to be disaffection in the spirit world. The patient may have violated a taboo. The spirits revenged by introducing into the body a demon, which had to be let out. Sir William Osler wrote, "[Trephination] was done for epilepsy, infantile convulsions, headache and various cerebral diseases believed to be caused by confined demons to whom the hole gave a ready method of escape."

Another cause of cerebral disorder was thought to arise from the loss of the ethereal image of man. Once separated from the body, illness followed. If there was no way for the spirit to return, the patient died. Horrax suggested that the afflicted may have suffered paralysis, **cerebral palsy,** severe depression, or mental retardation and that trephination would have been used to allow the spirit to return, thereby curing the disease.

There is no indication that any anesthetic beyond a mild intoxicant was used, perhaps potentiated by herbal preparations of datura, yuca, or coca. Sachs wrote that "the common practice of chewing the leaves of Erythroxylon coca . . . may have been used for its anesthetic effect." The most painful aspect, the scalp and periosteal incision, would have already occurred in cases of trauma. The operation may have been performed while the patient was in coma or shock.

Walker, Asenjo, Wilkins, and others have noted that the operation itself followed a definite sequence. The patient may have been in a sitting position or semireclining to reduce blood pooling and to increase the field of vision. The high frequency of **parietal craniectomies** may have been due to the accessibility of the area to the operator, who may have held the head fixed with his left arm or between his knees and then operated with his right hand. From the study of mummies with scalp scars, the incisions seem to have been linear. These were made with chisels of copper, silver, gold, or a mix of these three metals; knives and obsidian lances; or tumis (straight or crescentic blades with a short central T-shaped handle). The cranial openings were recti- or curvilinear, V-shaped in cross section and canoe-shaped as seen from a coplanar angle. They were broad and deep toward the middle and shallow and narrow at the edges. Bone elevation was done by applying a knife or other instrument in lever-like fashion as a fulcrum over one margin, resulting in the edge being splintered, crushed, or undercut. Rough margins were smoothed over by rasping or filing away the bone with an irregularly edged instrument. Modern neurosurgeons, repeating the procedure experimentally on postmortem adult skulls, estimated that one trephination took 30 minutes to an hour.

Three types of Peruvian trephination have been classified according to the shape of the craniectomy: rectangular, cylindrical-conical, and circular. A variation of the last method, the suprainion technique, is distinguished by its consistent location in the wormian "Inca bone." Taveras and Wood suggested that the term "Inca" was used to denote this bony anomaly because of its presumed frequency in Peruvian mummies.

Hemostasis may have been obtained by the application of extracts from the Andean *Ratania* root and *Pumachuca* shrub, rich in tannic acid. The surgeon may have applied beeswax to bone edges and compressed the scalp externally. Scalp margins were joined in some cases by tying the hair across both sides of the cut. The wound may have been sutured; metal needles and cotton thread have been found at burial sites. One 1500-year-old Peruvian skull with signs of recent trephining had a cotton bandage covering the wound.

Little is known about what these primitive surgeons did to prevent infection. Harvey Cushing noted that skulls had been found with gold or silver plates covering the craniectomy, but that the plates were not well tolerated. **Cranioplasties** of mate, coca, gourd, coconut, calabash, or other plants also failed. Few cases of osteomyelitis were found, however. Sachs wrote that the operations were done rapidly because little anesthetic was used. This speed may have played a key role in decreasing infection.

It is hard to believe that the ancient surgeons did not have some understanding of anatomy, as many of their patients survived. Horsley suggested that prehistoric surgeons may have had an idea of localized brain function because many openings were made over the **motor cortex,** "which when irritated gives rise to movements of the opposite side of the body." As noted by Gurdjian, "In some specimens the midline vertex bone is undisturbed as if the operator knew of possible dangers from working in the midline vertex." This understanding of vital brain regions may have been gained by experience when surgeons damaged the venous channels and caused hemorrhage and death. Perhaps such information was related to other operators or training centers in Cuzco or Paracas, where evidence of medical treatment has been found. There is no firm evidence that trephination was performed posthumously in Peru, but it has been suggested that the procedure was practiced by inexperienced surgeons on patients who had died of some cause other than that directly related to the trephination itself to give the young surgeon technical experience.

That trephination was practiced independently in several areas around the world implies that certain practices arise from similar human responses to ideology or need, irrespective of culture or environment. Possibly the people treating such cases recognized the relation between certain syndromes and lesions of the nervous system. Because primitive humans explained disease in magical

terms, critics have sought to discredit the knowledge of medicine that they may have possessed. As Asenjo noted, however, "even the most primitive peoples attributed to the brain the faculty of directing the spiritual and intellectual activity of man." Therapeutic methods often become acceptable depending on their results, whether or not they are understood. Once thought to be effective, they may be used routinely, as trephination is today in the practice of modern neurosurgery.

▲

What Did Our Ancestors Eat?

Stanley M. Garn, Ph.D., and William R. Leonard, Ph.D.

In an era of fast-food restaurants and highly processed foodstuffs, the modern-day diet of affluent societies is not necessarily the most healthy for the human body. Bookstores are full of volumes by proponents of this diet or that, who often base their theories on the premise that, in times past, humans ate more healthily. Thus, if we would only eat as our ancestors did, we would enjoy better health and nutrition. Such a premise is questionable, as this reading clearly states. Our ancestors—whether as far back as the australopithecines of two million years ago or the relatively recent inhabitants of pharaonic Egypt—did not necessarily eat well, and they often suffered from vitamin deficiencies, dental trauma from eating grit, and foodborne illnesses and parasites. The current dietary fads enjoining consumers to eat a more "primitive" and simple diet are based more on a romanticized view of the past than on a realistic appraisal of what our ancestors actually ate.

▲

It is a reasonable notion, consistent with the tenets of evolutionary biology, that the nutritional requirements and dietary needs of contemporary human beings were established in the prehistoric past. It follows that some dietary practices that may be "unhealthy" for contemporary human beings are disadvantageous because we are not adapted to such nutrient excesses or deficiencies. For these reasons we now witness considerable interest in what our ancestors ate

and various attempted reconstructions of the beneficial "diets" our ancestors presumably enjoyed. Inferences as to the diets of fossil hominids and fossil hominoids are equally cited by advocates of megavitamin therapy, by those who urge increased consumption of nondigestible fibers, and by advocates of a high-protein dietary regimen.

Some workers in human nutrition see us as the descendants of foraging and browsing and

Reprinted by permission of International Life Sciences Institute, from Stanley M. Garn and William R. Leonard, "What Did Our Ancestors Eat?" *Nutrition Reviews* 47, no. 11 (1989): 337–44.

fruit-eating ancestors, with a diet necessarily high in ascorbic acid. . . . Others working in the field of human nutrition view contemporary mankind as the recent descendants of animal-hunting, flesh-eating ancestors of the ice age, like the classic Neanderthals or the polar Eskimo, In consequence they view a daily intake of 1 g of quality protein/kg of body weight as far too low, even though it sustains life and allows growth. Still others draw attention to the presumed seed-eaters of our most distant past, or grubbers and gatherers still extant, with diets high in insoluble fiber and stool volumes of remarkable size.

These various dietary models cover a very considerable period in evolutionary time. For the gorilla-like browsing and foraging model, one must assign a time depth of 5–8 million years, before *Homo* and *Gorilla* and *Pan* diverged, according to DNA sequence calculations. That is a long time ago, and we may have made many dietary and nutritional adaptations in the interim. For the presumably seed-eating ancestral model, hominoids but not necessarily hominids, a time depth of 1–2 million years is now tenable, if we assume that they were our ancestors. For the animal-hunting, cold-climate Neanderthals, who were of our genus and even of our species, we assume a time depth of 50,000 years into the late Pleistocene. These are very different models and very different taxa, even assuming that they are all in our direct ancestral line. In the Holocene, i.e., the recent postglacial period, there have been ever so many groups of human beings, subsisting on very different dietaries. Now we ask, "Which are our 'ancestors' and what did they eat?"

Because our early ancestors lived before the days of commercial food processing and before the addition of preservatives, coloring agents, extenders, and antioxidants, their diets have been described as "simple," "natural," and "safe." Their dietaries, presumably of mixed animal and vegetable origin, have also been described as "prudent," a term of recent introduction. However, it is probable that pit-stored and pot-stored grains may not have been safe under all circumstances, nor were animal flesh and fish eaten by early humans free of parasites. Caloric adequacy cannot be presumed in all seasons, for all mankind, nor can we assume the postulated "dietary prudence" with respect to animal fats or vitamins A and C.

In theory, fossil dentitions should provide insight into dietary habits (and therefore the kinds of foods and their volume). In a way this theory is true, since the hominoids and early hominids had larger dental arcades than we do and far larger food-processing surfaces. However, even the *erectus* fossils did not have long, projecting gorilla-like canines or the highly convoluted wrinkled molar surfaces that suggest dependence on roots, shoots, and large leaves. Our dentitions now are at most indicative of an omnivorous but relatively soft diet and they are equally suitable for gnawing at bones, gorging on fruit, or consuming fried rice, boiled wheat, and unleavened cakes. However, and despite their more specialized dentitions, chimpanzees prove to be far more omnivorous in the wild than we had earlier reason to imagine. So we must turn to the faunal and floral remains associated with past hominids and hominoids to provide some partial answers.

Hominoids, Hominids, and Their Diets

The Australopithecines, from South Africa, were once viewed as proto-hominid hunters of game because of the animal bones found at some of their habitation sites. Now they are relegated to the status of scavengers, who dragged other kills back home and deposited the remains in rather untidy fashion. Moreover, studies of the microwear on their dentitions suggest a wide utilization of available foods, attested to by the scratches and abrasions on their dental enamel.

There were several kinds of Australopithecines, the larger and more robust forms . . . and the smaller and more gracile kinds. . . . The number of different Australopithecine genera and species is unknown, for they lived during a long period of rapid evolutionary change when species multiplied. Exactly which was most nearly ancestral to us is still a matter of reasonable debate, but some had unusually large brain size relative to body size and merged nicely into *erectus* proportions. They were erect-walking, unlike earlier primates, and had some capacity to use or fashion tools.

The Australopithecine diet can best be described as mixed, certainly impressing a heavy chewing load on their large dentitions and oversized dentofacial complexes. However, these hominids were not hunters but spent much of their time in search of food, including carcasses left by true predators. As "ancestors" they were much more recent than the chimpanzee-like ancestor of 5 million or more years ago and more nearly omnivorous. They certainly had the ability to masticate and digest a large variety of foods, and had a goodly proportion of grit in their diets. Inferences as to the Australopithecine diet come from observations of scavenging among modern hunter-gatherers and non-human primates and from analyses of animal bone assemblages found associated with early hominoid findings.

Our Genus but Not Our Species

Next in order of appearance, in physical characteristics and in relationships to us, came the *erectus* fossils of our genus but not of our species, which we first came to know as "Pithecanthropus" from Java. The time frame for *Homo erectus* is early Pleistocene, the original habit of *erectus* was Africa. . . . Below the neck they were nearly indistinguishable from us. Above the neck they had much larger brains than the Australopithecines, but their brain volume (1100 cc) was less than ours. Their large dentitions exceed those of any living group of humans, and their teeth were attached to jaws of comparable size, with muscle attachments well up on the cranium. . . .

Homo erectus was a hunter who used stone tools and had the ability to make fires and presumably to cook or roast in the flames or coals. We therefore grant the *erectus* fossils a considerable year-round supply of animal flesh, but we have no knowledge of how much vegetation was also dug, pulled, picked, or stripped. Wear on *erectus* dentitions, which is considerable, appears to have been heightened by grit in the diet; these observations suggest plant sources for much of the food and no great fastidiousness in dining.

Climatic data and faunal associations indicate that these earlier people of our genus were not browsers. They correspond to the notion of "early man" as hunters, at least in part, and their generous intakes of nonnutrient materials certainly included dirt and small gravel. It is only a guess as to whether they cooked or processed in any way whatever vegetation they collected.

Changing Diets of the Later Pleistocene

By the late Pleistocene *erectus* hominids had become extinct and people of our species (*Homo sapiens*) made successive appearances. They brought with them increasingly sophisticated technologies and distinctively different dietaries, ultimately including stone-ground wild grains and presumably some sort of hoe-cakes baked on rocks or ashes.

The Neanderthals . . . were rather widely distributed—from Germany and France, eastward into Russia and the Middle East, and thence to North Africa. They were cold-climate hunters of large game and presumably subsisted primarily on game during the coldest periods. They were the mighty hunters we once imagined, although the extent of dependence on fruits and roots in season is still problematic. They were big-brained hominids, often larger than we in brain size, and by no means were they devoid of the niceties of life, including (apparently) burial of the dead and the ability to care for the crippled and the elderly to a respectably advanced age.

Their cooking techniques appear to have included "earth-ovens" . . . constructed rather like a barbecue pit or a Hawaiian luau or a New England clambake. The Neanderthals . . . had the ability to slow-cook tough meat to chewability, and they did subsist on a diet rather high in animal protein. We presume that vitamin C may have been in short supply during the long, cold winters of the ice age.

After the Neanderthals, with or without genetic admixture, came the people of the Upper Paleolithic and the Mesolithic. . . . They hunted, though they sought small mammals more than did the Neanderthals; they dug and foraged and grubbed and picked berries. They also developed the capacity to gather wild grains by use of very serviceable wooden scythes set with little pointed flakes (microliths), thus taking advantage of the wild grains that ripened each summer. They ground these grains on stone grinding blocks, and presumably baked the coarse flour as cakes, scones, or unleavened bread.

These people of the Upper Pleistocene, and later those of the Mesolithic, were our immediate ancestors, no longer hunters exclusively and with whole-grain products and a variable amount of roots, fruits, leafy vegetables, and nuts in their diet. We must grant them a mixed diet, with animal fat providing a smaller proportion of their food energy than was probably true for the Neanderthals. They still lacked pottery and therefore the capacity to make gruel, or potage, but they may have employed stone-boiling (in animal skins) and may have made a kind of haggis (mixing meat products and cereal grains).

Advent of Agriculture and Diminution in Size

The advent of agriculture is lost in antiquity and so are the reasons why different groups took up the cultivation of roots, shoots, tubers, fruits, nuts, leafy vegetables, and seed grains. Since even before agriculture some wild grains were harvested with scythe and sickle and then sprouted close to habitation sites, it is reasonable to guess how formal grain-growing began. However, while the origins of agriculture are debated, the consequences are clear. Grain growing in particular allowed population expansion (in fact it demanded the cooperative behavior of entire groups). Villages, even

towns, grew with the grain fields, allowing the emergence of administrators and demanding defense forces for protection. While the sizes of populations grew, in permanent habitation sites the size of individuals often became smaller, a point that merits amplification. . . .

Grains, in particular, could be stored, providing a food reserve from one harvest to the next and assuring a more constant energy reserve year-round. Grain growing and many other forms of agriculture necessitated the cooperative labor of men, women, and children to plant, to weed, to protect against animals, and then to gather, grind, and store. Children formed an important part of the labor force, at cost to their own growth, as is true in many parts of the world today.

American archaeologists, in particular, observe a diminution in body size associated with the advent of maize agriculture and further deteriorations coincident with its intensive cultivation. They cite such evidence as an apparent increase in the number of radio-opaque (**Harris**) **lines** seen in the skeletons, . . . [which] may suggest iron-deficiency or diminished availability of vitamin C. There are also well-documented growth deficiencies, including protein-energy malnutrition, that stem from single-crop agriculture. We are aware of many problems of growth and reproduction that arise from the phytates in wheat and other grains, reducing the availability of iron and zinc. Sensitivity to wheat gluten is another problem, most prevalent now in Wales and Ireland.

Of course, agriculture itself is not to blame, but rather the departure from a mixed diet derived from a variety of sources. However, intensive single-crop agriculture is a natural response to growing population sizes and limited land, especially where the climate allows several crops each year. The answer to "What did our ancestors eat?" may be mostly maize or mostly wheat or mostly barley or mostly yams or mostly manioc, each with its own nutritional limitations.

The advantage of agriculture is also the ability to store grain, legumes, or other seeds in pits or pots against future need. In many parts of the

American Southwest a two-year reserve was considered necessary. However, pit-stored and pot-stored grains and legumes are subject to losses inflicted by insects and rodents. Furthermore, if such foods are improperly dried or exposed to unseasonable moisture, they are subject to fungal infestations and contamination by various toxins. **Ergotism** and **aflatoxin**-derived diseases are possible disadvantageous consequences of grain agriculture.

All of our great cultures or civilizations have come from an agricultural base. Some of us have been grain eaters for 10,000 years. Even today, few Americans gain nearly as much food energy from flesh and milk products as from processed grains. However, agriculture has had its price in diminished body size. . . . For those of us of European, Middle Eastern, or Asiatic ancestry, our ancestors ate mostly grain. The potato was a very recent introduction in Europe, and the Potato Famine of the [19th] century is a further lesson on the shortcomings of agricultural dependence on a single crop and on what happens when that crucial crop fails.

Drought, Famine, and Cyclical Starvation

Most readers . . . are quite insulated against seasonal and cyclical variations in food availability and in the intakes of specific nutrients. Only fresh berries and some fruits may be temporarily absent from our stores, but we can replace them with frozen or canned varieties. We do not have to eat much more in winter to compensate for heat lost from our bodies, and (except for the gardeners among us) we do not exert more energy in seasonal food gathering or agricultural labor. . . . However, third-world people still experience seasonal variations in food availability and in the intakes of specific nutrients, as did nearly all of our immediate ancestors and the hunting and gathering and foraging humans of the past.

We readers . . . are also well protected against cyclical variations in food availability due to drought, excessive rainfall, or occasional winter kill. Our foods come from many geographic areas, we import a surprisingly large proportion of our food, and our storage facilities hold a multiyear supply of grains. However, year-to-year differences in crop yields, recurrent dryness and floods, and extended runs of adverse weather make for precarious food supplies in much of the world as well as in our recent historic past. We recall crop failures in England, the "Little Ice Age" (which lasted until the mid-1800s), and the "Seven Lean Years" recounted in the Bible. Once verdant areas of the Southwest are now near-deserts. Arabia was once "Eden." Long-term changes in rainfall and temperature have affected all of our ancestors and their access to food.

When we report energy and nutrient intakes for any population, it is important also to record the season of the year. High-season intakes may be double those of the low season. Some nutrients, particularly ascorbic acid and the carotenoids in temperate climates, may be in short supply during part of the year. . . . Growth and development are obviously most affected by seasonal lows, and the low-season intakes may directly determine the size attained. Fertility, too, may be seasonal and most affected by low-season availability of food. Fewer conceptuses will come to term or reach a viable birthweight if food is restricted in the later months of pregnancy. Most agricultural peoples experience such seasonal variations in food availability, and so do hunters and gatherers. Bushmen in Africa lose considerable weight and fat during the rainy season and regain both when dry weather returns and there are more plants to gather and use. American Indians who lived by the hunt experienced seasonal differences in weight and so did the animals they hunted. Tropical forests are not equally productive of fruits and roots the year round. . . .

When we attempt to reconstruct the diets of hunters, hunter-gatherers, diggers, and foragers (hominid or hominoid), seasonal variations in food availability must be kept in mind, and so must seasonal and cyclical variations in fat weight or percentage fat and in the size of the lean body mass as well.

Poorer and Richer

In general, the more affluent or the politically favored had more access to food and were protected by rank, status, and wealth against seasonal variations in availability of food, especially animal fats and animal protein. Many recent studies . . . document the much smaller seasonal variability in foods consumed by the more affluent and the greater cyclic disparity in foods available to the poor. Size and growth rates of the children, therefore, reflect the low-season intakes of the poor. Although we cannot project backwards over the entire history of humankind, such differences surely existed in predynastic Egypt, in Meso-America, and in Asia. Dimensional differences between the nobility and the peasants are obvious in European skeletal material and apparently reached their maximum in early Victorian times. Burial mounds from Illinois to Tennessee also indicate the nutritional advantages of higher social status. The rich or the nobles did get the gravy, even in the prehistoric Americas.

The question of what our ancestors ate, therefore, represents more than just the level of food technology and the shift to food production rather than food gathering. Seasonal variations must be considered, including the length of the low season and the extent to which available resources were diminished. Human beings must have adapted, albeit imperfectly, to low-season dietary and nutritional deficits. Longer-term food restrictions, of climatic origin, must have had a major impact on the elderly, on the young, and on pregnant women. Moreover, we cannot assume that most populations were strictly egalitarian, allotting unto each according to his nutritional needs. By right of birth, accomplishment, or valor some were accorded an extra share (or took it by force). Some men had multiple wives, a custom allowing longer birth-spacing and therefore more viable progeny, each more likely to survive.

Our ancestors' diet, therefore, is not just a function of evolutionary time and of whether they hunted or gathered or planted, or whether they ate seeds or tubers or game, but also is a function of differences in food availability and of the duration of droughts and famines. Moreover, what the Neanderthals or the Australopithecines ate may be less relevant to our requirements than what was eaten in ancient Anatolia, Thessaly, Indonesia, the European city-states, or medieval towns. For some of us at least, when our ancestors acquired wheat instead of oats or barley may be far more relevant than whether we are most directly descended from hunters or gatherers or scavengers or whether we trace our ancestry to browsers and fruit eaters in some Miocene tropical forest.

What Natural, Healthy, or "Prudent" Diet?

. . . Even for the Neanderthal hunters of the late Pleistocene, who subsisted on a high-protein diet out of necessity, the amount of seasonal energy supplied by carbohydrates is conjectural, as is that supplied by animal fats. The game was lean by contemporary standards of the U.S. Department of Agriculture, but we do not know whether the Neanderthals gorged on the fat or trimmed it off. Eaton and Konner have published some estimates of the fossil diet, having decided first upon an arbitrary energy intake and then having assigned a "mixed" diet including fruits, flesh, and leaves. Not surprisingly, they then deemed their "primitive" diet both adequate and "healthy."

Obviously, most of the time (excluding famines, shortages, and off-season lows), the energy intake at most periods in the past was sufficient for growth and reproduction. . . .

How past dietaries bore on chronic and debilitating diseases is conjectural, given the abbreviated lengths of life. So we cannot assume that Australopithecines were free of colorectal cancer or that the people of the Mesolithic did not suffer from hypertension. Calcium intakes may have been low for the massive meat eaters, unless they chewed bones and ate fish whole. They may also have experienced symptoms of scurvy in the late winter; we know that the hunters of the North American plains showed signs of vitamin C deficiency.

The safety of the diets of our early ancestors is a further question, given animal parasites (and insufficient cooking), toxins resulting from poor storage of food, cycad neurotoxins, toxins and neurotoxins resulting from inadequate preparation of food, and the occasional inclusion of toxic plants mixed with those gathered in the wild. For the early miners of metals, ochre, and other pigments, heavy metal contaminations were an occupational hazard. Shellfish eaters of the past also had to contend with "red tides."

Although we think of early man as accustomed to a low-sodium intake, at least inland and at higher elevations, salt springs, salt outcroppings, and salt caves were discovered by human beings early and were exploited or mined for millennia. . . . Sea salt entered into trade channels early in the Neolithic and was traded hundreds of miles inland. Though wood ashes served as a low-sodium and high-potassium condiment for the Indians of the Southwest, some of our cultivated plants, including beets and carrots, do provide as much as 200 mg of sodium per edible portion. Some of our ancestors may have had a considerable sodium intake, even before salt was regularly used for the preservation of fish and meats.

It is part of our intellectual tradition to romanticize the past, both so-called Natural Man and an imaginary time in the past when people were presumably healthy and happy subsisting on unprocessed foods. Ever so many food regimens, including that suggested by Graham . . . and the natural-food regimen developed by Dr. Kellogg of the Battle Creek Sanatorium, have been hailed as a return to our early diets. In reviewing what we know about our ancestors of the more recent and more distant past, it is difficult to identify any one dietary that may represent our specific adaptation. In length of time, measured in millions of years, the diet of the scavenging Australopithecines may perhaps be designated as ours. . . . For most of us, originating in Europe or Asia, a diet high in carbohydrate and grain phytates (but low in animal protein and animal fat) may be the diet to which we had become accustomed, though not necessarily adapted. Except for the polar Eskimo, a diet high in animal fat is not in our gastrointestinal tradition, nor, except for the Aleut and Indians of the Northwest, is a diet high in fish oils with salmon at every meal.

Past foods may have been unprocessed and free from pesticides and additives, but they were not necessarily safe, before or after cooking. Parasites lurked in undercooked meats, fungal infestations contaminated grains in the fields and during storage, heavy metals leached out of decorated pottery, cooked legumes held their own dangers, and cyanides remained in poorly processed tubers. While our immediate ancestors were not exposed to cycad toxicity and its long-term neurologic consequences, they did not always enjoy enough food, an adequate protein intake, or reasonable levels of many vitamins the year-round. However, we can grant them a higher intake of fiber, with possible consequences to calcium availability and protein utilization.

▲

Disease in Antiquity

The Case of Cancer

Marc S. Micozzi, MD, PhD

One of the hotly contested topics in paleopathology is the existence and prevalence of cancer in premodern populations. Early research seemed to indicate that cancers could be detected in both

Reprinted from Marc S. Micozzi, "Disease in Antiquity," *Archives of Pathology and Laboratory Medicine* 115 (1991): 838–43.

bony and soft tissue remains, but those results are now questionable. Investigations into the antiquity of cancer showcase a number of the problems involved in diagnosing disease in ancient cultures. Original written sources have often been mistranslated, preservation of remains can be compromised by mineral leaching and decomposition, and differential diagnoses such as trauma and inflammation must be considered. In addition, an individual's socioeconomic status may influence everything from his or her age at death to the means of preservation, which makes generalizations precarious. As new technology and methodologies are developed, along with a better understanding of disease processes, earlier statements about the incidence of cancer appear to need to be revised.

▲

Many medical textbooks begin with words to the effect that cancer has been known since earliest times. . . . Such statements are based, for example, on Egyptian medical papyruses that date from 3000 BC, making reference to what has been translated by 19th century Victorian Egyptologists without medical training as "tumors." . . . Modern translations of Egyptian papyruses . . . often reveal not cancer at all, but tumors in the traditional Latin sense of the word "swelling," which can be due to any of a number of causes. . . . There is little or no hard evidence of cancer in antiquity.

. . . A frequent counterargument is that cancer is primarily a disease of old age . . . and since people did not live to old age in antiquity, they did not live long enough to get cancer. . . . If bone neoplasia were common in antiquity, we should observe it in ancient bones. . . . Regarding soft-tissue remains to detect other cancers, Egyptian mummies provide an abundant source of preserved soft tissues. . . . If cancer were common in antiquity, we should be able to detect it in ancient . . . mummies. . . .

Why Study Cancer in Antiquity?

. . . Dietary and life-style patterns of human populations that have changed through time are also thought to have significant implications for the health of human populations. Development of a **diachronic** perspective on the antiquity of cancer in human populations that are undergoing demographic transition provides additional descriptive information about the possible influences of diet, life-style, and other environmental factors on cancer through time.

How the Antiquity of Cancer Can Be Studied

Three types of descriptive observations are available to help build a diachronic perspective on the antiquity of cancer. The first category of evidence comes from human and animal remains, consisting primarily of skeletal remains that may or may not have undergone **diagenesis** (fossilization), as well as significant accumulations of soft-tissue remains. . . . Some of the so-called fossil evidence of ancient cancers, reported by luminaries in the new field of anatomic pathology in the 1800s, has not been borne out as representing examples of malignant neoplasms when reexamined with the use of modern techniques of diagnosis in the 20th century. . . .

The second category of evidence comes from ancient clay tablets, papyruses, texts, and other documents that purportedly report ancient cases of cancer therein. . . . [M]any of these texts, . . . [which] came under serious scrutiny in Europe . . . , were often acquired by Victorian gentlemen who either translated or had them translated by scholars of antiquity with little or no medical or scientific background or training. . . .

The third category of evidence comes from early demographic and statistical information. . . . Such medical and vital statistics, collected by the state for official purposes, may or may not have been accompanied by data on employment, housing, lifestyle, nutrition, etc. . . .

Preservation of Human and Animal Remains

. . . The study of skeletal remains provides information on diseases of bone, as well as non-bone diseases, provided they leave the slightest traces on the skeleton. . . . [S]keletal remains also provide a permanent record of primary bone **neoplasms,** as well as **metastatic** cancers from other primary sites. . . . In any case of unequivocal diagnosis, all ancient diseases have appeared to be morphologically similar to their modern forms throughout 20 years of paleopathologic studies. . . . It seems reasonable to assume that if cancer exists in ancient skeletal remains, we should know what it looks like when subjected to modern analysis. Such remains can be subjected to modern techniques of clinical diagnosis, including **roentgenography** and other imaging studies, . . . [and] microscopic and ultrastructural pathologic analysis, as well as trace element studies. . . .

In addition, . . . there are certain conditions under which soft tissues may also be preserved after death. . . . Post-mortem preservation of tissue is essentially a competition between decomposition and desiccation. Desiccation occurs naturally due to environmental conditions that commonly exist in . . . deserts [and] . . . can also be facilitated by freezing . . . and by cultural processes of **evisceration** and chemical treatment. . . .

Preservation of soft tissues also may occur under natural conditions, where tissues remain in which the diagnosis of cancer could be readily made if present. . . . Metastatic tumors are . . . preserved and remain recognizable. Therefore, if physical evidence of cancer exists in ancient human and animal remains, it should be preserved and relatively recognizable within the bone or soft tissue that remains.

Paleopathologic Evidence from Human and Animal Remains

Primary malignancies of bone have not been positively identified among extinct animals. . . . The earliest example of a suspected neoplasm came from the fossilized remains of a large dinosaur . . . from the . . . Mesozoic era. . . .

The next oldest example is a benign osteoma . . . of a mosasaur . . . from the later Cretaceous period. . . .

Perhaps the earliest example of a suspected malignant tumor in a hominid was described in the Kanam mandibular fragment from East Africa, probably of the Lower or Middle Pleistocene. . . . [H]owever, two noted authorities on paleopathology expressed serious reservations about a malignant diagnosis, favoring the possibility of trauma and low-grade inflammation. . . .

. . . [A]n osteosarcoma was diagnosed in the right ulna of an adult man from the Neolithic period. . . . Several reports relate to possible multiple **myeloma** in late Neolithic crania . . . ; however, insufficient description is given to render independent diagnosis. . . . The malignant character of two lesions of a skull from . . . France was questioned, based on gross and radiographic observation, . . . [and] "carcinomatous" destruction of bone in the temporal area of a skull from a Winchester (England) Saxon burial . . . , as well as multiple myeloma in a medieval youth from Scarborough, England, have all been attributed to postmortem **taphonomic** changes. . . .

Ancient Egypt and Nubia

. . . [M]eaningful occurrences of neoplasms in ancient Egypt have not been established. Initial diagnosis of an osteosarcoma in a femur from the cemetery of the Gizeh Pyramids . . . has been more recently reinterpreted as a benign osteochondroma. . . .

. . . In the relatively recent Byzantine Period, cases of malignant disease that involved the nasopharynx and rectum, respectively, were suggested by Elliot-Smith and Dawson on the basis of destructive lesions in the base of the skull and sacrum. . . .

Changes in disease patterns were observed in ancient Nubia from 350 BC to 1400 AD, with up to 12 malignant neoplasms reported for this later period.

Among 222 skulls that were collected from a vast Coptic cemetery near El-Barsha from the early Christian period in Egypt . . . , five lesions were observed that possibly were consistent with nasal, oral, and other carcinoma.

Ancient Middle East

A skull from the Tepe Hessar site of Iran (3500 to 3000 BC) showed destruction of the left maxillary alveolus and antral wall and was cited . . . as an example of primary carcinoma. . . .

The New World

. . . [T]he search for cancer in antiquity may be limited to the pre-Columbian period in the New World, since the arrival of Columbus was associated with dramatic changes in life-style and marked the beginning of an evolution into disease patterns that are associated with the modern world.

. . . Two cases of multiple myeloma have . . . been reported in skeletal remains of an adult male and of a 10-year-old child. It is more likely that the lesions of the child represented secondary **neuroblastoma** or another childhood disease. . . .

In a survey of the mummies of Ica, Peru, representing five different pre-Columbian cultures that dated from 600 BC, no evidence of malignant neoplasms was found. However, . . . investigators recorded a metastatic tumor in the skeleton of a female from the Tiahuanco period of Chile.

. . . The skeletons of several pre-Columbian mummies from Chancay, and Chongos, Ica, Peru, were thought to show evidence of malignant melanoma metastatic to bone, perhaps related to the high altitude of these sites in the Andes Mountains and increased exposure to UV solar radiation.

In Canada, the earliest known human remains (at least 7500 years ago) showed no evidence of primary or secondary bone tumors. . . .

. . . Steinbock found evidence for metastatic carcinoma in two Alaskan Eskimo skulls (500 to 1500 AD) held in the Smithsonian Institution, Washington, DC, and Cassidy observed probable malignant neoplasms in the mandible of a Sadlermiut Eskimo from the historic period.

Documentary Evidence for Cancer in Antiquity

. . . The Edwin Smith papyrus (approximately 1800 BC), Ebers papyrus (approximately 1550 BC), and Kahun papyrus (approximately 1750 BC) are representative of Egyptian medical papyruses. . . . The Ebers papyrus has a series of prescriptions that are believed to be the remains of a "book on tumors," which deals with tumors and swellings. These tumors appear to have consisted of benign ganglionic masses, polyps, sebaceous cysts, varicose veins, and aneurysms. . . . The word "tumor" appears frequently but always in the sense of swelling. The legendary rumor that malignant melanoma was described in the Ebers papyrus is apparently apocryphal. . . .

The Greek Dioscorides in the first century AD used a drug made from autumn crocus . . . and wrote that "the plant . . . should be soaked in wine and administered to dissolve tumors . . . and growths . . . not yet making pus." Dioscorides' terms . . . may have included malignant neoplasms, but their use clearly was not restricted to malignant conditions. Galen . . . and the Byzantine physicians used the term *onkos* to cover all types of swellings, tumors, and lesions. Galen's Greek term *karkinos* . . . could not have exclusively been applied to malignant neoplasms.

In ancient India, medical conditions were described in the ***Rigveda*** . . . , *Ayurveda*, ***Ramayana***, and other texts, . . . [but] . . . the writings in the ancient texts cannot be verified against material remains.

Neck tumors, mentioned in the ***Vedas***, were probably endemic goiter. . . . The physician Sushruta . . . compiled a surgical treatise in which a chapter is devoted to *arbuda*, ie, glands and tumors. Here, *arbuda* is a swelling with characteristics that may implicate a malignant process. . . .

. . . Sushruta described cancers of the lip, alveolus, tongue, palate, and pharynx, manifesting "lotuslike" growths. . . . Approximately 20 diseases of the female breast and genital organs are described, but none are consistent with cancer of the uterus, ovaries, or breast. . . .

Cancer in Modern Societies

Modern primate populations and contemporary societies around the world that follow a traditional life-style may also provide insights into the origins of human cancer. No cancer was observed among diseases of wild apes, for example. Several diseases are also characteristically uncommon among populations following a traditional life-style, including **myocardial infarction** and carcinoma of the lung. Adenocarcinoma . . . that involves the breast, colon, pancreas, and prostate also appears to be rare in traditional societies.

On the other hand, as reliable modern data were collected, it was recognized that oral and nasopharyngeal cancers are relatively common in parts of Africa and China. These patterns in contemporary Asian and African populations may be related to evidence for oral and nasopharyngeal cancers in ancient Egypt and India as documented in human remains and medical texts. However, ancient evidence for the modern so-called cancers of civilization remains elusive or simply nonexistent in examinations conducted around the world during the [late nineteenth to late twentieth] century.

Conclusion

Understanding postmortem preservation and transformation of human and animal remains is important in interpreting the case for cancer in antiquity. When historically suspected "cancer cases" are interpreted in light of current knowledge of postmortem artifacts, and utilizing modern diagnostic criteria, little evidence for malignant neoplasms in antiquity remains.

Those few cases of suspected malignancy that cannot be disproved are consistent with nasopharyngeal carcinoma or other cancers that remain common throughout the Third World today. Those cancers that are common in the modern industrialized world have left no traces of their existence in prehistory and early human civilizations. . . .

KEY TERMS

Aflatoxin, 14 • Cerebral palsy, 8 • Coprolites, 1 • Cranioplasties, 9 • Diachronic, 17 • Diagenesis, 17 • Diploë, 8 • Ergotism, 14 • Evisceration, 18 • Harris lines, 13 • Hemostasis, 9 • Metastatic, 18 • Motor cortex, 9 • Myeloma, 18 • Myocardial infarction, 20 • Neoplasms, 18 • Neuroblastoma, 19 • Osteitis, 8 • Paleopathology, 1 • Parietal craniectomies, 9 • *Ramayana,* 19 • *Rigveda,* 19 • Roentgenography, 18 • Spina bifida, 4 • Subdural hematomas, 8 • Taphonomic, 18 • Trephining, 7 • *Vedas,* 19

QUESTIONS TO CONSIDER

1. What is compassion? Is it culturally defined? Can its definition change with time? Or, is it a universal concept that crosses barriers of time, space, and culture? Can an act considered compassionate in one culture be considered uncompassionate in another? Is

compassion a luxury affordable only in affluent societies? Can you think of a compassionate act, as judged by contemporary society, that might have been deemed a lack of compassion in the past?

2. A procedure as tricky as opening a human skull and exposing the brain would not have been performed without careful consideration. Even today, such a procedure is not undertaken lightly. What reasons might the ancient Peruvians have had for trephining? To what would you credit their high success rate? Does knowledge of this procedure change your mental picture of the medical and surgical abilities of early humans? How?

3. Having read the articles in this chapter, what do you see as the greatest pitfalls in the attempt to shed light on the epidemiological picture of early humans? How can researchers avoid such problems?

4. A question nonhistorians often ask about various controversies over the interpretation of historical facts is "So what?" The same question might be asked about debates in forensic anthropology or medicine over the identity of ancient diseases. What is the importance of ascertaining the presence of cancer in prehistoric humans? What are the ramifications of finding cancer in these populations? Is this question purely intellectual, or relevant to the real world?

5. In the reading on cancer in antiquity, the author raises the criticism that nineteenth-century publications on the topic were not written by men with medical backgrounds. Does this fact alone invalidate their findings? Can the history of medicine be written only by medical doctors? What does the historian, often without a solid grounding in anatomy, physiology, or pathology, bring to the advancement of medical history?

RECOMMENDED READINGS

Aufderheide, Arthur C., and Conrado Rodriguez-Martin. *The Cambridge Encyclopedia of Human Paleopathology*. Cambridge: Cambridge University Press, 1998.

Cockburn, Thomas Aidan, Eve Cockburn, and Theodore A. Reyman, eds. *Mummies, Disease & Ancient Cultures*. 2nd ed. Cambridge: Cambridge University Press, 1998.

Diamond, Jared. *Guns, Germs, and Steel: The Fates of Human Societies*. New York. Norton, 1999.

Greenblatt, Charles, and Mark Spigelman, eds. *Emerging Pathogens: Archaeology, Ecology and Evolution of Infectious Disease*. Oxford: Oxford University Press, 2003.

Majno, Guido. *The Healing Hand: Man and Wound in the Ancient World*. Cambridge, MA: Harvard University Press, 1975.

Roberts, Charlotte, and Keith Manchester. *The Archaeology of Disease*. 3rd ed. Ithaca, NY: Cornell University Press, 2005.

Chapter Two

The Middle East in Antiquity

Introduction

The great civilizations of the ancient Fertile Crescent are famous for their urban development, their complex religious traditions, and, above all, their writing. Medical practices developed alongside the other advances, which produced in Egypt, Mesopotamia, and Palestine a concrete set of rules and formulas by which to treat the sick and injured. In Egypt and Mesopotamia, the practice of medicine combined elements of religious beliefs and empirical methods, and, in both cultural areas, physicians were highly regarded. Among the Hebrews, the religious explanation of disease predominated; thus, the physician was relegated to a social status well below that of the priest. In all three cultures, however, concern for the ill existed, and a body of professionals treated medical problems according to their best understanding of the ailments.

Written sources from this time and place provide considerable insight into medical practices. In Egypt, several medical papyri have survived, including the Edwin Smith papyrus on surgery, the Ebers papyrus listing many remedies for a variety of problems, and the Kahun papyrus on obstetrics and gynecology. In Mesopotamia, the Nippur clay tablets document healing traditions dating to the Sumerians and describe many recognizable medical syndromes. One of the Babylonians' most significant writings, Hammurabi's famous code of law, sets forth a number of rules by which doctors were to practice their trade, together with a harsh set of punishments for errors. The Judaic writings of the Old Testament clearly state that illness and suffering came from God, to be accepted rather than treated, and in particular address one of the most feared diseases of the ancient world: leprosy.

Medicine in the ancient world dealt with battlefield injuries, work-related trauma, and the infectious diseases that spread through increasingly closely packed populations. In addition, physicians addressed reproductive problems, blindness and deafness, and the myriad minor ailments afflicting the human body. Treatments included prayer, incantation, and divination; simple remedies such as bathing, rest, and nutrition; and an impressive array of animal, vegetable, and mineral substances all designed to appease the gods and alleviate human suffering. Medicine was clearly becoming a specialized and full-time profession.

TIME LINE

ca. 2980 B.C.E.*	Birth of Imhotep, Egyptian demigod of medicine
2000–1950 B.C.E.	Physicians begin forming an important professional group in Babylon and Syria
1800–1700 B.C.E.	Code of Hammurabi is written sometime during this time span
ca. 1700 B.C.E.	Ebers papyrus is written, based on information from texts dating to about 2640 B.C.E.
1550–1500 B.C.E.	Edwin Smith papyrus is written, a copy of a manuscript written about 2500 B.C.E.
1479–1224 B.C.E.	Ten plagues of Egypt occur sometime during this span
ca. 1440 B.C.E.	Book of Leviticus is probably written

*B.C.E., "before the common era."

▲

The Holy Bible

A number of passages in the Bible deal with what the writers called leprosy, *a condition that caused considerable concern among the ancient Hebrews. However, the term did not refer to modern leprosy, or* **Hansen's disease,** *but rather to a variety of skin problems such as eczema and dermatitis, as well as various forms of molds found on houses and fabrics. The image of "unclean" that was attached to the leper related not to a sense of filth or contagion, but rather to a spiritual uncleanliness that had to be removed ritually. Nevertheless, the subsequent figure of the leper as feared, hated, and untouchable, which dominated Western thought from the Middle Ages to the twentieth century, largely dates from the scriptural mandates and stories of the Bible.*

▲

Exodus 4:6–8

[6] Again, the LORD said to him, "Put your hand into your bosom." And he put his hand into his bosom; and when he took it out, behold, his hand was leprous, as white as snow. [7] Then God said, "Put your hand back into your bosom." So he put his hand back into his bosom; and when he took it out, behold, it was restored like the rest of his flesh. [8] "If they will not believe you," God said, "or heed the first sign, they may believe the latter sign."*

Leviticus 13:2–3, 45–46

[2] "When a man has on the skin of his body a swelling or an eruption or a spot, and it turns into a leprous disease on the skin of his body, then he shall be brought to Aaron the priest or to one of his sons the priests, [3] and the priest shall examine the diseased spot on the skin of his body; and if the hair in the diseased spot has turned white and the disease appears to be deeper than the skin of his body, it is a leprous disease; when the priest has examined him he shall pronounce him unclean. . . .

[45] "The leper who has the disease shall wear torn clothes and let the hair of his head hang loose, and he shall cover his upper lip and cry, 'Unclean, unclean.' [46] He shall remain unclean as long as he has the disease; he is unclean; he shall dwell alone in a habitation outside the camp."

2 Kings 7:3–4

[3] Now there were four men who were lepers at the entrance to the gate; and they said to one another, "Why do we sit here till we die? [4] If we say, 'Let us enter the city,' the famine is in the city, and we shall die there; and if we sit here, we die also. So now come, let us go over to the camp of the Syrians; if they spare our lives we shall live, and if they kill us we shall but die."

2 Chronicles 26:20–21

[20] And Azari'ah the chief priest, and all the priests, looked at him, and behold, he was leprous in his forehead! And they thrust him out quickly, and he himself hastened to go out, because the LORD had smitten him. [21] And King Uzzi'ah was a leper to the day of his death, and being a leper dwelt in a separate house, for he was excluded from the house of the LORD. And Jotham his son was over the king's household, governing the people of the land.

Matthew 8:1–4

[1] When he came down from the mountain, great crowds followed him; [2] and behold, a leper came to him and knelt before him, saying, "Lord, if you will, you can make me clean." [3] And he stretched out his hand and touched him, saying, "I will; be clean." And immediately his leprosy was cleansed. [4] And Jesus said to him, "See that you say nothing to any one; but go, show yourself to the priest, and offer the gift that Moses commanded, for a proof to the people."

---

*The first sign occurred when God told Moses to throw a staff onto the ground, whereupon it turned into a serpent. Then God told Moses to pick the serpent up by its tail, and when Moses did, the serpent turned back into a staff. Moses was supposed to use these signs to prove to others that God had appeared to him.

The Edwin Smith Papyrus
The Surgical Treatise

Discovered by a British Egyptologist in 1862, the Edwin Smith papyrus is one of the oldest known written records of medical procedures. The papyrus is dated at approximately 1500 B.C.E., but it is apparently a copy of a document written about a thousand years earlier. The papyrus consists of forty-eight case histories, each classified by its verdict. After examination, the physician pronounced each case to be either treatable, not treatable, or one with which he would "contend," meaning one with an uncertain prognosis that he would attempt to treat. Treatments consisted of surgical intervention, use of external remedies, or both. Many of the injuries described were probably the result of normal life and work, but a number of them were undoubtedly inflicted in battle. The papyrus reveals a unique picture of the rational side of ancient Egyptian medicine, in contrast to the more frequent ancient linkage of medicine and religion.

CASE SEVEN
III 2–IV 4

A Gaping Wound in the Head Penetrating to the Bone and Perforating the Sutures

TITLE

Instructions concerning a gaping wound in his head, penetrating to the bone, (and) perforating the **sutures** of his skull.

EXAMINATION

[If thou examinest a man having a gaping wound in his head, penetrating to the bone, (and) perforating the sutures of his skull], thou shouldst palpate his wound, (although) he shudders exceedingly. Thou shouldst cause him to lift his face; if it is painful for him to open his mouth, (and) his heart beats feebly; if thou observe his spittle hanging at his two lips and not falling off, while he discharges blood from both his nostrils (and) from both his ears; he suffers with stiffness in his neck, (and) is unable to look at his two shoulders and his breast, . . .

FIRST DIAGNOSIS

Thou shouldst say regarding him: "One having a gaping wound in his head, penetrating to the bone, (and) perforating the sutures of his skull; the cord of his **mandible** is contracted; he discharges blood from both his nostrils (and) from both his ears, while he suffers with stiffness in his neck. An ailment with which I will contend."

FIRST TREATMENT

Now as soon as thou findest that the cord of that man's mandible, his jaw, is contracted, thou shouldst have made for him something hot, until he is comfortable, so that his mouth opens. Thou shouldst bind it with grease, honey, (and) lint, until thou knowest that he has reached a decisive point.

Reprinted by permission of the University of Chicago Press, from James Henry Breasted, ed., *The Edwin Smith Surgical Papyrus*, vol. 1 (Chicago: University of Chicago Press, 1930), 435–36, 447, 458. Copyright © 1930.

SECOND EXAMINATION

If, then, thou findest that the flesh of that man has developed fever from that wound which is in the sutures of his skull, while that man has developed *ty'* from that wound, thou shouldst lay thy hand upon him. Shouldst thou find his countenance is clammy with sweat, the ligaments of his neck are tense, his face is ruddy, his teeth and his back [-], the odor of the chest of his head is like the *bkn* (urine) of sheep, his mouth is bound, (and) both his eyebrows are drawn, while his face is as if he wept, . . .

SECOND DIAGNOSIS

Thou shouldst say regarding him: "One having a gaping wound in his head, penetrating to the bone, perforating the sutures of his skull; he has developed *ty'*, his mouth is bound, (and) he suffers with stiffness in his neck. An ailment not to be treated."

THIRD EXAMINATION

If, however, thou findest that that man has become pale and has already ⌈shown exhaustion⌉.

THIRD TREATMENT

Thou shouldst have made for him a wooden brace padded with linen and put into his mouth. Thou shouldst have made for him a draught of *wh*-fruit. His treatment is sitting, placed between two supports of brick, until thou knowest he has reached a decisive point. . . .

CASE TWENTY-ONE
VIII 6–9

A Split in the Temporal Bone

TITLE

Instructions concerning a split in his temple.

EXAMINATION

If thou examinest a man having a split in his temple, shouldst thou find a swelling protruding on the outside of that split, while he discharges blood from his nostril and from his one ear having that split, (and) it is painful when he hears speech, because of it, . . .

DIAGNOSIS

Thou shouldst say concerning him: "One having a split in his temple, while he discharges blood from his nostril and his ear having that injury. An ailment with which I will contend."

TREATMENT

Thou shouldst put him at his mooring stakes, until thou knowest he has reached a decisive point. . . .

CASE THIRTY-NINE
XIII 3–12

Tumors or Ulcers in the Breast Perhaps Resulting from Injury

TITLE

Instructions concerning tumors with prominent head in his breast.

EXAMINATION

If thou examinest a man having tumors with prominent head in his breast, (and) thou findest that the swellings have spread with pus over his breast, (and) have produced redness, while it is very hot therein, when thy hand touches him, . . .

DIAGNOSIS

Thou shouldst say concerning him: "One having tumors with prominent head in his breast, (and) they produce ⌈cists⌉ of pus. An ailment which I will treat with the fire-drill."

TREATMENT

Thou shouldst burn for him over his breast (and) over those tumors which are on his breast. Thou shouldst treat him with wound treatment. Thou shouldst not prevent its opening of itself, that there may be no *mnhy-w* in his wound (sore?). Every wound (sore ?) that arises in his breast dries up as soon as it opens of itself. . . .

⊼

The Ebers Papyrus

Remedies for Common Complaints

*In the ancient world as in the modern, a significant amount of physicians' time was spent addressing relatively minor ailments. The Ebers papyrus, dated about 1550 B.C.E. but written much earlier, listed 811 remedies for the Egyptian doctor to use for myriad medical problems and is the earliest known pharmaceutical list. The 110-page papyrus is haphazardly divided into sections on specific ailments, with individual paragraphs on individual remedies. Many of the potions were **polypharmacological,** with an often-long list of animal, plant, and mineral components, and the resulting concoctions were used as gargles, inhalations, enemas, poultices, pills, lotions, and infusions. The papyrus also included magical elements in the form of several incantations to improve the efficacy of the potions. The primary focus, however, was on empirical medicine rather than on magical medicine, with a largely accurate description of the function of the heart and circulatory system, and even a description of "despondency" that easily matches the modern picture of clinical depression.*

⊼

Diseases of the Alimentary System

Remedy to Clear Out the Body and to Get Rid of the Excrement in the Body of a Person

Berries-of-the-Castor-oil-tree	1

Chew and swallow down with Beer in order to clear out all that is in the body. . . .

[Remedy to Stop the Diarrhoea]

Figs	$\frac{1}{8}$
Grapes	$\frac{1}{8}$
Bread-dough	$\frac{1}{32}$
pit-corn	$\frac{1}{32}$
Fresh Lead-earth	$\frac{1}{64}$

Onions	$\frac{1}{32}$
Elderberry	$\frac{1}{8}$

SING:　O, Hetu!
AGAIN:　O, Hetu! . . .

Ready Remedy to Drive Indigestion Out of the Body

Figs	$\frac{1}{8}$
sebesten	$\frac{1}{8}$
Grapes	$\frac{1}{16}$
Caraway	$\frac{1}{64}$
Resin-of-Acanthus	$\frac{1}{32}$
Writing-fluid	$\frac{1}{64}$
Peppermint	$\frac{1}{32}$
gengent-beans	$\frac{1}{8}$
Sweet Beer	

Keep moist and take for four days. . . .

Reprinted from Cyril P. Bryan, trans., *The Papyrus Ebers* (New York: Appleton, 1931), 44, 48–49, 52, 60, 68–71, 89.

Minor Medicine

Remedy to Drive Out the Pain in the Head

Inner-of-Onions	1
Fruit-of-the-am-tree	1
Natron	1
setseft-seeds	1
Bone-of-the-Sword-fish, cooked	1
Redfish, cooked	1
Skull-of-the-Crayfish, cooked	1
Honey	1
abra-ointment	1

Smear the Head therewith for four days. . . .

Minor Surgery

To Prevent Burn Wounds

A Frog

Warm in Oil and rub therewith. . . .

[A More Elaborate Remedy] Against Burns

To Use on the First Day

Black amat-juice
Put thereto.

Another on the First Day

Elderberries
uah-corn
Cat's dung

Mix into one in Cake-water and apply thereto.

To Use on the Second Day

Goat's dung

Burn, crush, rub in Yeast-that-is-fermenting, and put thereto.

To Use on the Third Day

Thorns-of-Acanthus, dried

Crush them in cooked durra-corn and Onions, put in Oil, and apply as a plaster.

To Use on the Fourth Day

Wax
Roasted Cow's Fat
Palm-fibres

Make into one in uah-corn, and apply as a plaster.

To Use on the Fifth Day

Onions
Read-lead
Fruit-of-the-am-tree

Crush, rub in Copper-splinters, make into one, and apply as a plaster.

Incantation for a Burn

'O son, Horus! There is Fire in the Land! Water is not there and thou art not there! Bring Water over the River-bank to quench the Fire.'

To be spoken over Milk-of-a-Woman-who-has-Borne-a-Son. . . .

Diseases of the Skin

To Allay Itching

Cyperus-from-the-Meadow
Onion-meal
Incense
Wild Date-juice

Make into one and apply to the scurvy place.

> LOOK TO IT BECAUSE THIS IS THE TRUE REMEDY.
> IT WAS FOUND AMONG THE PROVEN REMEDIES IN THE TEMPLE OF THE GOD, OSIRIS.
> IT IS A REMEDY WHICH DRIVES AWAY THE SCURF IN EVERY LIMB OF A PERSON.
> YES, IT HEALS AT ONCE.
> YOU SEE. . . .

▲

An Epidemiological Analysis of the Ten Plagues of Egypt

John S. Marr and Curtis D. Malloy

The Bible is both the seminal document of Judeo-Christian belief and a historical document. Modern researchers continue to find corroborating historical evidence of many stories in both the Old Testament and the New. One of the best-known stories is the Exodus account of Moses and the plagues of Egypt, with its powerful message about the might of Yahweh. Most of the plague events have remained mysteries to historical researchers: The tenth plague, the death of the firstborn, is the most inexplicable. In the analysis in the following table, the authors not only make a concerted effort to pair ancient sources and modern biology to discover the nature of each of the plagues, but also propose convincingly that each misery built on the previous plagues, all culminating with the final destruction of the firstborn and the devastation of Egypt.

▲

Reprinted by permission of John S. Marr, M.D., Free Union, VA, and Curtis D. Malloy, M.P.H., Seattle, WA, from John S. Marr and Curtis D. Malloy, "An Epidemiological Analysis of the Ten Plagues of Egypt," *Caduceus* 12, no. 1 (1996): 12–13.

SUMMARY OF INTERPRETATIONS GIVEN TO THE TEN PLAGUES OF EGYPT

Plague ARAMAIC HEBREW	1. Water to Blood DAM דס	2. Swarm of Frogs TS'-FAR-DEI-A צפררע	3. Plague of Lice KI-NIM בניס	4. Swrams of Flies A-ROV ערוב
Biblical Passage	"Stretch out thine hand upon the waters of Egypt: upon their streams, upon their rivers, upon their ponds, upon their pools of water, that they may become blood."	"Stretch forth thine hand with thy rod over the streams, over the rivers, and over the ponds, and cause frogs to come up upon the land of Egypt."	"Aaron stretched out his hand with his rod, and smote the dust of the earth, and it became lice in man, and in the beast; all the dust of the land became lice, through the land of Egypt."	"[T]here came a grievous swarm of flies into the house of the Pharaoh, and into his servants' houses, and into all of the land of Egypt; the land was corrupted by reason of the swarm of flies."
Chapter, Verse	Exodus 7:19	Exodus 8:5	Exodus 8:16	Exodus 8:24
Ipuwer Papyrus	"Lo, the river is blood. As one drinks of it one shrinks from the people. And thirsts to water."	"Towns are ravaged. Upper Egypt became wasteland. Lo, crocodiles gorge on their catch.*"		
Interpretation				
Bryant England/1810	"tainted and polluted streams"	Frogs (a deity) and their death are emblematic of a prophetic influence	Lice: "vermin . . . pediculi"	(House?) flies representing "Zebub"
Blanc United States/ 1890	—	Anthrax (*Bacillus anthracis*), infected and killed frogs	Flies transmitting anthrax	Flies transmitting anthrax

*Some rabblnical acholars have Interpreted the Habraic text as possibly meaning amphiblans in general.

5. Animal Murrain *DE-VER* דבר	6. Boils and Blains *SH'HIN* שח'ן	7. Hailstorms *BA-RAD* ברד	8. Locusts *AR-BEH* ארבה	9. Darkness *HOSHEKH* חשׁר	10. Death of Eldest *MA-KAT B'KHO-ROT* פבת בבנבנת
"Behold the hand of the Lord is upon thy cattle which is in the field, upon the horses, upon the asses, upon the camels, upon the oxen, and upon the sheep: there will be a grievous murrain."	"Take to you handfuls of ashes of the furnace, and let Moses sprinkle it toward the heaven in the sight of the Pharaoh. And it shall become small dust in all the land of Egypt, and shall be a boil breaking forth with blains upon man, and upon beast, throughout all the land of Egypt."	"Stretch forth thine hand toward heaven, that there will be hail in all the land of Egypt, upon man and upon beast, and upon every herb of the field, throughout the land of Egypt."	"[W]hen it was morning, the east wind brought the locusts. And the locusts went up over all the lands of Egypt, and rested in all the coasts of Egypt; very grievous were they; before them there were no such they, neither after them shall be such."	"Moses stretched forth his hand toward heaven; and there was a thick darkness in all the land of Egypt three days: They saw not one another, neither rose from any of his place for three days; but all the Children of Israel had light in their dwellings."	"About midnight I will go out into the middle of Egypt: And all the first-born in the land of Egypt shall die, from the firstborn of Pharaoh that sitteth upon his throne, even unto the first born of the maid-servant that is behind the mill; and all the firstborn of the beasts."
Exodus 9:3	Exodus 9:8	Exodus 9:22	Exodus 10:13	Exodus 10:22	Exodus 11:4
"Lo, all beasts, their hearts shall weep, Cattle bemoan the state of the land."	"Plague is throughout the land. Blood is everywhere."	"Lo, hearts are violent, storms sweep the land."	"Birds find neither fruit nor herbs . . . Trees are destroyed. No fruit nor herbs are found."	"Lo, the desert claims the land . . . Those who had shelter are in the dark of the storm. . . . Egypt will not be given over [to] sand. . . . The land is not light."	"Ladies suffer like maidservants . . . Then he who would have smitten the evil stretched out his arm against it, would have de-stroyed their seed and their heirs."
"the distemper"	"That where any atom of this dust be whiffled might be entailed, but with a different intention . . . a plague and a curse."	"thunder, hail, fire" destroy crops	Locusts caused famines	"a preternatural state of night"	Confluence of God's will
Anthrax	Anthrax	Hail	Locusts	Locust swarms	Anthrax

(continued)

Summary of Interpretations Given to the Ten Plagues of Egypt

Plague *ARAMAIC* *HEBREW*	1. Water to Blood *DAM* דם	2. Swarm of Frogs *TS'-FAR-DEI-A* צפרדע	3. Plague of Lice *KI-NIM* כנים	4. Swrams of Flies *A-ROV* ערוב
Velikovsky USSR/1950	The fall of red meteorite dust from a comet polluting waters	—	—	—
Hort Netherlands/ 1957	Red silt, flagellated protozoa *Euglena sanguina, Haematococcus pluvialis*	Anthrax (*Bacillus anthracis*) infected and killed frogs	Mosquitos (Culex species)	Stable Flies (Stomoxys calcitrans) transmitting Plagues 5 & 6
Schoental United States/ 1980	Microfungi and *Fusarium roseum* contaminating waters	Frogs killed by dinoflagellates producing soluble poisons	"vermin"	"flies"
Schmidt Germany/1990	Water contaminated by dead fish	Frogs	—	Horseflies
Jacoby United States/ 1990	Nile (a deity) waters made undrinkable secondary to dead fish	Frogs	"Sand fleas," not gnats	"An insect akin to a winged ant"
Hoyte Australia/1993	**Dinoflagellates** *Gymnodiuium* and *Glenodinium* (unnamed species)	Dehydration and dessication killed escaping frogs	"Midges" (*Culux antennatus*)	Stable flies *Stomoxys calcitrans* (see Hort)
Ceccarelli Italy/1994	**Dinoflagellates** *Gymnodiuium* and *Glenodinium* species (after Hoyte)	Frogs	"Midges" *Culex antennatus* (after Hoyte)	Streptococcal and Staphylococcal infections; **Babesiosis**
Marr, Malloy United States/ 1996	Freshwater **cyanobacteria** causing river to turn red, and killing fish.	Frogs leave deoxygenated water and die, contributing to Plague 3	*Culicoides* appears de novo from pupae hatching in sand (Hoyte) transmitting Plague 5	Stable flies (Hort and Hoyte) transitting Plague 6

5. Animal Murrain *DE-VER* דבר	6. Boils and Blains *SH'HIN* שח"ן	7. Hailstorms *BA-RAD* ברר	8. Locusts *AR-BEH* ארבה	9. Darkness *HOSHEKH* חשׁר	10. Death of Eldest *MA-KAT B'KHO-ROT* פבת בבנבנת
Secondary skin infections from comet dust	Boils secondary to dusts, blisters from flaming naptha	Dust, gravel, and burning naptha from a comet	—	Cinder dust from a comet	An earthquake
Anthrax	Anthrax	Hailstorms destroyed flax and barley but not wheat or spelt	Locusts	Sandstorms (khamsin)	Famine secondary to destruction of wheat and spelt harvests
Mycotoxins	2° bacterial infect. due to immunosuppression by **trichothecenes**	Hail	—	—	Mycotoxin-induced death from moldy feeds
—	—	—	Locusts	—	—
—	"herpes-like infection"? "bubonic infection"? "inflammation of sexual organs"?	Hail	Locusts	Darkness?	—
Surra (debab) (*Trypanasoma evansi*)	**Ecthyma** (Group A hemolytic *Streptococcus pyogenes*)	Crops ruined by hailstorms	Locusts ruined crops	Sandstorms	Typhoid fever and **salmonellosea** (*S. Typhl* and enteriditis).
Babesiosis (*Babesia bigemini*)	Babesiosis (*Babesia bigemini*)	Hail	—	—	—
African horse sickness; **Bluetongue;** Epizootic hemorrhagic disease	**Glanders** (fancy) *Pseudomonas mallei*	Hail destroying established crops and dampening stored foods	*Schistocerca gregaria* eat all remaining vegetation, including sprouts and seedlings	Sandstorms (khamsin) cover existing food stands and stored food supplies	Mycotoxins specific to stored grains preferentially killed first to access store

⋀

Babylonian Medicine, Managed Care and Codex Hammurabi, Circa 1700 B.C.

Allen D. Spiegel, PhD, MPH, and Christopher R. Springer

Managed care is a fact in modern U.S. health-care delivery. With it come many regulations dealing with everything from price caps and provider lists to patients' rights and sanctions for providers who violate the rules. Yet, the idea of controlling medical care is not new, as this reading suggests. Even as far back as 1700 B.C.E., physicians and other health-care providers were governed by laws regulating their actions. The Code of Hammurabi, the oldest known written law code, with its "eye-for-an-eye, tooth-for-a-tooth" philosophy, established fee schedules and meted out harsh justice, all within the context of a social hierarchy that determined both fees and punishments on the basis of the patient's socioeconomic class. The regulation of medical care under Hammurabi differed substantially in detail from modern practices, but in both cases, the result—professional regulation—was accomplished.

⋀

With the reform of the health care delivery system uppermost in the minds of strategic health planners, managed care has emerged as the new consensus choice for resolving cost containment problems. Uniquely, managed care integrates the following health care system attributes: reasonable fee schedules for professional services; standards to monitor the quality of care rendered; assurance of patient's rights and satisfaction; and competitively marketed health care services.

Amazingly, health care reformers need not have labored to reinvent the wheel! More than 4,000 years ago, at the dawn of civilization, a number of nomadic Semite tribes had already documented the creation of managed care techniques that applied to their health care delivery system.

Codex Hammurabi

Managed care concepts were enduringly inscribed in the written clay tablet compilations by Urukagina of Lagash (2400 B.C.), Eshnunna (2100 B.C.) and Lipit-Ishtar of Isin (1800 B.C.). When writing letters on clay tablets some 4,000 years ago, wellness wishes frequently appeared as divine beseechments to the gods: "May Shamash and Marduk give thee health." During the golden age of King Hammurabi of Babylon, he adapted managed care prerogatives from these earlier written codes and documented the following managed care precepts in stone in the Codex Hammurabi:

- Rate setting of specific fees for general surgery, eye surgery, setting fractures, curing diseased muscles, and other specific health care services.

Reprinted by permission of Kluwer Academic/Plenum Publishers, and Allen D. Spiegel, Ph.D., M.P.H., and Christopher R. Springer, SUNY Downstate Medical Center, Brooklyn, NY, from Allen D. Spiegel and Christopher R. Springer, "Babylonian Medicine, Managed Care and Codex Hammurabi, Circa 1700 B.C.," *Journal of Community Health* 22, no. 1 (1997): 69–70, 73–74, 76–88.

- Fees were set according to a sliding scale based on ability to pay.
- Owners were required to pay for the health care for their slaves.
- Objective outcome measurement standards assured the quality of care.
- Outcomes information management included data collection and evaluation.
- Consumer and patient's rights were publicized, explained and known to all.
- Marketing and advertising promoted the adoption of the plan.

There is no consensus as to the dates when Hammurabi ruled even though most agree that he was the sixth king of the first or Amorite dynasty of Babylon. Experts have placed his 43 year reign within periods ranging from 2123–2080 B.C., or 1948–1905 B.C. or 1728–1685 B.C. A comparison of eight different authorities places Hammurabi's reign at different dates between 2067–1669 B.C. Regardless of the exact date, managed care principles were literally set in stone and inscribed on clay tablets between the 17th and 21st centuries B.C., eons before health care evolved from priestly incantations, magical applications, omens and evil demons. Despite the dominating presence of supernatural deities, Babylonian society was cultured and sophisticated. Babylonian society, medicine and managed care are all interrelated. . . .

Medicine in Babylonia

Illness was believed to be caused by the intervention of extraneous metaphysical forces such as demons, evil spirits, ghosts of the dead, or the wrath of the gods. People became ill for committing a sin or by being victimized by outside agents such as cold, dust or a bad smell. Ashakku was the demon of consumption, Irra the spirit of pestilence, Alu caused blindness, Nergal gave a fever, Tiu caused headaches, and Namtar was the evil spirit responsible for the plague. With these beliefs, it is not surprising that medicine belonged to the priestly class and was largely magico-religious with three types of healers; diviners, exorcists, and physicians. In addition, veterinarians and barbers are mentioned in the Code. Barbers (**gallabu**) performed plastic surgery as they marked slaves or removed slave brandings, and performed surgical procedures such as dental operations.

Diviners (**Baru**), essentially internal medicine specialists, interpreted omens and foretold the course of the illness. Since the Semitic peoples believed that the liver was the seat of the soul and the center of vitality, Barus practiced **hepatoscopy**. A sick person breathed into the nostrils of a sheep, the animal was sacrificed, and the Barus compared a concisely coded clay model to the sheep's liver to make a diagnosis. Ezekiel the prophet refers to Babylonian medical foretelling when he noted that "he looketh at the liver."

Exorcists (**Ashipu**) inquired about the nature of the offense to the gods. After discovering the transgression, the Ashipu drove out the evil spirits causing the disease with incantations, prayers, recitations, sacrifices, and ceremonial rituals beseeching the gods for a cure. A typical exorcist prayer was as follows:

> Whoever or whatever you are, evil ghost or evil devil, evil god or evil fiend, or sickness or death, or a phantom or wrath of the night, a fever or deadly pestilence, whatever or whoever you are— get out! Take yourself off before me! Get out of this house! For I am the priest of EA, I who recite the incantation for the relief of the man who is sick. Be exorcised by heaven! Be exorcised by earth! *Get out!*
>
> [EA was the god of waters, spells and incantations]

Both Ashipu and Baru used physical examinations to discover signs and omens.

Physicians (**Azu**) were educated in priestly administered schools associated with the temples and the students learned from the recorded clay tablets and practical experience. In keeping with the religious site of their schooling, an Azu worshipped Gula, the goddess of medicine and healing, and her husband, Ninurta. Ninazu was the lord doctor, the patron of physicians, and his son, Ningishzida, a healing god, carried a round staff with a double-sexed two headed serpent named Sachan. An Azu discovered the illness by listening to the patient's accounts, not by physical examination. Many hundreds of clay tablets recorded descriptions of ailments such as abscesses, apoplexy, appetite control, colic, constipation, cough, ear, eye, fevers, gallbladder trouble, heart disease, intoxication, nose and throat disease, **phthisis,** plague, rectal **prolapse,** rheumatism, skin disease, tumors, and venereal disease. Forty tablets dealt with interpreting dreams and avoiding nightmares. After the diagnosis, the Azu prescribed drugs and medications, performed surgery, set fractures, palliated visible sores, and treated snakebites. Medical instruments included bronze lancets, metal tubes to blow remedies into bodily orifices, tubes for catheters and spatulas. More than 250 medicinal plants, 120 mineral substances and 180 other drugs were used in combination with alcoholic beverages, bouillon, fats, honey, milk in various forms, oils, wax, and parts and products of animals. Medications were prepared by grinding, straining, and filtering substances for ointments or plasters to spread on a piece of thin leather to apply. External medication applications used solvents from bark, flowers, fruit skins and juices, plants, resins, sea-kelp, seeds or turpentine dissolved in beer or milk and mixed with wine, fats and honey. Narcotics came from hemp, **mandragora,** opium and solium temulentum. Prescriptions could specify administration via enemas, laxatives, lotions, ointments, pessaries, pills, poultices, powders, salves, and suppositories. A patient's prescription could be "enveloped in the aroma of burning feathers and liberally dosed with dog dung and pig's gall." When they set up practice, Azus created their own seals with inscriptions such as: "O Edinmagi, Servant of the god Girra, who helps mothers in childhood, Ur-Lugaledina the physician is your servant."

Within this Babylonian society and culture of medicine, the stele with the inscribed Codex Hammurabi emerged as a unifying force throughout the nation. . . .

Codex Hammurabi and Managed Care Comparisons

Key managed care precepts are concerned with a number of commonalities: control of care by management; defining the population covered; establishment of a fee schedule for provider health care services; an administrative division of labor; a credentialing process for providers; deselection of providers; specialty referrals, consultations, and denial of care; pharmaceutical benefits; medical records documentation; patient rights and satisfaction; disenrollment; and quality assessment including practice criteria, outcome measurement, and penalties; and marketing the product.

Managed Care Control

By modern standards, would Hammurabi's government be considered as regulators of medical care? In 1981, the *Stewart v. Midani* ruling defined management control. This court identified factors that determined whether an institution affected a physician's judgment or behavior. Specific elements in the relationship between the physician and the institution focused upon the answers to eight questions regarding the services of physicians: Who directly supervises their work?; Did a contract specify their tasks or services?; Who controlled their work time? Who was authorized to inspect their work?; Who provided their supplies and/or facilities?; Who could terminate the contract?; Who could evaluate their degree of skill?; and Who determined the payment method?. If a preponderance of these variables proved a relationship, the court claimed that the physician was under the influence of the employer. In effect, the employer was, at least, partially responsible.

Based on the medical related sections of the Code of Hammurabi, the Babylonian government did have the right to inspect the physician's work, if the care was questioned by the patient. In addition, the government set forth the amount of payment for services and penalties for malpractice. However, evidence from clay tablets indicates that the physicians of Babylon were frequently independent of the government. In practice, the physicians handled their own patient contracts as well as the specific services and supplies utilized.

Applying the eight questions in the court ruling, Hammurabi and his government could not be held accountable for the actions of a physician. Furthermore, the Babylonian government did not hold itself out as a caregiver, did not receive money from the patients for the physicians' services, and did not limit the patient's choice of a physician. In effect, the Code of Hammurabi presents a mixed bag as a controlling edict from a managed care organization. Nevertheless, as a 4,000 year old document, the Codex Hammurabi still stands as an innovative testament to the origin of managed care concepts.

Defining the Population Coverage

Everybody in Babylonia, including the people in the conquered nations, were covered by the health care system specifically identified in the Code. All of the 282 edicts were applicable within the unequal distinctions based upon the three social classes. In addition to the 15 sections that mentioned physicians, veterinarians, barbers, or wet-nurses, there were about 20 others that dealt with injuries in an affray such as damaging an eye, breaking a bone, knocking out a tooth, striking a cheek, causing a miscarriage, or blows resulting in a death. However, those sections do not mention health care services but incur monetary fines or "eye for an eye" penalties. A Medicaid-type coverage was in force for slaves as their owners were required to pay for their health care services.

Establishment of a Fee Schedule

To contain the costs, managed care organizations employ health care providers who agree to accept set fees or salaries for their services. Similarly, Codex fees were based upon the patient's social class and the ability to pay in addition to the seriousness of the procedure. **Awelum** paid the most, **mushkenum** less, and the **wardum's**

owner paid the least as illustrated in the precise language of the Codex's scheduled fees:

§215   If a surgeon has made a deep incision in the body of a gentleman with a lancet of bronze and saves the man's life or has opened a caruncle in the eye of a man with a lancet of bronze and saves the eye, he shall take ten shekels of silver.

§216   If the patient is a freeman, he shall take 5 shekels of silver.

§217   If the patient is a slave, the master of the slave shall give 2 shekels of silver to the surgeon.

A comparative examination of Hammurabi's Code quickly reiterates the successful and unsuccessful fee setting and penalties methodology. Fees are possibly omitted for unsuccessful bone setting and sinew mending because the outcome is usually not fatal and the operation can be repeated until the result is satisfactory. A reasonable explanation for the omission of fees for the general and eye operation on Mushkenum is that the scribe somehow or the other skipped a section. Based upon other comparable sections of the Codex, it is likely that a monetary penalty would be applied.

For a comparable economic understanding of the fee, a free craftsman earned 5–8 grains of silver per day and had to work about one year to earn 10–14 shekels. A wooden door cost one to two shekels, earthenware jars sold for from $^{1}/_{4}$ to $^{2}/_{3}$ of a shekel, and a wooden tray for carrying on the head, $^{1}/_{2}$ shekel. A middle class dwelling rented for five shekels a year. Based on these comparisons, it is obvious that physicians were well paid for their services. Additional specified medical care fees included the following:

§206   If a man strikes a freeman in an affray and inflicts a wound on him, that man may swear "Surely I did not strike him willingly" and he shall pay the surgeon.

§221   If a physician set a broken bone for a man or cure his diseased bowels, the patient shall pay five shekels of silver to the physician.

§222   If he be a freeman, he shall give three shekels of silver.

§223 If it be a man's slave, the owner of the slave shall give two shekels of silver to the physician.

§224 If a veterinary physician operate on an ox or an ass for a severe wound and save its life, the owner shall give to the physician 30 grains of silver.
(180 grains of silver = 1 shekel).

Documentation from surviving clay tablet business contracts indicates that employer and employee considered the prevailing economy and deviated from the established fee schedules in the Codex. It is also possible that the fees in Hammurabi's code applied to people working for the King or the temple priests. Furthermore, the fees in the code may have included food and lodging or similar benefits.

In today's terms, the Code of Hammurabi established a uniform fee-for-service schedule with a sliding scale based upon ability to pay. Considering the relative lack of specific diagnoses mentioned, the Code may have initiated the first **Diagnosis Related Groups (DRGs)** used to calculate reimbursements as currently applied in the U.S. Medicare program. There was no **capitation**. Because of the sliding fee-for-service, there was no level of uncompensated care. This eliminated the need for physicians to apply the Robin Hood payment technique of overcharging the upper classes to cover the cost of care for the needy and indigent. Similar to current payment schedules, the established fees caused the physician to absorb any additional expenses of treatment beyond the set fee. Obviously, it is not a modern problem for the physician to be forced to be cost-conscious while treating patients.

Though there was no utilization review by any voluntary or governmental regulatory body, the Code forced Babylonian physicians to constantly be reminded of the need for efficient operations. Efficiency and effectiveness still haunts physicians today as many managed care organizations withhold a portion of the physician's compensation until their practice patterns can be analyzed. "Pricing cannot compensate for ineffi-

cient delivery of services. . . . Providers will eventually be penalized for inefficient operations." Cost based reimbursements cannot be expected; neither in Hammurabi's Babylon, nor in the modern day American health care marketplace.

Administrative Division of Labor

Managed care organizations utilize a variety of ancillary providers to render care to their enrolled population. In like fashion, the Code of Hammurabi set out a division of labor. Priestly health care providers, Baru and Ashipu, rendered internal medicine care through their divining and exorcisms. Azu took care of ailments that were unrelated to divine or mystical causation using non-magical means such as the "bronze lancet" or manipulation. Barbers engaged in plastic surgery by removing branding marks from slaves. A veterinary surgeon, literally "the doctor of an ox or an ass," tended to the animals. A wet-nurse could be classified as a nutritionist or dietitian. Particular duties were identified for each provider in the various sections of the Code, except for the priestly physicians, the Baru and the Ashipu.

Credentialing of Providers

Physicians were educated in schools run by the temple priests. There were many textbooks consisting of clay tablets with recorded descriptions of diseases, prescriptions, and remedies. In addition, the physicians made rounds and learned from practical experience. Critics of managed care argue that "any willing provider" should be allowed to participate in a plan's program. With the risk of death or dismemberment in Hammurabi's Code, how willing would any provider be to participate? According to Herodotus' much disputed description of Babylon's medical system, sick people were brought to the marketplace where passers-by who had experienced a similar affliction could give advice to those lying in the marketplace. In fact, it was an obligation for passers-by to inquire about the sick person's condition. Anybody advising the sick could be considered a "willing provider" without worrying about the threat of punishment that accompanied the responsibility of treatment.

Exclusion of Providers

Hammurabi's Code created the harshest form of exclusion possible. If the physician erred through omission or commission, his fingers or hands were cut off. Immediately, that physician was stopped from seeing any more patients. This severe punishment for negligence easily weeds out those physicians incapable of delivering adequate care. In addition, the punishment insures that the physicians will not practice again in a different locality. That certain risk that accompanied every procedure probably helped to stave off any physician surplus. Notwithstanding, the belief in illness caused by demons and magic allowed physicians to invoke that alibi to make a plea for the court to evaluate in unsuccessful treatments. How could a court be satisfied that a death was not the result of divine intervention and was not the surgeon's fault?

Specialty Referrals, Consultations and Denial of Care

There did not appear to be any limitation on making referrals or seeking consultations. Kings and aristocrats assured themselves of the services of the most renowned physicians, loaned the doctors to their allies, and sent them "to visit the courtesans whom they loved." Certainly, there were no financial incentives for physicians to limit specialty consultations. Baru, Ashipu and Azu freely interacted and readily exchanged treatment regimens. Since the health care services were on a fee-for-service schedule, there was no denial of care because the procedure was considered experimental. There is no mention of refusing to care for a patient although one clay tablet text warned medical students "not to touch a patient who is likely to die." That advice seemed reasonable when a negative outcome could result in bodily mutilation for the caregiver. By today's medical malpractice standards, such refusal constitutes

unprofessional conduct but today's lawsuits involve insurance policies and dollar amounts.

Pharmaceutical Benefits

Payments for health care did not add extra charges for materials used in the huge pharmacopeia of minerals, vegetables, animal parts, liquids, or unguents. All patients needing medications of any type received them from the health care provider. Similar to today's therapies, traditional family remedies were supplied as well by grandparents, parents, distant relatives and strangers passing by.

Medical Records Documentation

Thousands of clay tablets recovered by archaeologists document that medical care data were collected and recorded about ailments, causes, treatments, and therapy outcomes. Information management was systematic and routinely entered including the physician's name and constitutes a report card of sorts.

Patient Rights and Satisfaction

In the U.S., the American Hospital Association's "Bill of Rights" for patients is posted in hospitals and distributed to new inpatients. Complaints about managed care indicate "there is a pattern of dissatisfaction with choice and quality of doctors, access to specialty and emergency care, and waiting time for appointments." Efforts by the American Medical Association promote a "Patient Protection Law" to assure patients their choice and to allow managed care physicians to be "ungagged" and to tell their patients about medical care alternatives.

Hammurabi's Code anticipated these communication problems and commanded providers to follow the edicts on the stele. But communication is a two way street and there had to be assurance that patients knew their rights. In addition to the huge stele erected on the grounds of the major temple in Babylon for everybody to read, the Codex was duplicated on clay tablet copies and distributed throughout the nation. Certainly, the population was aware of the code and the ramifications. Furthermore, the king specifically called attention to all those seeking justice that the code would tell them what to expect.

> Let the oppressed man who has a cause, come before my statute called "King of Justice" and then have the inscription on my monument read out and hear my precious words, that my monument may make clear his cause to him, let him see the law which applies to him, and let his heart be set at ease!

No one was left wondering if they received a fair value in their treatment since it actually was inscribed in stone. Reading the Code sections, patients learned what to expect from health care providers beforehand and could seek justice from a legal system if not satisfied. However, there is no evidence of either prosecution or defense lawyers in Babylonia.

In an effort to create an ideal conception of the physician-patient relationship, modern researchers devised a normative standard based around the six C's: choice, competence, communication, compassion, continuity, and conflict of interest. While communication and compassion might be difficult to research, Codex Hammurabi strictly enforced competence through severe penalties. As far as continuity and choice, since the Codex fees were the same no matter what physician the patient saw, there is no reason to believe that these aspects would be impeded. With the fees established, both patient and physician knew what to expect and both could refuse the treatment, which should have eliminated any conflict of interest. Babylonians appear to have been adequately prepared regarding the concept of the ideal physician-patient relationship.

Patient Disenrollment

While there was no managed care organization from which to disenroll, Babylonians could move up or down the social class ladder and thereby change their level of health care.

Quality Assessment, Practice Criteria, Outcomes Measurement, and Penalties

Nonsurgical intervention was not subject to quality of care controls or to malpractice verdicts. A Baru or Ashipu could not be held responsible for illness or outcomes that were caused by the gods, demons or evil spirits. However, when an Azu used a "bronze lancet" or other means to heal a patient, that provider was accountable for direct human error or aggression. If a patient died or was seriously damaged, the objective measurement was easily observable and the "eye for an eye" penalty imposed. Significantly, the judges regularly omitted any references to the Code in their recorded decisions and appear to have been guided by tradition, public opinion, and common sense. Quality of care edicts in Hammurabi's code left no margin for error on the part of the provider of care. Physicians and other health care providers had to be flawless or lucky. Conditional clauses in the code such as the following could certainly make physicians uncomfortable, to say the least.

§194   If a man gives his child to a nurse and the child die in her hands, but the nurse unbeknown to the father and mother nurse another child, then they shall convict her of having nursed another child without the knowledge of the father and mother and her breasts shall be cut off.

     [A wet nurse was paid about 3 shekels]

§218   If a physician operate on a man for a severe wound with a bronze lancet and cause the man's death; or open an abscess in the eye of a man with a bronze lancet and destroy the man's eye, they shall cut off his fingers.

§219   If a physician operate on the slave of a freeman for a severe wound with a bronze lancet and cause his death, he shall restore a slave of equal value.

§220   If he open an abscess in his eye with a bronze lancet, and destroy his eye, he shall pay silver to the extent of one-half his price.

     (Average prices for male slaves ranged from 16–30 shekels)

§226   If a barber has excised a slave's mark without the knowledge of his owner so that he cannot be traced, they shall cut off the fore-hand of that barber.

§227   If a man has constrained the barber and he excises the slave's mark so that he cannot be traced, they shall put that man to death and shall hang him at his own door; the barber may swear "Surely I excised it unwittingly" and he then goes free.

Throughout the code, there were 32 decrees with the death penalty administered by burning, drowning, hanging, or impalement on a stake. Other penalties included bodily mutilation and monetary fines. As with the set fees, the quality of care penalties were adjusted by social class with the higher class able to escape death or mutilation by paying a monetary fine.

Managed care organizations and their management must balance their cost containment efforts with patient expectations as they provide quality leadership to maintain the delivery of a high quality of care. Quality assessment includes multiple factors such as standardized practice criteria, measurement of therapy outcomes, and corrective actions to resolve deviations. Babylonian medicine also was concerned with these variables. King Hammurabi left no doubt as to his leadership and repeatedly told his subjects that he was the wisest, the most just, and the most caring. Practice standards were written on the clay tablets and taught by the temple schools. Outcome measurements were specifically identified in sections of the Code as were the severe corrective actions for improving the practice of medicine. How much more total can Total Quality Management be than to "cut off the hands" of the offending health care provider?

Marketing and Advertising the Codex

In the introduction to the Code, Hammurabi lavishly applied the ancient advertising rule that if you say something loud enough, often enough and in grandiose language, your audience will believe

it. Hammurabi evoked the gods and repeatedly glorified his magnanimous actions undertaken for the benefit of his subjects:

> Anum and Illil . . . called me by name Hammurabi . . . to make justice to appear in the land, to destroy the evil and wicked that the strong might not oppress the weak. . . . When Marduk commanded me to give justice to the people of the land and to let them have good governance, I set forth truth and justice throughout the land and prospered the people. . . . My words are choice, my deeds have no rival; only for the unwise are they vain, and for the profoundly wise they are worthy of all praise.

Continuing his self-glorification, Hammurabi proclaimed his being: "a god amongst kings endued with knowledge and wisdom"; the "bountiful provider of holy feasts"; a gatherer of "abundance and plenty" bringing "overflowing wealth"; the provider of "abundant waters for his people"; a philanthropist giving out "abundant riches"; a military hero and "a warrior whom none can resist" who "stormed the four quarters of the world" and brought them "to obedience"; a ruler who "magnifies the fame of Babylon." Despite the high powered hyperbole, Hammurabi was actually "a formidable warrior, an astute diplomat, and a diligent, meticulous manager with a sincere interest in the well being of his subjects." In addition, he was an above average communicator. His image gave weight to his self-praise and by syllogism to the mandates in the code. In addition, in a society of multiple deities, the impact of his blessings and curses surely influenced the population. Hammurabi's code had 16 lines of blessings and 282 lines of calamitous curses for those who did not abide by his doctrines.

Modern Medicine and Codex Hammurabi

Some immensely aggrieved modern health care consumers may wish for a return to the harsh "eye for an eye, tooth for a tooth" penalties in the name of justice and/or simply for revenge. However, with the rush toward endorsing managed care as the modal type of health care provider, our society may be re-entering the realm of a 4,000 year old medical care system. Anybody reading the popular literature and newspapers and listening to radio or watching TV realizes that natural remedies and holistic therapies are the "in-thing." It is possible that the clay tablet prescriptions could re-emerge in the *Materia Medica* of family practitioners. In the late 1980s, Babylonian clay tablet cookbooks from 1700 B.C. resurfaced to reveal "a cuisine of striking richness, refinement, sophistication and artistry." Hammurabi's advice might call attention to the fact that he collected the best medical decisions, the wisest, the most sagacious, the most worthy, and that it would be advantageous to follow such dictums. In the prologue and epilogue, Codex Hammurabi even presents lofty moral and ethical goals for managed care organizations to emulate with appropriate changes in health care delivery terminology.

> . . . to cause justice to prevail in the land, to destroy the wicked and the evil, to prevent the strong from oppressing the weak, to go forth like the Sun over the Black Head Race [Babylonians], to enlighten the land and to further the welfare of the people . . . I brought health to the land; I made the populace to rest in security; I permitted no one to molest them . . . I restrained them that the strong might not oppress the weak, and that they should give justice to the orphan and the widow. . . .

KEY TERMS

Ashipu, 35 • Awelum, 37 • Azu, 35 • Babesiosis, 32 • Baru, 35 • Bluetongue, 33 • Capitation, 38 • Cyanobacteria, 32 • Diagnosis Related Groups (DRGs), 38 • Dinoflagellates, 32 • Ecthyma, 33 • Gallabu, 35 • Glanders, 33 • Hansen's disease, 23 • Hepatoscopy, 35 • Mandible, 25 • Mandragora, 36 • *Materia Medica,* 42 • Mushkenum, 37 • Mycotoxins, 33 • Phthisis, 36 • Polypharmacological, 27 • Prolapse, 36 • Salmonellosea, 33 • Surra, 33 • Sutures, 25 • Trichothecenes, 33 • Wardum, 37 •

QUESTIONS TO CONSIDER

1. We can find examples of prejudice and fear based on incorrect information throughout history. One of the most enduring images in the history of Western culture is the hideously disfigured and loathsome body of a leper. Yet, the principal source of the attitude toward leprosy is based on an erroneous label perpetuated in the Bible. Consider the stigma and stereotypes surrounding the modern-day individual with AIDS. Are not these conceptions also often the result of misinformation? Have similar fates befallen other diseases and medical conditions? If so, name some.

2. Trying to discern correctly the nature of various diseases in the past can be tricky, but as more information becomes available, perhaps historians can gain a clearer picture of actual events. Evaluate critically the evidence in the selection on the plagues of Egypt. Are the authors' conclusions valid? Do gaps in their argument exist? Consider, too, whether knowing the specific nature of these events is important or whether they should simply be regarded as illustrations of a larger theological lesson.

3. One difficulty in translating ancient documents such as the Ebers papyrus is the many references to substances unknown to the modern reader. Some of the ingredients in the remedies are totally unknown, such as setseft seeds and the fruit of the am tree. Nevertheless, many of the ingredients are recognizable: castor oil, onions, gruel, and caraway. Modern readers often scoff at such remedies and point to the vast improvement in even over-the-counter remedies. However, should we discard all these remedies out of hand? Can you recognize any ingredients that might have had some beneficial effects? Or, was the placebo effect simply at work to make patients and doctors think that such substances provided relief?

4. The case studies in the Edwin Smith papyrus provide some clear insights into the medical ethics of the ancient Egyptians. Some cases were simply beyond help, given the limited knowledge and resources of these people, and the physician was under no pressure to treat incurable wounds. Such ideas are generally repugnant to modern physicians, who are bound to do whatever possible to treat trauma and relieve suffering. Can you think of instances in which the modern-day physician would, or should, make such decisions about whether to treat a patient?

RECOMMENDED READINGS

Adamson, P. B. "The Influence of the King on Medical Practices in Ancient Mesopotamia." *Medicina nei Secoli* 1 (1989): 13–22.

Filer, Joyce. *Disease.* Austin: University of Texas Press, 1995.

Hamarneh, Sami K. "Practical Ethics in the Health Professions. Pt. 1: The Hammurabi and Hippocratic Codes." *Hamdard Medicus* 3, no. 1 (1993): 11–24.

Kottek, Samuel J. "Concepts of Disease in the Talmud." *Koroth* 9, nos. 1–2 (1985): 7–32.

Miller, R. L. "Paleoepidemiology, Literacy, and Medical Tradition Among Necropolis Workmen in New Kingdom Egypt." *Medical History* 35 (1991): 1–24.

Morsy, Tosson A. "Cutaneous Leishmaniasis in Egypt: History, Background, and Current Knowledge." *Journal of the Egyptian Society of Parasitology* 13, no. 2 (1983): 597–611.

Prioreschi, Plinio. *History of Medicine.* Vol. 1, *Primitive and Ancient Medicine.* Lewiston, NY: Edwin Mellen Press, 1991.

Rosner, Fred. *Medicine in the Bible and the Talmud: Selections from Classical Jewish Sources.* New York: Ktav, 1977.

Chapter Three

China and India in Antiquity

INTRODUCTION

The great ancient civilizations of China and India each had a sophisticated and effective medical tradition, both of which have survived largely intact. These traditions are based on the importance of balance and harmony, and they share the basic precept that maintaining good health is more important than curing disease. Neither tradition is based on physical anatomy as it is taught in the West, but rather on the balance and function of all parts of the body. Eastern medicine is not as invasive as Western and has a philosophical base entirely different and separate from Western traditions. For centuries confined to Asia and the subcontinent, Eastern medicine has begun to have a considerable increase in Western followers.

In the Chinese medical tradition, as based on the classic **Nei Ching** and the scholar-physicians, disease is explained as the result of an imbalance of **yin and yang,** the dualism of all known existence, which in turn upsets the balance of the **Five Elements** (fire, earth, metal, wood, and water). This imbalance causes a malfunction of the corresponding organs. Although in both traditions a correct diagnosis is emphasized, traditional Chinese medicine strongly relies on the importance of the pulse in detecting internal problems. Discussed at length in the *Nei Ching* are some fifty pulses, with more than two hundred variations, the theory being that irregularities in the heartbeat can explain chronic, acute, even incipient illness in any organ system.

One of the best-known aspects of Chinese traditional medicine is **acupuncture.** It is based on the theory that twelve channels are responsible for moving energy throughout the body, each associated with a particular organ system. Some 160 points located along these channels are described in the *Nei Ching,* locations where insertion of specifically shaped needles made of various materials would open the channel to restore the free flow of energy and thus rebalance yin and yang. A related method, **moxibustion,** involves causing small burns along such channels.

The other great Eastern medical tradition comes from India and is generally known as **Ayurvedic** medicine. Its basic premise is that the principal cause of disease is either a magical element such as sin or a disturbance of the three humors, or **doshas** (wind, bile, and phlegm), which, along with blood, control all bodily functions. The Indian physician uses natural remedies to restore the humoral balance and thus good health. In a system similar to

Chinese acupuncture, Ayurvedic medicine focuses on **chakras,** or energy points, along the spine, where nerves from elsewhere in the body join the spinal cord and along which energy flows. Many Ayurvedic treatments involve restoring the flow of energy throughout the chakras, often with the use of acupuncture.

In both ancient China and ancient India, different types of health-care providers practiced their profession. The formally trained physicians in both cultures enjoyed considerable status, even wealth, but were not available to the majority of the population. The average Chinese or Indian was far more likely to depend on less well-trained healers who attended the sick.

TIME LINE

2500 B.C.E.	Earliest evidence of cranial surgery **(trepanation)** in India
2100–1600 B.C.E.	**Shang oracle bones** and other carvings in China show references to headaches, abdominal and eye problems, and parasites
800 B.C.E.–647 C.E.*	Post-Vedic period of Indian history; Ayurvedic medicine develops
700–221 B.C.E.	*Nei Ching* is written sometime during this period (actual date highly controversial, between 4600 B.C.E. and 1 C.E.)
700–600 B.C.E.	Bian Que lives, in China—earliest physician for whom we have reliable biographical information; known as "The Master of Pulse Therapy"
ca. 585 B.C.E.	*Sushruta Samhita* is written in India
551–479 B.C.E.	K'ung Fu-tzu (Confucius) lives, in China; greatest Chinese philosopher
525 B.C.E.	*Charaka Samhita* is written in India
145–208 C.E.	Famous surgeon Hua-To lives, in China
200–300 C.E.	Wang Shuhe compiles writings on pulse therapy, produces *The Pulse Classic,* systematizing pulse theory
ca. 400 C.E.	Ayurvedic medical texts are translated into Chinese; by 700 C.E. Chinese scholars are studying in India
643 C.E.	Death of the physician Chen Ch'uan in China—first person to note that diabetes symptoms include thirst and sweet urine
1151 C.E.	Standardization of medications by first ministry of medicine in China
1596 C.E.	Posthumous publication of Li Shi-Zhen's massive *Materia Medica*—more than ten thousand prescriptions made from nearly two thousand substances
1914 C.E.	Chinese Nationalists abolish traditional medicine; do not allow its practice until 1953, when Mao Zedong orders its reinstitution

*C.E., "the current era."

A

The Sushruta Samhita

SUSHRUTA

Sushruta was the greatest surgeon of ancient India, and his collected writings, known as the Sushruta Samhita, *describe a number of the procedures that made him famous. Probably the surgical procedure for which he is most famous is **rhinoplasty**, in which he successfully restored severed noses, or ears—usually the result of punishment for adultery or other crimes. He also practiced **couching**, by which cataracts were displaced to allow much-improved vision. In addition, he is known for performing surgeries for fractures, amputations, hernias, and the removal of various growths. In his **Samhita**, Sushruta described 120 surgical instruments, some of them specialized, and more than 300 surgical procedures. Together, the* Charaka Samhita *and the* Sushruta Samhita *form the foundation of Ayurvedic medicine in India.*

In this selection from his Samhita, *Sushruta explains the meaning and significance of **marmas**. One of the best-known aspects of Ayurvedic, or Indian, medical theory, marmas are described as junctions of channels of energy—various structures such as ligaments, blood vessels, joints, and nerves. He described 107 marmas in the human body, each a vital point that can cause disease, suffering, and even death if pierced or otherwise damaged. Conversely, massage of these points can greatly relieve pain and swelling. Marma therapy is still an important part of contemporary Ayurvedic medical practice.*

A

Chapter VI.

Now we shall discourse on the Śáriram which specifically treats of the Marmas* or vital parts of the body. . . .

Classification of Marmas

There are one hundred and seven Marmas (in the human organism), which may be divided into five classes, such as the Mánsa-Marmas, Śirá-Marmas, Snáyu-Marmas, Asthi-Marmas and the Sandhi-Marmas. Indeed there are no other Marmas (vulnerable or vital parts) to be found in the body than the preceding ones.

Their Different Numbers

There are eleven Mánsa-Marmas (vulnerable muscle-joints); forty-one Śirá-Marmas (similar veins, anastomosis); twenty-seven Snáyu-Marmas (vital ligament-unions); eight Asthi-Marmas (bone-unions) and twenty Sandhi-Marmas (vulnerable joints).

Their Locations

Of these, eleven are in one leg, thus making twenty-two in the two lower extremities. The

---

Reprinted from Sushruta, *An English Translation of the Sushruta Samhita*, vol. 2, trans. and ed. Kaviraj Kunjalal Bhishagratna (Varanasi, India: Chowkhamba Sanskrit Series Office, 1963), 172, 176–82, 188–90.

---

*Places where veins, arteries, ligaments, joints and muscles unite and an injury to which proves generally fatal.

same number counts in the two hands. There are twelve Marmas in the regions of the chest and the abdomen (Udara); fourteen in the back; and thirty-seven in the region of the neck (Grivá) and above it. . . .

Names and Descriptions of Marmas

. . . Firm unions of Mánsa (muscles), Śirá (veins), Snáyu (ligaments), bones or bone-joints are called Marmas (or vital parts of the body) which naturally and specifically form the seats of life (Prána), and hence a hurt to any one of the Marmas invariably produces such symptoms as arise from the hurt of a certain Marma.

The Marmas belonging to the Sadyah-**Pránahara** group are possessed of fiery virtues (thermogenetic); as fiery virtues are easily enfeebled, so they prove fatal to life (in the event of being any way hurt); while those belonging to the Kálántara-Pránahara group are fiery and lunar (cool) in their properties. And as the fiery virtues are enfeebled easily and the cooling virtues take a considerable time in being so, the Marmas of this group prove fatal in the long run (in the event of being any way hurt, if not instantaneously like the preceding ones). The Viśalyaghna Marmas are possessed of Vátaja properties (that is, they arrest the escape of the vital **Váyu**); so long as the dart does not allow the Váyu to escape from their injured interior, the life prolongs; but as soon as the dart is extricated, the Váyu escapes from the inside of the hurt and necessarily proves fatal. The Vaikalyakaras are possessed of Saumya (lunar properties) and they retain the vital fluid owing to their steady and cooling virtues, and hence tend only to deform the organism in the event of their being hurt, instead of bringing on death. The Rujákara Marmas of fiery and Vátaja properties become extremely painful inasmuch as both of them are pain-generating in their properties. Others, on the contrary, hold the pain to be the result of the properties of the five material components of the body (Páncha-bhautika).

Different Opinions on the Marmas

Some assert that Marmas, which are the firm union of the five bodily factors (of veins, ligaments, muscles, bones and joints), belong to the first group (Sadyah-Pránahara); that those, which form the junction of four such, or in which there is one in smaller quantity, will prove fatal in the long run, in the event of their being hurt or injured (Kálántara-Pránahara). . . .

But the fore going theory is not a sound one, inasmuch as blood is found to exude from an injured joint which would be an impossibility in the absence of any vein, ligament (Snáyu) and muscle being intimately connected with it. Hence every Marma should be understood as a junction or meeting place of the five organic principles of ligaments, veins, muscles, bones and joints.

Metrical Text

This is further corroborated by the fact that the four classes of Śirá or vessels (which respectively carry the Váyu, Pitta, Kapha and the blood) are found to enter into the Marmas for the purpose of keeping or maintaining the moisture of the local ligaments (Snáyu), bones, muscles and joints and thus sustain the organism. The Váyu, aggravated by an injury to a Marma, blocks up (those four classes of vessels) in their entire course throughout the organism and gives rise to great pain which extends all over the body. All the internal mechanism of a man (of which a Marma has been pierced into with a shaft or with any other piercing matter) becomes extremely painful, and seems as if it were being constantly shaken or jerked, and symptoms of syncope are found to set in. Hence a careful examination of the affected Marma should precede all the foregoing acts of extricating a Śalya from its inside. From that similar aggravated conditions and actions of the Pitta and the Kapha should be presumed in the event of a Marma being any way injured or pierced into.

A Marma of the Sadyah-Pránahara type being perforated at its edge brings on death at a later time (within seven days), whereas a deformity of the organ follows from the piercing of a Kálántara-Máraka Marma at the side (instead of in the centre). Similarly, an excruciating pain and distressful after-effects mark a similar perforation of a Marma of the Visályaghna group. And a Marma of the Rujákara class produces an excruciating pain (instead of a sharp one) in the event of its being pierced at the fringe.

An injured Marma of the Sadyah-Pránahara type terminates in death within seven days of the injury, while one of the Kálántara type, within a fortnight or a month from the date of hurt (according to circumstances). A case of injured Kshipra-Marma seldom proves fatal before that time (seven days). An injured Marma of the Visályaghna or Vaikalyakara group may prove fatal in the event of its being severely injured.

Marmas of the Extremities

Now we shall describe the situation of every Marma. The Marma, known as the *Kshipra,* is situated in the region between the first and the second toes (Tarsal articulation), which, being injured or pierced, brings on death from convulsions. The Marma, known as the *Tala-Hridaya,* is situated in the middle of the sole of the foot in a straight line drawn from the root of the middle toe. An injury to this Marma gives rise to extreme pain which ends in death. The Marma, known as the *Kurchcha,* is situated two fingers' width above from the Kshipra one on each side of the foot. An injury to this Marma results in shivering and bending in of the foot. The Marma called *Kurchcha-Sirah* is situated under the ankle-joints, one on each side of the foot (Gulpha-Sandhi); an injury to it gives rise to pain and swelling of the affected part. A perforation of the *Gulpha-Marma,*

which is situated at the junction of the foot and the calf, results in pain, paralysis and maimedness of the affected leg.

An injury to the Marma which is situated in the middle muscle of the calf to the distance of between twelve and thirteen fingers' width from the ankle, and known as the *Indravasti-Marma,* results in excessive hæmorrhage which ends in death.

An injury to or piercing of the *Jánu-Marma,* situated at the union of the thigh and the knee, results in lameness of the patient.

A piercing of the *Áni-Marma,* situated on both the sides above three fingers' width from the Iánu (knee-joint), brings on swelling and paralysis (numbness) of the leg.

A perforation of the *Urvi-Marma,* situated in the middle of the Uru (thigh), results in the atrophy of the leg, owing to the incidental hæmorrhage. An injury to the *Lohitáksha-Marma,* situated respectively a little above and below the Urvi-Marma and the Vankshana (groin-joint), and placed near the thigh, is attended with excessive hæmorrhage and causes paralysis (of the leg).

An injury to the *Vitapa-Marma,* situated between the Scrotum and the Vankshana (inguinal region), brings on loss of manhood or scantiness of semen. Thus the eleven *Sakthi-Marmas* of one leg have been described; those in the other being of an identical nature with the preceding ones. The Marmas in the hands are almost identical with those of the legs, with the exception that *Manivandha, Kurpara* and *Kakshadhara* Marmas occur in the place of the Gulpha, Iánu and Vitapa Marmas respectively. As the Vitapa-Marma is situated between the scrotum and the Vankshana (inguinal region), so the Kakshadhara-Marma is situated between the Vaksha (chest) and the Kaksha (armpit). An injury to these causes supervening symptoms. An injury to the Manivandha-Marma (wrist-marma) results specially in inoperativeness (Kuntha) of the affected hand; an injury to the Kurpara-Marma ends in dangling (Kuni) of the hand; and an injury to the Kakshadhara results in **hemiplegia**. Thus the forty-four Marmas of the upper and the lower extremities have been described. . . .

Memorable Verses

. . . Men, versed in the science of surgery, have laid down the rule that, in a case of surgical operation, the situation and dimension of each local Marma should be first taken into account and the incision should be made in a way so as not to affect that particular Marma, inasmuch as an incision, even extending or affecting, in the least, the edge or the side of the Marma, may prove fatal. Hence all the Marma-Sthánas should be carefully avoided in a surgical operation.

The amputation of a hand or a leg may not prove fatal whereas a wound in any of the Marmas situated therein is sure to bring on death. The vessels become contracted in the case of a cut in the leg or in the hand of a man, and hence the incidental bleeding is comparatively scantier. Therefore it is that a cut in any of these parts of the body, however painful, does not necessarily prove fatal, like the lopping off of the branches of a tree. On the contrary, a man pierced into in any such Marmas, as the Kshipra or the Tala, suffers from excessive hæmorrhage (from the affected part) and attended with an excruciating pain, owing to the derangement of the Váyu, and meets his doom like a tree whose roots have been severed. Hence, in a case of piercing or of injury to any of these Marmas, the hand or the leg should be immediately amputated at the wrist or at the ankle (respectively).

The medical authorities have described the Marmas to have covered half in the scope of Śalya Tantra (Surgery), inasmuch as a person hurt in any of the Marmas dies presently (i. e., within seven days of the hurt). A deformity of the organ is sure to result from an injury to one of these Marmas, even if death be averted by a course of judicious and skillful medical treatment.

The life of the patient is not to be despaired of even in the case of fracture or crushing of a bone of the Koshtha, Śirah and Kapála or perforation of the intestines etc., if the local Marmas are found not to be in any way hurt or affected. Recovery is common in cases of cuts (pierce) in the Sakthi, Bhuja, Páda and Kara or in any other part of the body and even where a whole leg or band is found to be severed and carried away if the Marmas are not in any way hurt or affected.

These Marmas form the primary seats of the Váyu, the Soma (lunar) and Tejas (fiery principles of the organism), as well as of the three fundamental qualities of Satva, Rajas and Tamas, and that is the reason why a man, hurt in any of the Marmas, does not live.

An injury to a Marma of the Sadyah-Pránahara class (in which death occurs within a day) is attended with the imperfection of the sense organs, loss of consciousness, bewilderment of Manah (mind) and Buddhi (intellect) and various kinds of pain. An injury to a Marma of the Kálántara group (of a person) is sure to be attended with the loss of Dhátus (blood etc.) and various kinds of supervening symptoms (Upadrava) which end in death. The body of a person, hurt in any of the Vaikalyakara Marmas, may remain operative only under a skillful medical treatment; but a deformity of the affected organ is inevitable. An injury to any of the Viśalyaghna Marmas ends in death for the reasons mentioned above. An injury to any of the Rujákara Marmas gives rise to various kinds of pain in the affected organ, which may ultimately bring about a deformity of the same, if placed under the treatment of an ignorant and unskillful Vaidya (Surgeon).

An injury to the adjacent part of a Marma, whether incidental to a cut, incision, blow (Abhigháta), burn, puncture, or to any other cause exhibits the same series of symptoms as an actually affected one. An injury to a Marma, whether it be severe or slight, is sure to bring deformity or death.

The diseases which are seated in the Marmas, are generally serious, but they may be made to prove amenable with the greatest care and difficulty. . . .

⋏

Epilepsy in Ancient India

Bala V. Manyam

*Epilepsy has been recognized as a serious medical problem in many cultures for a long time. This selection and the next demonstrate that both the ancient Chinese and the ancient Indian physicians were well acquainted with its various manifestations. In each culture, epilepsy was described in the context of the physicoanatomical and philosophical constructs of the culture, and in both, physicians accurately recorded the clinical manifestations of the disease. Their explanations of the etiology of the disease diverge widely, one in terms of the balance of yin and yang and the Five Elements, and the other in terms of the **homeostasis** of the three humors that control all bodily functions. Both explanations are widely variant from the explanation of the causes of epilepsy offered by modern Western medicine. **Treatment modalities** in both Indian and Chinese medicine are classified on the basis of symptomology and perceived cause, and in both cultures, epilepsy was regarded as a serious problem.*

⋏

The ancient Indian medical system, called *Ayurveda,* or "science of life," in Sanskrit (*ayu,* life—combined state of body, senses, mind and soul; *veda,* science), was developed on sound scientific principles and is the oldest system of medicine in the world. The basic concepts of Ayurveda were refined and advanced further as they evolved during the Vedic period (4500–1500 B.C.). Literature in Ayurveda is divided into two groups—the major trio (*Brhattrayi*) and the minor trio (*Laghutrayi*). The major trio includes *Charaka Samhita, Susruta Samhita,* and **Astanga Hrdaya.** The second group includes three relatively smaller and later volumes: *Madhava Nidana, Sarangadhara Samhita,* and *Bhavaprakasa.* These six volumes form the backbone of Ayurvedic literature.

According to Ayurvedic concepts, there are three fundamental systems of [the] body; namely, doshas, dhatus, and malas. *Doshas* (humors), of which there are three, govern the physiological and physiochemical activities of the body: vata, pitta, and kapha. **Vata** is responsible for all movements

and sensations including motor actions. *Pitta* is responsible for all physiochemical activities in the form of metabolism (production of heat and energy). **Kapha** is the substance that maintains compactness or cohesiveness in the body by providing the fluid matrix. In a healthy person, these doshas are in a state of homeostasis. Any disturbance of the homeostasis of doshas can lead to disease. The type of disease or syndrome depends on the type of disturbance. For example, nervous and mental disorders are said to originate from a disturbance of vata humor. In Ayurveda, neurologic diseases ate generally studied under vata rogas (*roga,* disease).

Epilepsy is referred to as *Apasmara* in Ayurveda. The prefix *apa* means negation or loss of, and *smara* means consciousness or memory. Apasmara is described in *Charaka Samhita, Madhava Nidana,* and to some extent in *Susruta Samhita.*

The etiology of epilepsy was considered to be due to both **endogenous** and **exogenous** factors. Among the exogenous factors are internal hemorrhage; high fever; excessive sexual intercourse;

Reprinted by permission of *Epilepsia,* and Bala V. Manyam, MD, from Bala V. Manyam, "Epilepsy in Ancient India," *Epilepsia* 33, no. 3 (1992): 473–74.

disturbances of the body due to fast running, swimming, jumping, or leaping; eating of foods that are contaminated; nonhygienic practices; or extreme mental agitation caused by anger, fear, lust, or anxiety. An endogenous disturbance refers to a metabolic derangement in the form of a disturbance of doshas that are aggravated and lodged in the channels of *hrt,* or brain. It was also recognized that epilepsy could arise as a result of other diseases.

An attack of seizures is said to occur when the patient sees nonexistent objects (visual hallucinations), falls down, and has twitching in the tongue, eyes, and eyebrows with jerky movements in the hands and feet. In addition, there is excessive salivation. After the paroxysm is over, the patient awakens as if from sleep.

Aura was recognized and was called *Apasmara Poorva Roopa. Charaka* lists a large number of symptoms: seeing nonexistent objects, subjective sensation of sounds, a feeling of delusion, a sense of darkness, vertigo, dream-like state, constricting sensation in the chest, dribbling of saliva, body ache, and trembling.

Epilepsy was classified into four types, the first three being caused by defects in one of the three doshas (vata, pitta, and kapha) and the fourth type by a combination of disturbances in all three doshas.

The *Vatika* type, due to the disturbance of vata, is characterized by frequent fits with uncontrollable crying, unconsciousness, trembling, gnashing of teeth, and rapid breathing. Upon regaining consciousness, the patient has a headache.

In *Pattika* epilepsy, there is a disturbance of pitta in which the patient becomes agitated, has sensations of heat and extreme thirst, and has an aura of the environment being on fire followed by frequent fits accompanied by groaning and frothing at the mouth and often striking against the earth. The froth is yellow.

In *Kaphaja* epilepsy, in which there is a disturbance of kapha, the onset of convulsions is delayed and is preceded by an aura during which the patient feels cold and heavy and sees objects as white. The seizure is accompanied by falling and frothing at the mouth. In this type the froth is whitish.

The fourth type, *Sannipatika,* is due to a combination of disturbances in all three humors. This type is incurable, occurs in older people, and results in emaciation.

It was reported that if an epileptic person has violent convulsions, becomes excessively emaciated, has frequent eyebrow movements, and has eyes that are twisted in different ways, death will result. The periodicity of epilepsy was considered to be intervals of 2 weeks, 12 days, 1 month, or some other period of time.

The physician should treat the curable epileptic person cautiously with strong evacuative measures and respective pacificatory ones. When epilepsy was thought to be caused by an exogenous factor in addition to a disturbance of a dosha, the physician prescribed a general treatment to alleviate the exogenous cause. In addition, a more specific treatment was directed at correcting the disturbances of the dosha, as the goal in Ayurveda was correcting the whole body—physical, mental, and spiritual—not just treating a symptom. However, the physician was directed to first take steps for the "awakening of the heart" (meaning waking the patient from unconsciousness) by using drastic measures to clear those doshas that block channels of the mind. He was instructed to treat the *Vatika* type predominately with enema, the *Pattika* with purgation, and the *Kaphaja* type mostly with emesis; the *Sannipatika* type remained the most difficult to treat.

After the patient was cleansed by all means, drug formulations to alleviate epilepsy were administered. Several formulations, including the amount of each ingredient and method of preparation, are mentioned. The ingredients of these preparations included *gandhaka* (sulfur), aged *ghee* (butter fat), and many herbs such as *Achyranthes aspera, Holarrhena antidysenterica, Alstonta scholaris,* and *Ficus carica.* Blends of herbal formulations such as *Pancamula* and *Triphala* were also named. Pharmaceutical processes and preparations involving fermenting, extracting, preparing inhalable substances, filtrating, heating in a closed cavity, purifying, and pill-making are described. Many of these preparations are not specific for epilepsy; they were also used for treatment of insanity, intermittent fever, and other conditions. Epileptic persons, like the insane, were to be kept away from dangerous situations;

namely, water, fire, treetops, and hills. General measures to correct exogenous factors such as proper hygiene and balanced diet were recommended. Epilepsy was considered chronic, but treatable with difficulty.

⅄

History of Epilepsy in Chinese Traditional Medicine

CHI-WAN LAI AND YEN-HUEI C. LAI

⅄

The history of epilepsy in Western medicine can be traced to the era of Hippocrates (~460–377 B.C.), when it became accepted that epilepsy was not caused by supernatural forces. The history of epilepsy in ancient Chinese medicine, on the other hand, is not well known in the Western world. . . .

. . . The description of epilepsy first appeared in *The Yellow Emperor's Classic of Internal Medicine, Huang Di Nei Jing* . . . , an early Chinese medicine book, written as a dialogue between Qi Po . . . and the Yellow Emperor, Huang Di . . . , who discuss a theory of humans in health and in disease and a theory of medicine. The true author (or authors) of this book can no longer be confirmed, but it is believed to be a collective work of a group of Chinese physicians, around the period of Warring States (~770–221 B.C.). The book consists of two volumes: *Shu-Wen* and *Ling-Shu*. In the *Shu-Wen* volume, a short passage describes emotional shock of the pregnant mother as a cause of her child's epilepsy. The *Ling-Shu* volume provides a vivid description of an epileptic attack compatible with "grand mal."

Recurrent attacks as a definition of epilepsy can be traced back to the *Shu-Wen* volume of

Huang Di Nei Jing, which states: ". . . Initially the sickness occurs once a year. If not treated, then it will occur once a month. If not treated, then four or five times a month. Then this is called Dian."

. . . In Chinese traditional medicine, epilepsy sometimes tends to be confused with psychosis or mania. This ambiguity stems from the fact that the word "Dian" sometimes refers to epilepsy and at other times refers to insanity. The word "Dian" is used sometimes with the word "Kuang . . ." (mania) or "Feng" (psychosis) to form the compound word "Dian-Kuang," or "Feng-Dian," a practice that further blurs the distinction between epilepsy and psychosis.

A differentiation between epilepsy and madness (mania), however, can be found as early as around 200 B.C. during the period of Warring States in a medicine text, *Nan Jing* . . . , possibly authored by the famous physician, Bian Que. . . . The "59th Difficult Issue" states:

During the initial development of madness, one rests only rarely and does not feel hungry. One will (speak of) oneself as occupying a lofty, exemplary position. One will point out one's special wisdom, and one will behave in an arrogant and haughty

Reprinted by permission of *Epilepsia,* and Chai-Wan Lai, MD, from Chi-Wan Lai and Yen-Huei C. Lai, "History of Epilepsy in Chinese Traditional Medicine," *Epilepsia* 32, no. 3 (1991): 299–302.

way. One will laugh—and find joy in singing and making music—without reason, and one will walk around heedlessly without break. During the initial development of falling sickness, one's thoughts are unhappy. One lies down and stares straight ahead. The yin and the yang (movements in the) vessels are full in all three sections.

Wang Ken Tang (A.D. 1549–1613, Ming Dynasty) in his medicine textbook, *Zheng Zhi Zhun Sheng* . . . , further elaborated the differences between psychosis and epilepsy. He emphasized that the epileptic attacks usually consisted of convulsions with loss of consciousness, frothing, and vocalization, whereas patients with psychosis or mania did not have such symptoms. Unfortunately, despite his efforts to differentiate these disease entities, he still misled the readers by discussing psychosis, mania, and epilepsy in the same chapter.

. . . The description of an epileptic attack was very vivid and accurate in the early account in *Huang Di Nei Ching*. In the *Ling-Shu* volume, under the title of "Dian-Kuang," the following description is given:

> In the beginning of an epileptic attack, the patient suddenly becomes moody, notes a heavy sensation and pain in the head, stares with eyes widely open and turning red. The patient then feels agitated. . . . Then the epileptic attack takes off and the patient cries out, and gasps, . . . Sometimes, the attack starts out with stiffening, then the patient develops back pain (spasm?). . . .

Subsequent descriptions of epileptic attacks in other medical texts were more detailed, but all appeared to be confined to generalized convulsions (grand mal) as manifested by **tonic-clonic** movements, "staring" eyes, frothing at the mouth, tongue biting, vocalization, unconsciousness, and urinary and fecal incontinence. The characteristics of epileptic attacks, recurrent with sudden onset of spontaneous recovery, were recognized.

Status epilepticus was probably first described in Chinese medicine by Shen Jin Ao . . . in his book, *Shen Shi Zun Sheng Shu* . . . (A.D. 1773, Qing Dynasty). He stated:

During the epileptic attacks, the patient makes unusual noises, and froths at the mouth. When the patient is about to awaken, the epileptic attacks begin again, and the cycle occurs again and again and never stops. . . .

In chapter 68 of a book entitled, *Qi Xiao Liang Fang* . . . (A.D. 1470, Ming Dynasty), Fang Xian . . . described a different kind of epileptic attack:

> The patient suddenly sees a ghost-like subject, and smells an awful odor, falls to the ground with both fists clenched, limbs become cold and then the patient becomes unconscious. . . .

The description is highly compatible with a complex partial seizure which becomes secondarily generalized as defined in the International Classification of Epileptic Seizures. We have not been able, however, to find any description of true absence seizures under the category of epilepsy in Chinese medicine books. Such a nonconvulsive epileptic seizure may have been classified under psychiatric diseases or simply was not recognized as a medical condition.

. . . The first attempt to classify epileptic seizures was probably made by Cao Yuan Fang . . . , the author of an authoritative medicine textbook, *Zhu Bing Yuan Hou Lun* . . . (A.D. 610, Sui Dynasty). This book deals with etiology, mechanism, and pathology of various diseases and covers 67 diseases and 1,729 symptoms and signs. Cao first used age of onset to define two types of seizure, "Jian is a seizure occurring before the age of 10, and Dian one after the age of 10." He further proposed five types of epilepsy on the clinical observation of the symptoms and/or the "presumed causes":

I. "Yang Dian . . ." (Yang epilepsy): "During the attack, the patient appears as if dead, becomes incontinent, and then recovers spontaneously in a few moments."

II. "Yin Dian . . ." (Yin epilepsy): ". . . caused by having been given several baths during neonatal stage before the wounds of the severed umbilical cord were healed."

III. "Feng Dian . . ." (wind epilepsy): "During the attack eyes are fixed, limbs sustained in tonic contraction, and a goat-like crying occurs. The recovery ensues in a few moments . . . caused by being sweaty and exposed to the wind or having indulged in excessive sexuality or alcohol . . . causes stress, shortness of breath, and palpitation."

IV. "Shi Dian . . ." (wet epilepsy): ". . . frontal headache and heaviness of the body . . . caused by shampoo without drying of the hair; consequently the brain sweat can not leave the head."

V. "Lao Dian . . ." (labor epilepsy): "During the attack, eyes deviate upward, mouth shuts tightly, both arms and legs are sustained in tonic contraction, and the body feels hot."

Subsequent classifications have been proposed, the most fascinating being one based on the "noises" the patient makes during epileptic attacks. This classification was described in *Qian Jin Yao Fang* . . . (A.D. 682, Tang Dynasty) by Sun Si Miao . . . , who named epileptic attacks after various animals whose cry the "epileptic cry" resembled. It divided epileptic attacks into six types, "Yang Dian" (goat epilepsy), "Ma Dian" (horse epilepsy), "Zhu . . . Dian" (pig epilepsy), "Niu Dian" (cow epilepsy), "Qi . . . Dian" (chicken epilepsy), and "Gou . . . Dian" (dog epilepsy). The terminology used in this classification probably has had an adverse effect on the way Chinese society perceives epilepsy, as shown in the colloquial expression of epilepsy as "Yang-Dian-Feng" which can be translated literally as "goat-falling sickness-psychosis."

In the same book, Sun Si Miao also classified epilepsy alternatively according to the visceral organs believed to cause the disease. The groups consisted of "Xin . . . Xian" (heart epilepsy), "Gan . . . Xian" (liver epilepsy), "Pi Xian" (spleen epilepsy), "Fei Xian" (lung epilepsy), "Shen Xian" (kidney epilepsy), and "Chang . . . Xian" (intestine epilepsy). The ways of differentiating these various types of epilepsy were complex and were based on the Chinese philosophy of medicine. . . .

The brain was not even considered as the organ involved in epilepsy!

The concept of classifying epileptic seizures as either partial (focal) or generalized does not appear in Chinese traditional medicine. Even in a recently published traditional medicine textbook on this subject, only epileptic attacks with loss of consciousness are included.

. . . The earliest description of etiology of epilepsy appears to be that recorded in *Huang Di Nei Ching*. . . . In this account, Qi Po answers Huang Di's question as to the cause of epilepsy, as follows: "Epilepsy is a congenital illness. The baby contracts epilepsy inside its mother's womb when the mother experiences an emotional shock. . . ." Since then, many causes, derived from various theories, have been proposed. Some of them are currently considered incorrect by Western medicine. . . .

. . . The philosophy of treatment of diseases in Chinese traditional medicine is different from that of Western medicine. In general, traditionalist doctors are convinced that:

> [L]ife is the result of a combination in specific proportions of YANG energy from the sun and YIN energy from the earth. Human activity, health and sensitivity are nothing other than the refraction of the vital force through the body, which is itself a condensation and materialization of cosmic energy.

It is believed that when the balance between Yin and Yang is disturbed, diseases will follow. Another doctrine, "Wu Xing . . ." (Five Elements), consists of the belief that the human body is made up of a harmonious mixture of five primordial substances:

> . . . metal, wood, water, fire, and earth. The five elements also interact, resulting in five "generators" and five "subjugators." Corresponding to these five elements are the five organs—spleen, liver, heart, lungs and kidneys—which are further related in a complex system of arrangements of the planets, color, taste, climate, etc. . . . So long as the proportions remain proper, health results; if the balance is disturbed, disease follows.

The treatments are designed to restore the balance by a variety of means.

A recent text of Chinese traditional medicine suggests a general principle of "Bian Zheng Lu Zi" (to differentiate the symptoms/signs, and then determine the therapy), and proposes eight rules in treating epilepsy. These include the following:

> [E]xpel the wind . . . expel the phlegms . . . calm the patient . . . bring down the fever . . . relieve the stagnation of food . . . activate the blood circulation (for cases of posttraumatic epilepsy or epilepsy secondary to birth trauma), energize the spleen (when epileptic attack becomes less frequent), energize the kidney (when it is a congenital epilepsy).

The therapy includes herbs, acupuncture, "Mai Yao" (injection of herbs into the acupuncture points), "Mai Xien . . ." (burying a piece of goat intestine into the acupuncture points), or massage.

Several general guidelines in dealing with epileptic patients were summarized in a published Chinese traditional medicine textbook:

1. Physicians should see patients as frequently as possible.
2. A description of the epileptic attack should be given by an observer.
3. Physicians may change the treatment if epileptic attacks continue to recur.
4. Physicians should ask for any precipitating factors and circumstances under which epileptic attacks occurred.

▲

Huang Ti Nei Ching Su Wên

The Yellow Emperor's Classic of Internal Medicine

ILZA VEITH, TRANS.

The Yellow Emperor's Classic of Internal Medicine, or Huang Ti Nei Ching Su Wên, *is the greatest of the classic texts on traditional Chinese medicine. Its origins are unclear, but it is believed to have been written during the time of the Warring States (770 B.C.E.–221 C.E.) as a compilation, by several authors, of a great deal of older information. The* Nei Ching *is organized as two series of questions by the Yellow Emperor, answered by his physician, Chi'Po; one series is designated as "simple" questions, the other as "difficult." In addition to addressing purely medical matters, the text presents ethical, religious, and philosophical considerations, all of which have enormously influenced the practice of traditional Chinese medicine.*

One example of the principles of such practice appears in this selection on pulse therapy. In traditional Chinese medicine, an accurate analysis of pulses is the most important diagnostic tool available to the physician. While the pulse was recognized as the "storehouse

Reprinted by permission of the University of California Press, from Ilza Veith, trans., *Huang Ti Nei Ching Su Wen: The Yellow Emperor's Classic of Internal Medicine* (Berkeley: University of California Press, 1949), 159–67. Copyright © 1947 1975 Ilza Veith.

*of the blood," it reflected far more than the simple heartbeat: It was believed to demonstrate
the health of internal organs such as the liver, stomach, and kidneys. Mastering the art
of pulse therapy required much training and skill, and this type of therapy remains an essential part of traditional Chinese medicine.*

▲

Treatise on the Importance of the Pulse and the Subtle Skill of its Examination

The Yellow Emperor asked: "What is the way of medical treatment?"

Ch'i Po answered: "The way of medical treatment is to be consistent. It should be executed at dawn when the breath of Yin [the female principle in nature] has not yet begun to stir and when the breath of Yang [the male principle of life and light] has not yet begun to diffuse; when food and drink have not yet been taken, . . . when vigor and energy are not yet disturbed—at that particular time one should examine what has happened to the pulse.

"One should feel whether the pulse is in motion or whether it is still and one should observe attentively and with skill. One should examine the five colors and the **five viscera,** whether they suffer from excess or whether they show an insufficiency, and one should examine the six bowels whether they are strong or weak. One should investigate the appearance of the body whether it is flourishing or deteriorating. One should use all these five examinations and combine their results, and then one will be able to decide upon the share of life and death.

"The pulse is the store-house of the blood. When the pulse beats are long and the strokes markedly prolonged . . . , then the constitution of the pulse is well regulated; when the pulse beats are short and without volume . . . , then the constitution of the pulse is out of order. When the pulse is quick, and contains six beats to one cycle of respiration . . . , then it indicates heart trouble; and when the pulse is large . . . the disease becomes grave.

"When the upper pulse is abundant then its impulse is strong; when the lower pulse is abundant then it indicates flatulence. When the pulse is irregular and tremulous and the beats occur at irregular intervals . . . , then the impulse of life fades; when the pulse is slender [smaller than feeble, but still perceptible, thin like a silk thread] . . . , then the impulse of life is small. When the pulse is small and fine, slow and short like scraping bamboo with a knife . . . , then it indicates that the heart is irritated and painful.

"When the force of the pulse is **turbid** and the color disturbed like a bubbling well, it is a sign that disease has entered the body, the color has become corrupted and the constitution delicate. And when the constitution is delicate it will be broken up like the strings of a lute and die. . . ."

The Emperor asked: "Is not the pulse influenced by the four seasons? How can one know where the disease is located? How can one know the changes a disease may undergo? How can one know whether a disease is at first located in the interior? How can one know whether it may not at first be located at the outside? I beg you to answer these five questions."

Ch'i Po answered: "Please bear in mind that the power of Heaven is great and that it can change ill luck for the better. Outside of all living creation and within the Universe are transformations brought about by Heaven and Earth and by the interrelation of Yin and Yang. . . ."

"If it were not for excellent technique and the subtlety of the pulse one would not be able to examine it. But the examination must be done according to a plan, and the system of Yin and Yang [the two principles of nature] serves as [a] basis for examination. When this basis is established one can investigate the twelve main vessels and the five elements that generate life. Life itself follows a pattern that was set by the four seasons. . . .

"The feeling of the pulse should be done according to method: for when it is slow and quiet it acts as protector and guardian. In days of Spring the pulse is superficial, like wood floating on water . . . or like a fish that glides through the waves. . . .

"Hence it is said: Those who wish to know the inner body feel the pulse and have thus the fundamentals for diagnosis. . . .

"When the heart pulse beats vigorously . . . and the strokes are markedly prolonged, the corresponding illness makes the tongue curl up and makes the patient unable to speak. . . .

"When the pulse of the lungs beats vigorously and long, the corresponding illness produces blood in the sputum; when the pulse beats are soft and scattered, the corresponding illness produces torrents of sweat which up till the present time cannot be absorbed and be issued again.

"When the pulse of the liver beats vigorously and long and the complexion is not grayish green, the corresponding illness produces a sinking sensation as though one were fatally stricken, and the blood within the ribs and flanks descends presently, leaving people panting and exhausted. When the pulse beats are soft and scattered and the complexion shining and glossy, the corresponding illness requires abundant drinking, thirst is violent and requires more drinking, and changes befall the flesh and the skin and are transmitted to the outside through the stomach and the bowels.

"When the pulse of the stomach beats vigorously and long, the complexion turns red and the corresponding illness causes bent or broken thighs. When the pulse beats are soft and scattered, the resulting illness causes great pains while eating food.

"When the pulse of the spleen beats vigorously and long and the complexion turns yellow, the corresponding illness produces a shortness of breath and reduced force of life. When the pulse beats are soft and scattered and the complexion is not glossy and shining, the corresponding illness produces swelling of the coccyx and of the feet, which assume the appearance as though they contained water. . . ."

The Emperor said: "When one examines the pulse of the heart and finds it hasty, what sickness is then indicated? And what form does this illness take?"

Ch'i Po answered: "The name of the disease is 'rupture of the heart' . . . , and it is in the small intestines where the disease becomes visible."

The Emperor asked: "How can you describe the disease?"

Ch'i Po answered: "The heart acts as bolt of the door to the store house; the small intestines act as messengers; therefore one says that the small intestines are the place where the disease becomes manifest."

The Emperor inquired: "When, upon examination, one finds that the pulse of the stomach indicates disease, what does then happen?"

Ch'i Po answered: "When the pulse of the stomach is full and slightly tense . . . it indicates **dropsical** swellings; when it is empty slow and compressible . . . it indicates a leakage. . . .

". . . When there is proof that the pulse is reduced and that the complexion is not violated, then the disease is a recent one. But when there is proof that the pulse is not discordant yet the complexion is affected, then the disease is chronic. When there is proof that the pulse and the five colors (of the complexion) are all equally disturbed, then again the disease is chronic. When upon investigation it is found that the pulse and the five colors are equally undisturbed, then the disease is of recent date. . . .

"The inner pulses in the arms both denote the state of adjacent regions; they denote the state of the short ribs. . . . The outer pulses of the arms denote the state of the kidneys. When the pulses of the arms are examined for the interior, they indicate that which goes on within the stomach. Furthermore, the left outer pulse of the arm denotes the state of the liver, while the left inner pulse indicates the state of the diaphragm. The right outer pulse denotes the condition of the stomach and the right inner pulse indicates the state of the spleen. Moreover, the upper right pulse of the outside denotes what goes on within the thorax, whereas the upper left pulse of the outside denotes the condition of the heart and the upper left pulse of the inside indicates what goes on within the middle of the thorax. . . .

"When the pulse is dense and coarse and large its content of Yin elements is insufficient, and there is a surplus of Yang elements which causes fevers within the body.

"When an illness has arrived and departs very slowly and the upper pulse is full and large and the lower pulse is empty and slow, these symptoms indicate madness. When the disease which has arrived slowly departs and when the upper pulse is slow and empty, and the lower pulse is full and large, it indicates evil influences. Thus, it is found that Yang suffers evil influences within the body.

"When the pulse beats are heavy the examiner should make a careful count, for the (the region of the) lesser Yin is rebellious. When the pulse beats are heavy and upon careful examination are found to be scattered and irregular, they indicate chills and fevers. When the pulse beats are light and floating and also scattered and irregular, they indicate dizziness and blurred vision and people are apt to fall down prostrate.

"When the pulse beats are all light and floating and not hasty, then they all stem from the (region of) Yang and thus they indicate fever.

"When the pulse beats are small and heavy then they all stem from (the region of) Yin and

thus they indicate aching bones. When the pulse is calm and quiet the disease is indicated by the pulse of the foot. . . .

"All those who excel in the art of feeling the pulse find that when it is fine, slow, and short, there is an excess of Yang and when the pulse is slippery, like pebbles rolling in a basin, there is an excess of Yin.

"When there is an excess of Yang the body is hot and feverish and there is no perspiration. When there is an excess of Yin there is too much perspiration and colds and chills. . . ."

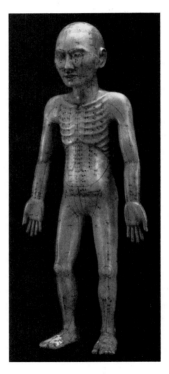

FIGURE 3–1   Acupuncture Chart
Although the practice of acupuncture predates the writing of the *Nei Ching*, the second volume of that work focused on the practice, describing the meridians, types of needles, needling techniques, and locations of some 160 points. Models made of clay, jade, and other materials were used as references for practitioners, such as this one made of lacquered cardboard, dating from the Qing Dynasty. (Art Resource/Reunion des Musees Nationaux).

▲

Medicine Is a Humane Art

The Basic Principles of Professional Ethics in Chinese Medicine

DAQING ZHANG AND ZHIFAN CHENG

Western medical ethics, or, more properly, bioethics, *have evolved since Hippocrates told his students, "First, do no harm." Heavily influenced by the Enlightenment and philosophers such as Immanuel Kant and John Locke, bioethics is now regarded as the basic rules by which all Western medicine must be practiced. However, many Western doctors are unaware that a parallel tradition of ethics in medicine existed in China even earlier than when Hippocrates was practicing in Greece. Chinese medical ethics are most commonly associated with the teachings of K'ung-Fu-tzu (***Confucius***), but as this selection shows, it has been a dynamic and evolving tradition from Confucius's time to the present. Given the strong differences in the principles of Chinese and Western medical practices, the two ethical traditions might be expected to vary. Yet, as this reading clearly reveals, both are based on common principles of beneficence, autonomy, nonmaleficence, and justice.*

▲

The value system of medical ethics in China has a long tradition that can be traced back to ancient times. Those values are reflected in the (Confucian) precept that "medicine is a humane art." That is, medicine is not only a means to save people's lives, but also a moral commitment to love people and free them from suffering through personal caring and medical treatment. Although this precept has been well accepted as the basic principle of professional ethics [and] a general principle that emphasizes doctors' self-accomplishment and self-restraint, there has never been a universally accepted professional code and binding principles in Chinese medicine comparable to the *Hippocratic Oath* in western medicine.

. . . As in ancient Greek medicine, the professional values of ancient Chinese medicine arose with the development of medical professionalism itself. In ancient China, "profession" meant one's duties. During the Zhou Dynasty (from 1065–771

B.C.E.), an independent medical profession and medical system took shape, built around four aspects: dietetic, internal, surgery, and veterinary. Standards for evaluating, and paying, doctors were established. Thus the *Rites of the Zhou Dynasty* records that "at the end of each year, doctors are paid according to their medical performance, the highest payment to those who got 100 percent cure rate, the payment for 90 percent cure rate ranks the second, 80 percent the third, and so on."

During the Spring and Autumn Period (770–476 B.C.E.) and the Warring States (475–221 B.C.E.), medicine began to divorce itself from witchcraft and became an experience-based knowledge and a professional skill. At the same time, professional physicians emerged as a distinct social class, no longer seen as wizards with superman skills but as ordinary technicians, whose relationship with patients and among themselves were being redefined. Codes of ethics and standards concerning medicine arose, and the emergence of schools of medicine laid the foundation for the development of formalized medical ethics.

In ancient China, folk physicians didn't have fixed clinics or hospitals but went from one place to another practicing medicine freely. They hadn't formal training and weren't licensed, but performed their work by their own skills and consciences. As a result, there were deceitful quacks as well as experienced, good-hearted physicians. Physicians also ran tremendous risks while practicing medicine. For instance, in the *Code of Hammurabi* (1700 B.C.E.), there were severe punishments for physicians' wrongdoings. Wenzhi, a 5th century B.C.E. physician, lost his life for failing to cure Emperor Qi's illness. To preserve their own reputations and distinguish themselves from quacks and to protect themselves, value emerged among physicians and between physicians and their disciples, such as emphasis on prognosis and observation of codes of conduct. These values gradually formed the foundation of early medical ethics.

Unschuld identifies three protective mechanisms for physicians in medical history: sorcery, prognosis, and medical ethics. We agree with Unschuld but we also think that these mechanisms are basically stages in the development of medical ethics. However, the evolution of these three stages isn't simply a substitute of one for another; there are overlaps among them and even coexistence of them. The first mechanism, sorcery, hinges on a belief in ghosts and gods and supernatural power to effect treatment; it is the domain of wizards and magicians.

The second mechanism, prognosis, rests on the advancement of medical knowledge and therapies and changes in people's conceptions about illness to believe that natural and reasonable factors cause disease. As physicians distinguished themselves from wizards and medicine lost the protective aura of magic, prognosis became the new protective mechanism. Ancient physicians paid great attention to prognosis and accumulated rich experience, codified in ancient medical books such as the *Canon of Medicine* and *Classic on Medical Problems.* By judging whether a patient was curable or incurable, a physician decided whether to accept the case for treatment.

The third mechanism is formal professional codes, which function as guidance for physicians' behaviors and as a standard for distinguishing excellent doctors from quacks. And they enable the public to believe that when the code is adhered to, bad outcomes will be regarded as the work of gods or beyond human beings' control.

According to the 1st century *Han Dynasty Records: Crafts,* from the eighth through the third centuries there existed seven schools of medicine as will as many other kinds of health-related practical schools. The various schools of medicine were both academic schools and professional groups, the germ of nongovernmental medical organizations. Some popular doctors, such as Bianque and Canggong, had a number of disciples. Bianque is said to have put forward the following standards for medical practice:

> medicine should not be offered in six circumstances, namely, to (1) people who have unreasonable arrogance and indulgence, (2) people who appreciate riches more than life, (3) people who cannot even keep body and soul together, (4) people who suffer from interlocking Yin and Yang, (5) people who are too weak to take medicines, and (6) people who don't believe in medicine but in sorcery.

Although Bianque's "six taboos" are framed as practical guidance, they implicitly set standards for professional conduct and values and therefore can be regarded as a sort of medical ethics and code of conduct for ancient Chinese doctors. In this respect, Bianque's code had much in common with the ancient western medical codes.

. . . As more effective therapies were developed and physicians' professional status was consolidated, the protective function of professional medical ethics gradually weakened and its proscriptive function steadily strengthened. From the Han Dynasty (206 B.C.E.–220 C.E.) forward, Confucianism shaped the core values of Chinese culture. In medicine, the influence of the Confucian school is embodied in the precept that "medicine is a humane art" with its emphasis on caring about patients and on physicians' self-cultivation in virtue.

Confucian Medicine

Benevolence is the core of **Confucian ethics.** In Confucianism "benevolence" means, "to love the people." Confucianists saw medicine as a means to save people's lives by love. In the "Miraculous Pivot" of the *Canon of Medicine,* it was noted that a man who mastered medicine could keep the ordinary people as well as himself in good health, so that a harmonious society could be formed and maintained. A prestigious physician of the East Han Dynasty, Zhongjing Zhang (150–219) said that only if they grasped medical theories and paid attention to medical treatment could the Confucianists realize their ambition of "loving the people." Throughout the Song, Jin, and Yuan (10th–13th centuries) dynasties, many Confucianists rushed into the field of medicine and "benevolence" became the theoretical foundation of medical ethics.

The Confucian principle of "loving the people" enjoins three fundamental commitments. First, it calls for veneration of human life—the *Canon of Medicine* notes that there is nothing in the world more precious than human beings. Confucianism required doctors to be very cautious and responsible in the course of diagnosis and prescription in order to avoid mistakes that would harm patients. The philosopher Mencius said: "In medicine, benevolence means causing no harm to patients."

Second, the Confucian principle also calls for respect for patients. The *Canon of Medicine* emphasized that doctors should not pose as those who bestowed favor, nor should they take advantage of their profession for benefits such as money or sex. Instead, they should fully respect their patients.

Third, the principle calls for "universal love," that is, to treat every patient equally, regardless of social status, family background, appearances, age,

etc. In *The Essential Prescriptions Worth a Thousand Gold* the Tang dynasty physician Simiao Sun instructed, "Whoever comes to seek cure must be treated like your own relatives regardless of their social status, family economic conditions, appearances, ages, races, and mental abilities." And Tingxian Gong, a doctor of the Ming Dynasty (1368–1644), severely denounced those doctors who treated patients unequally according to their family backgrounds.

However, it was not the formulation of strict laws and regulations but individuals' cultivation of virtue that Confucianists valued: saving people by love reflected one's own virtue. In their eyes, conscience was the foundation of medical virtue, doctors should have a sense of pity, of shame, of respect, and of right and wrong. The "sense of pity" requires doctors to cherish life, to relieve patients' pains, and to keep them in good health. The "sense of shame" means that physicians should think of patients' interests first and be ashamed to serve their own interests; to reach a diagnosis without performing the four physical examination methods (observation, **auscultation** and olfaction, interrogation, and pulse feeling and palpation) is a shameful means to abuse medicines and to deceive patients.

The "sense of respect" requires physicians to respect patients. The "sense of right and wrong" requires doctors not to do things that will damage patients' interests. Because doctors and patients are not equals, Confucianism also emphasizes that doctors should behave properly even without others' supervision and should not do to others what they wouldn't do to themselves. Tianchen Li of the Ming Dynasty said: "We should treat the patients as our mothers." Boxiong Fei (1800–1879), a doctor famous during the Qing Dynasty, described the virtuous physician: "If I am sick, what kind of doctor do I expect to see? If my parents, my wife, or children are sick, what kind of doctor do I expect to meet? See from the patient's point of view, then the self-serving desires will vanish." This emphasis on doctors' ethical cultivation is the major component of Chinese medical ethics.

Taoism and Buddhism in Relation to Medical Ethics

Taoism and Buddhism also influenced the development of medical ethics in China, themselves vigorously promoting the practice of medicine as a means of doing good. Taoism favors life and resents death. It regards being alive as the happiest thing and pursues immortality. Taoists pursue long life in either of two ways: by taking special medicines made from plants, animals, or minerals and by doing good deeds that benefit others. Five commandments are at the heart of Taoist religious codes. A Taoist is forbidden to kill any living thing, eat any meat or drink any alcohol, behave dishonestly, steal, or be sexually promiscuous. Central values in Taoism include loyalty, **filial piety,** politeness, trust, and humanity.

Buddhism is also a very important thread in the fabric of traditional Chinese medical ethics. To alleviate suffering and transcend the cycle of fate *(karma)* and rebirth, many Buddhists practiced good deeds by means of practicing medicine. Among China's early physicians were many well-known Buddhist monks, like Jianzhen of the Tang Dynasty who was not only a famous monk but also an outstanding doctor of great attainments.

The commandments of Taoism and Buddhism were introduced to the medical profession, and to some extent promoted the establishment of medical ethics and helped popularize doctors' codes of conduct.

Thus Chinese medical ethics came into existence in the course of conflict and convergence of many cultures: In medical ethics, as a discipline of applied ethics, various ethical theories and principles are fully embodied in medical treatment. Hence the major religions and philosophical systems of ancient China—Confucianism, Taoism, and Buddhism—had great influence on the formation and development of Chinese medical ethics. But its traditionally important position made Confucianism the core of medical ethics. Even so, and despite the fact that many doctors promulgated ethical standards over the history of Chinese medicine, a single, universally accepted code of ethics in medicine did not come into existence.

Traditional Chinese Medical Ethics

Chinese culture pays special attention to moral evaluation. This is fully characterized by showing filial obedience, being amicable to others, respecting ordinary people, and appreciating morality. Confucius taught that everyone had a sense of right and wrong; people could tell what they should do from what they should not do. Confucianism instructed people to tell right from wrong by self-examination rather than by proposing standards or codes of conduct to restrict people's behavior. Under the influence of the Confucian tradition, self-examination, self-criticism, and self-restriction became the core components of doctors' moral self-cultivation. Many believed that only with such right conduct and moral self-cultivation could the physician cure. Just for this reason, in ancient Chinese medical ethics it is hardly possible for us to find unified and legislative ethical standards like those in the Western world.

Traditional Chinese medical ethics also emphasized individual self-cultivation over uniform standards, in part because the traditional system of medicine was composed mainly of private physicians. There was no unified administrative system. Early China was mainly an agricultural society, in which families were the productive units. Although there were trade organizations similar to those of the Western world, they were much less steady and less influential—Shuming Liang, a famous philosopher, thought that ancient China lacked organizations. Thus medical education and practice were characterized by individualism and familism, with medical associations or organizations lagging behind. And because doctors had no close connections or contact with one another, and their economic interests were not seen to be in conflict, competition in the medical profession was not severe. Thus there was no need to formulate universally accepted and binding codes of ethics; doctors' self-discipline sufficed.

Another important characteristic of Chinese traditional medical ethics lies in its medical education. Medical education in China developed very early in the historical period, but its main purpose was to train doctors for royal courts, where they worked as servants to the nobility. Under this condition, the theories and practice of medical ethics could not achieve any normal development. Those who were going to practice medicine for ordinary people were trained mainly by families or through apprenticeship.

These differences meant that the issues which concerned Western and Chinese medicine were also quite different. All in all, where Western medical ethics emphasized the standardization and systemization of medical practice, ancient Chinese medical ethics focused more on personal virtues.

. . . From a cross-cultural perspective, the early medical ethics of the West and China share many similarities. The evolution of medical ethics has passed from prognosis to code of conduct and then to values. With the development of medical professionalism and the establishment of medical systems influenced by different religious and philosophical ideas, the development of Chinese medical ethics also differed in many features from that of Western medicine. Under the domination of Confucianism, "medicine is a humane art" became the basic principle of early medical ethics in China, resting on doctors' individual self-cultivation of doctors. Later, with the introduction of Western medicine and the establishment of modern medical systems, people in the medical field began to attach more importance to the construction of a popular code of medicine that nonetheless preserved inherited medical ethical values. . . . Yet no matter how rapidly medical technologies develop and no matter how greatly health care systems change, the concept of medicine as a humane art will continue to flourish in China. It is possibly the very essence of medicine.

KEY TERMS

Acupuncture, 44 • *Astanga Hrdaya,* 50 • Auscultation, 61 • Ayurvedic, 44 • Charaka, 45 • Chakras, 45 • Confucian ethics, 61 • Confucius, 59 • Couching, 46 • Doshas, 44 • Dropsical, 57 • Endogenous, 50 • Exogenous, 50 • Filial piety, 62 • Five Elements, 44 • Five viscera, 56 • Hemiplegia, 48 • Homeostasis, 50 • Kapha, 50 • Marmas, 46 • Moxibustion, 44 • *Nei Ching,* 44 • Pitta, 50 • Pránahara, 47 • *The Pulse Classic,* 45 • Rhinoplasty, 46 • *Samhita,* 46 • Shang oracle bones, 45 • Sushruta, 46 • Taoism, 62 • Tonic-clonic, 53 • Treatment modalities, 50 • Trepanation, 45 • Turbid, 56 • Vata, 50 • Váyu, 47 • Yin and yang, 44

QUESTIONS TO CONSIDER

1. It is often said that the earliest doctors were good observers but were not good at diagnosis. Is this statement valid in the case of India and China? To what extent were accurate diagnoses and treatments possible, given the lack of anatomical knowledge as it is taught in the West? Or, in fact, were Ayurvedic and traditional Chinese physicians far more accurate than practitioners of Western medicine are generally willing to acknowledge?

2. Consider Sushruta's description of marmas in the human body; then compare them to the acupuncture points shown in Figure 3–1. Do you see any common points of reference? Do you see any connection to Western anatomical studies, or do the Eastern body systems demonstrate entirely different approaches to medicine?

3. Practitioners of Western medicine have been slow to acknowledge the value of the Chinese and Ayurvedic traditions; only since about the 1970s have Western-trained physicians considered techniques such as acupuncture to have any validity. Why? What is at the root of their resistance? Why has recognition come so slowly?

4. If you were a practicing physician today, how would your faithful adherence to established principles of bioethics affect your treatment of patients? If you were treating Asian American patients, how would your ethical decisions be changed by focusing on Confucian rather than Western concepts?

RECOMMENDED READINGS

Conrad, Lawrence I., and Dominik Wujastyk, eds. *Contagion: Perspectives from Pre-modern Societies.* Burlington, VT: Ashgate, 1988.

Furth, Charlotte. *A Flourishing Yin: Gender in China's Medical History, 960–1665.* Berkeley: University of California Press, 1999.

Kendall, Donald E. *The Dao of Chinese Medicine: Understanding an Ancient Healing Art.* Oxford: Oxford University Press, 2002.

Meulenbeld, G. Jan, and Dominik Wujastyk, eds. *Studies on Indian Medical History.* Delhi, India: Motilal Banarsidass, 2001.

Unschuld, Paul, trans. *Forgotten Traditions of Ancient Chinese Medicine: A Chinese View from the 18th Century.* Brookline, MA: Paradigm, 1998.

———. *Medicine in China: A History of Ideas.* Berkeley: University of California Press, 1988.

Veith, Ilza, trans., and Ken Rose, ed. *The Yellow Emperor's Classic of Internal Medicine.* Berkeley: University of California Press, 2002.

Zysk, Kenneth G. *Religious Medicine: History and Evolution of Indian Medicine.* New Brunswick, NJ: Transaction, 1993.

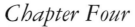

Chapter Four

Greece

INTRODUCTION

The practice and art of medicine underwent a sea change during the civilization of ancient Greece. Although elements of the magical explanation of the causes and cures of disease continued, particularly in the cult of Asklepios, Hippocrates of Cos, often referred to as "The Father of Western Medicine," and his followers introduced a new logical and rational approach. The ages-old reliance on the supernatural to explain illness was a self-limiting concept that did not lend itself easily to exploration of new ideas or challenge of old notions. Once an individual accepts that the gods cause and can cure disease, not much can be added. The rational model begun by the Greeks removed such limitations. With the basic premise that disease is caused by changes within the body, medical practitioners could begin the long road to discovering what the changes were and how to prevent or treat them. The new emphasis on patient history, observation of symptoms, diagnosis, and treatment all put medicine on a much more accurate footing.

Even with such advances, however, physicians remained unable to treat many problems successfully. Warfare erupted periodically, beginning with the legendary Trojan War described in Homer's *The Iliad,* and including the wars with Persia for control of the Aegean, and the Peloponnesian War, which pitted the great city-states of Athens and Sparta against each other. Weaponry was becoming more sophisticated, causing severe wounds and subsequent infections that doctors were powerless to treat. Infectious diseases were widespread and common, often occurring in conjunction with the wars, and little could be done to prevent their spread. One of the most famous epidemics of the ancient world, known as the *Plague of Athens,* occurred during the Peloponnesian War. Although the famous historian Thucydides carefully reported the outbreak, his description of the symptoms has never led to a definitive diagnosis of the disease, and the plague remains a mystery to this day. What was clear from Thucydides' account was that the mortality rate was high in the heavily overcrowded city under siege, which resulted in the loss of potential military and political leaders and was instrumental in the ultimate defeat of Athens. The Plague of Athens is only one of a number of medical events throughout the ages that have affected the overall course of history.

TIME LINE

ca. 1200 B.C.E.	Trojan War; Battle of Troy
776 B.C.E.	First Olympian games
600 B.C.E.–400 C.E.	Heyday of Asclepian temples and cures
580–489 B.C.E.	Pythagoras founds school at Croton; earliest studies on anatomy and physiology
ca. 492–c. 450 B.C.E.	Empedocles lives—believed to have accomplished several medical miracles; states that the heart is the center of the vascular system and the seat of emotions
479–388 B.C.E.	Golden Age of Greece, Age of Pericles
470 B.C.E.	Alcmaeon of Croton is doing dissections—first person known to do so
ca. 460–377 B.C.E.	Hippocrates of Cos, "The Father of Western Medicine" lives—writes *Hippocratic Corpus,* Hippocratic oath; emphasizes holistic care; encourages separation of religion and medicine
431–404 B.C.E.	Peloponnesian War
430–427 B.C.E.	Plague of Athens—recorded by eyewitness Thucydides in his *History of the Peloponnesian Wars*
420 B.C.E.	Approximate date of Hippocratic oath; date of earliest known Hippocratic writings
384–322 B.C.E.	Aristotle lives—believes that science can develop from careful observation, experimentation, and study of cause and effect; does nonhuman dissections, teaches comparative anatomy, and uses findings to support his biomedical theories
ca. 330–260 B.C.E.	Herophilus lives—first true anatomist; does public dissections at Alexandria; describes major internal organs and nervous system; believes the brain is the center of learning and emotions
ca. 304–ca. 250 B.C.E.	Erasistratus lives—contemporary anatomist with Herophilus; teaches at Alexandria
ca. 240–ca. 180 B.C.E.	Diocles lives—writes the first books on anatomy and herbal remedies
219 B.C.E.	Archagathus, traditionally considered the first Greek doctor to go to Rome, is given Roman citizenship
146 B.C.E.	Rome conquers Greece, which becomes a Roman province

The Peloponnesian War

The Second Book

THUCYDIDES

The Greek historian Thucydides is generally considered the first modern historian. Not content to merely report events and chronologies, he dealt with causes, effects, and relationships in historical events. His history of the Peloponnesian War is a classic, describing the struggle between Athens and Sparta for supremacy.

The Athenian defeat may have been caused in part by a mysterious epidemic that swept the city in 430 B.C.E. However, even with the clearly written descriptions of the plague by Thucydides, who was an eyewitness, the specific nature of the disease remains unknown. Many possible candidates have been suggested, from bubonic plague (which it clearly was not) to typhus. Whatever disease it was, the Plague of Athens killed a large number of people who had crowded into the city for protection. It returned twice—in 429 and finally in 427–426—which further reduced the population and military strength. Among the hardest-hit groups were the young adults, who could have provided political and military leadership during the war. The defeat of Athens ushered in a period of chaos and the decline of classical Greek civilization, which ultimately led to the era of Alexander the Great. Had it not been for the Plague of Athens, the history of Europe might have been far different.

47. . . . In the very beginning of summer the Peloponnesians and their confederates, with two-thirds of their forces as before, invaded Attica under the conduct of Archidamus the son of Zeuxidamas, king of Lacedaemon, and after they had encamped themselves, wasted the country about them. They had not been many days in Attica when the plague first began amongst the Athenians, said also to have seized formerly on divers other parts, as about Lemnos and elsewhere; but so great a plague and mortality of men was never remembered to have happened in any place before. For at first neither were the physicians able to cure it through ignorance of what it was but died fastest themselves, as being the men that most approached the sick, nor any other art of man availed whatsoever. All supplications to the gods and enquiries of oracles and whatsoever other means they used of that kind proved all unprofitable; insomuch as subdued with the greatness of the evil, they gave them all over.

48. It began, by report, first in that part of Ethiopia that lieth upon Egypt, and thence fell down into Egypt and Africa and into the greatest part of the territories of the king. It invaded Athens on a sudden and touched first upon those that dwelt in Piraeus, insomuch as they reported that the Peloponnesians had cast poison into their

Reprinted from Thucydides, *The Peloponnesian War,* vol. 1, trans. Thomas Hobbes, ed. David Grene (Ann Arbor: University of Michigan Press, 1959), 115–19.

wells (for springs there were not any in that place). But afterwards it came up into the high city, and then they died a great deal faster. Now let every man, physician or other, concerning the ground of this sickness, whence it sprung, and what causes he thinks able to produce so great an alteration, speak according to his own knowledge. For my own part, I will deliver but the manner of it and lay open only such things as one may take his mark by to discover the same if it come again, having been both sick of it myself and seen others sick of the same.

49. This year, by confession of all men, was of all other, for other diseases, most free and healthful. If any man were sick before, his disease turned to this; if not, yet suddenly, without any apparent cause preceding and being in perfect health, they were taken first with an extreme ache in their heads, redness and inflammation of the eyes; and then inwardly, their throats and tongues grew presently bloody and their breath noisome and unsavoury. Upon this followed a sneezing and hoarseness, and not long after the pain, together with a mighty cough, came down into the breast. And when once it was settled in the stomach, it caused vomit; and with great torment came up all manner of **bilious** purgation that physicians ever named. Most of them had also the hickyexe [possibly "the dry heaves"] which brought with it a strong convulsion, and in some ceased quickly but in others was long before it gave over. Their bodies outwardly to the touch were neither very hot nor pale but reddish, livid, and beflowered with little pimples and whelks, but so burned inwardly as not to endure any the lightest clothes or linen garment to be upon them nor anything but mere nakedness, but rather most willingly to have cast themselves into the cold water. And many of them that were not looked to, possessed with insatiate thirst, ran unto the wells, and to drink much or little was indifferent, being still from ease and power to sleep as far as ever. As long as the disease was at its height, their bodies wasted not but resisted the torment beyond all expectation; insomuch as the most of them either died of their inward burning in nine or seven days whilst

they had yet strength, or, if they escaped that, then the disease falling down into their bellies and causing there great exulcerations and immoderate looseness, they died many of them afterwards through weakness. For the disease, which took first the head, began above and came down and passed through the whole body; and he that overcame the worst of it was yet marked with the loss of his extreme parts; for breaking out both at their privy members and at their fingers and toes, many with the loss of these escaped; there were also some that lost their eyes. And many that presently upon their recovery were taken with such an oblivion of all things whatsoever, as they neither knew themselves nor their acquaintance.

50. For this was a kind of sickness which far surmounted all expression of words and both exceeded human nature in the cruelty wherewith it handled each one and appeared also otherwise to be none of those diseases that are bred amongst us, and that especially by this. For all, both birds and beasts, that use to feed on human flesh, though many men lay abroad unburied, either came not at them or tasting perished. An argument whereof as touching the birds is the manifest defect of such fowl, which were not then seen, neither about the carcases or anywhere else. But by the dogs, because they are familiar with men, this effect was seen much clearer.

51. So that this disease (to pass over many strange particulars of the accidents that some had differently from others) was in general such as I have shown, and for other usual sicknesses at that time no man was troubled with any. Now they died some for want of attendance and some again with all the care and physic that could be used. Nor was there any to say certain medicine that applied must have helped them; for if it did good to one, it did harm to another. Nor any difference of body, for strength or weakness, that was able to resist it; but it carried all away, what physic soever was administered. But the greatest misery of all was the dejection of mind in such as found themselves beginning to be sick (for they grew presently desperate and gave themselves over without making any resistance), as also their

dying thus like sheep, infected by mutual visitation, for the greatest mortality proceeded that way. For if men forebore to visit them for fear, then they died forlorn; whereby many families became empty for want of such as should take care of them. If they forbore not, then they died themselves, and principally the honestest men. For out of shame they would not spare themselves but went in unto their friends, especially after it was come to this pass that even their domestics, wearied with the lamentations of them that died and overcome with the greatness of the calamity, were no longer moved therewith. But those that were recovered had much compassion both on them that died and on them that lay sick, as having both known the misery themselves and now no more subject to the danger. For this disease never took any man the second time so as to be mortal. And these men were both by others counted happy, and they also themselves, through excess of present joy, conceived a kind of light hope never to die of any other sickness hereafter.

52. Besides the present affliction, the reception of the country people and of their substance into the city oppressed both them and much more the people themselves that so came in. For having no houses but dwelling at that time of the year in stifling booths, the mortality was now without all form; and dying men lay tumbling one upon another in the streets, and men half-dead about every conduit through desire of water. The temples also where they dwelt in tents were all full of the dead that died within them. For oppressed with the violence of the calamity and not knowing what to do, men grew careless both of holy and profane things alike. And the laws which they formerly used touching funerals were all now broken, every one burying where he could find room. And many for want of things necessary, after so many deaths before, were forced to become impudent in the funerals of their friends. For when one had made a funeral pile, another getting before him would throw on his dead and give it fire. And when one was in burning, another would come and, having cast thereon him whom he carried, go his way again.

53. And the great licentiousness, which also in other kinds was used in the city, began at first from this disease. For that which a man before would dissemble and not acknowledge to be done for voluptuousness, he durst now do freely, seeing before his eyes such quick revolution, of the rich dying and men worth nothing inheriting their estates. Insomuch as they justified a speedy fruition of their goods even for their pleasure, as men that thought they held their lives but by the day. As for pains, no man was forward in any action of honour to take any because they thought it uncertain whether they should die or not before they achieved it. But what any man knew to be delightful and to be profitable to pleasure, that was made both profitable and honourable. Neither the fear of the gods nor laws of men awed any man, not the former because they concluded it was alike to worship or not worship from seeing that alike they all perished, nor the latter because no man expected that lives would last till he received punishment of his crimes by judgment. But they thought there was now over their heads some far greater judgment decreed against them before which fell, they thought to enjoy some little part of their lives.

54. Such was the misery into which the Athenians being fallen were much oppressed, having not only their men killed by the disease within but the enemy also laying waste their fields and villages without. In this sickness also (as it was not unlikely they would) they called to mind this verse said also of the elder sort to have been uttered of old:

A Doric war shall fall,
And a great plague withal.

Now were men at variance about the word, some saying it was not *loimos* [plague], that was by the ancients mentioned in that verse, but *limos* [famine]. But upon the present occasion the word *loimos* deservedly obtained. For as men suffered, so they made the verse to say. And I think if after this there shall ever come another Doric war and with it a famine, they are like to recite the verse accordingly. There was also reported by such as knew a certain answer given by the oracle to the Lacedaemonians when they inquired whether they should make this war or not: *that if they warred with all their power, they should have the victory, and that the God himself would take their parts.* And thereupon they thought the present misery to be a fulfilling of that prophecy. The Peloponnesians were no sooner entered Attica but the sickness presently began, and never came into Peloponnesus, to speak of, but reigned principally in Athens and in such other places afterwards as were most populous. And thus much of this disease.

▲

On the Sacred Disease

HIPPOCRATES

Probably the most famous name in the history of medicine is Hippocrates of Cos, who is generally regarded as "The Father of Western Medicine." Although he is a historical figure, evidence strongly suggests that no individual person wrote the sixty-some works that make up the Hippocratic Corpus, *the collected Hippocratic writings. The* Corpus *was mainly written from 430 to 330 B.C.E., and the final compilation covers such topics as pathology, diagnosis and prognosis, treatment, gynecology, surgery, and ethics.*

The teachings and writings of Hippocrates and his colleagues provide a major watershed in the history of medicine because the medical arts became a rational discipline, based on careful observation of symptoms and treatments created individually for each patient. To the Hippocratics, disease was not the result of divine action, but was due to an imbalance or a disturbance of the natural health of the body, with both internal and external causes, and the physician's role was to help nature heal the problem. Diet and exercise were essential parts of any treatment, as well as a number of natural remedies, but often all a doctor could do was make the patient as comfortable as possible, not make the situation worse, and let nature take its course. Although many diagnoses were incorrect by modern standards, the new, nonmagical approach to healing the sick clearly made a permanent mark on the practice of medicine.

▲

It is thus with regard to the disease called Sacred: it appears to me to be nowise more divine nor more sacred than other diseases, but has a natural cause from which it originates like other affections. . . . The quotidian, tertian, and quartan fevers, seem to me no less sacred and divine in their origin than this disease, although they are not reckoned so wonderful. . . .

But this disease seems to me to be no more divine than others; but it has its nature such as other diseases have, . . . and it is curable no less than the others. . . . Its origin is hereditary, like that of other diseases. . . .

But the brain is the cause of this affection, as it is of other very great diseases. . . . The brain of man, as in all other animals, is double, and a thin membrane divides it through the middle, and therefore the pain is not always in the same part of the head; for sometimes it is situated on either side, and sometimes the whole is affected; and veins run toward it from all parts of the body, many of which are small, but two are thick,—the one from the liver, and the other from the spleen. And it is thus with regard to the one from the liver: a portion of it runs downward through the parts on the right side, near the kidneys . . . , to the inner part of the thigh, and extends to the foot. It is called vena cava. The other runs upward by the right veins and the lungs, and divides into branches for the heart and the right arm. . . . [I]ts thickest, largest, and most hollow part ends in the brain, another small vein goes to the right ear, another to the right eye, and another to the nostril. . . .

By these veins we draw in much breath. . . . For the breath cannot be stationary, but it passes upward and downward, for if stopped and intercepted, the part where it is stopped becomes powerless. . . .

This malady, then, affects phlegmatic people, but not bilious. It begins to be formed while the foetus is still *in utero*. . . . If the secretion (melting) from the whole brain be greater than natural, the person, when he grows up, will have his head diseased, and full of noises, and will neither be able to endure the sun nor cold. . . . Or, should **depuration** not take place, but congestion accumulate in the brain, it necessarily becomes phlegmatic. And such children as have an eruption of ulcers on the head, on the ears, and along the rest of the body, with copious discharges of saliva and mucus,—these, in after life, enjoy best health; for in this way the phlegm which ought to have been purged off in the womb, is discharged and cleared away, and persons so purged, for the most part, are not subject to attacks of this disease. But such as have had their skin free from eruptions, and have had no discharge of saliva or mucus, nor have undergone the proper purgation in the womb, these persons run the risk of being seized with this disease.

But should the **defluxion** make its way to the heart, the person is seized with palpitation and asthma, the chest becomes diseased, and some also have curvature of the spine. For when a defluxion of cold phlegm takes place on the lungs and heart, the blood is chilled, and the veins, being violently chilled, palpitate in the lungs and heart, and the heart palpitates. . . . And if the de-

fluxions be more condensed, the epileptic attacks will be more frequent. . . .

And if . . . its defluxion be determined to the veins I have formerly mentioned, the patient loses his speech, and chokes, and foam issues by the mouth, the teeth are fixed, the hands are contracted, the eyes distorted, he becomes insensible, and in some cases the bowels are evacuated. And these symptoms occur sometimes on the left side, sometimes on the right, and sometimes in both. The cause of every one of these symptoms I will now explain. The man becomes speechless when the phlegm, suddenly descending into the veins, shuts out the air, and does not admit it either to the brain or to the vena cava, or to the ventricles, but interrupts the inspiration. For when a person draws in air by the mouth and nostrils, the breath goes first to the brain, then the greater part of it to the internal cavity, and part to the lungs, and part to the veins, and from them it is distributed to the other parts of the body along the veins; and whatever passes to the stomach cools, and does nothing more; and so also with regard to the lungs. . . . [W]hen the veins are excluded from the air by the phlegm and do not receive it, the man loses his speech and intellect, and the hands become powerless, and are contracted, the blood stopping and not being diffused, as it was wont; and the eyes are distorted owing to the veins being excluded from the air. . . . And the bowels are evacuated in consequence of the violent suffocation; and the suffocation is produced when the liver and stomach ascend to the diaphragm, and the mouth of the stomach is shut up. . . . All these symptoms he endures when the cold phlegm passes into the warm blood, for it congeals and stops the blood. And if the deflexion be copious and thick, it immediately proves fatal to him, for by its cold it prevails over the blood and congeals it. . . .

Of little children who are seized with this disease, the greater part die, provided the defluxion be copious and humid. . . . But if the phlegm be in small quantity, and make a defluxion into both the veins, or to those on either side, the children survive, but exhibit notable marks of the disorder; for either the mouth is drawn aside, or an eye, the neck, or a hand, wherever a vein being filled with phlegm loses its tone, and is attenuated, and the part of the body connected with this vein is necessarily rendered weaker and defective. . . .

. . . [W]hen this disease attacks very old people, it therefore proves fatal, or induces paraplegia, because the veins are empty, and the blood scanty, thin, and watery. When, therefore, the defluxion is copious, and the season winter, it proves fatal. . . . For the blood being thin, cold, and scanty, cannot prevail over the phlegm. . . .

. . . When a person has passed the twentieth year of his life, this disease is not apt to seize him, unless it has become habitual from childhood, or at least this is rarely or never the case. For the veins are filled with blood, and the brain consistent and firm, so that it does not run down into the veins, or if it do, it does not master the blood, which is copious and hot. . . .

. . . [T]hey [who are subject to this disease] are attacked during changes of the winds, and especially south winds, then also with north winds, and afterwards also with the others. These are the strongest winds, and the most opposed to one another, both as to direction and power. . . . [A]nd so in like manner also, all the winds which arise from the sea and other waters. . . .

Men ought to know that from nothing else but the brain come joys, delights, laughter and sports, and sorrows, griefs, despondency, and lamentations. . . . And by the same organ we become mad and delirious, and fears and terrors assail us, some by night, and some by day, and dreams and untimely wanderings, and cares that are not suitable, and ignorance of present circumstances, desuetude, and unskilfulness. All these things we endure from the brain, when it is not healthy, but is more hot, more cold, more moist, or more dry than natural, or when it suffers any other preternatural and unusual affection. And we become mad from its humidity. . . .

As long as the brain is at rest, the man enjoys his reason, but the depravement of the brain arises from phlegm and bile, either of which you may recognize in this manner: Those who are mad from phlegm are quiet, and do not cry out nor make a noise; but those from bile are vociferous, malignant,

and will not be quiet, but are always doing something improper. If the madness be constant, these are the causes thereof. But if terrors and fears assail, they are connected with derangement of the brain, and derangement is owing to its being heated. And it is heated by bile when it is determined to the brain along the blood-vessels running from the trunk, and fear is present until it returns again to the veins and trunk, when it ceases. He is grieved and troubled when the brain is unseasonably cooled and contracted beyond its wont. This it suffers from phlegm, and from the same affection the patient becomes oblivious. He calls out and screams at night when the brain is suddenly heated. . . .

In these ways I am of the opinion that the brain exercises the greatest power in the man. This is the interpreter to us of those things which emanate from the air. . . . For inasmuch as it is supplied with air, does it impart sense to the body. It is the brain which is the messenger to the understanding. For when the man draws the breath into himself, it passes first to the brain, and thus the air is distributed to the rest of the body, leaving in the brain its acme, and whatever has sense and understanding. . . .

. . . Since, then, the brain, as being the primary seat of sense and of the spirits, perceives whatever occurs in the body, if any change more powerful than usual take place in the air, owing to the seasons, the brain becomes changed by the state of the air. . . .

And the disease called the Sacred arises from causes as the others, namely, those things which enter and quit the body, such as cold, the sun, and the winds, which are ever changing and are never at rest. And these things are divine, so that there is no necessity for making a distinction, and holding this disease to be more divine than the others, but all are divine, and all human. . . . Thus, then, the physician should understand and distinguish the season of each, so that at one time he may attend to the nourishment and increase, and at another to abstraction and diminution. And in this disease as in all others, he must strive not to feed the disease, but endeavor to wear it out by administering whatever is most opposed to each disease, and not that which favors and is allied to it. . . .

▲

Of the Epidemics

HIPPOCRATES

▲

CASE IV

The woman affected with **quinsy,** who lodged in the house of Aristion: her complaint began in the tongue; speech inarticulate; tongue red and parched. On the first day, felt chilly, and afterwards became heated. On the third day, a rigor, acute fever; a reddish and hard swelling on both sides of the neck and chest, extremities cold and livid; respiration elevated; the drink returned by the nose; she could not swallow; alvine and urinary discharges suppressed. On the fourth, all of the symptoms were exacerbated. On the fifth she died of the quinsy. . . .

CASE V

In Larissa, a man, who was bald, suddenly was seized with pain in the right thigh; none of the things which were administered did him any good. On the first day, fever acute, of the ardent type, not agitated, but the pains persisted. On the second, the pains in the thigh abated, but the fever increased; somewhat tossed about; did not sleep; extremities cold; passed a large quantity of urine, not of a good character. On the third, the pain of the thigh ceased; derangement of the intellect, confusion, and much tossing about. On the fourth, about noon, he died. An acute disease. . . .

CASE VIII

In Abdera, Anaxion, who was lodged near the Thracian Gates, was seized with an acute fever; continued pain of the right side; dry cough, without expectoration during the first days, thirst, insomnolency; urine well colored, copious, and thin. On the sixth, delirious; no relief from the warm applications. On the seventh, in

a painful state, for the fever increased, while the pains did not abate, and the cough was troublesome, and attended with **dyspnea.** On the eighth, I opened a vein at the elbow, and much blood, of a proper character, flowed; the pains were abated, but the dry coughs continued. On the eleventh, the fever diminished; slight sweats about the head; coughs, with more liquid sputa; he was relieved. On the twentieth, sweat, apyrexia; but after the crisis he was thirsty, and the expectorations were not good. On the twenty-seventh the fever relapsed; he coughed, and brought up much concocted sputa: sediment in the urine copious and white; he became free of thirst, and the respiration was good. On the thirty-fourth, sweated all over, apyrexia, general crisis. . . .

CASE XI

In Thasus, a woman, of a melancholic turn of mind, from some accidental cause of sorrow, while still going about, became affected with loss of sleep, aversion to food, and had thirst and nausea. She lived near the Pylates, upon the Plain. On the first, at the commencement of night, frights, much talking, despondency, slight fever; in the morning, frequent spasms, and when they ceased, she was incoherent and talked obscurely; pains frequent, great, and continued. On the second, in the same state; had no sleep; fever more acute. On the third, the spasms left her: but coma, and disposition to sleep, and again awaked, started up, and could not contain herself; much incoherence; acute fever; on that night a copious sweat all over: apyrexia, slept, quite collected: had a crisis. About the third day, the urine black, thin, substances floating in it generally round, did not fall to the bottom; about the crisis a copious menstruation. . . .

CASE XIV

Cyzicus, a woman who had brought forth twin daughters, after a difficult labor, and in whom the lochial discharge was insufficient, at first was seized with an acute fever, attended with chills; heaviness of the head and neck, with pain; insomnolency from the commencement; she was silent, sullen, and disobedient; urine thin, and devoid of color; thirst, nausea for the most part; bowels irregularly disordered, and again constipated. On the sixth, towards night, talked much incoherently; had no sleep. About the eleventh day was seized with wild delirium, and again became collected; urine black, thin, and again deficient, and of an oily appearance; copious, thin, and disordered evacuations from the bowels. On the fourteenth, frequent convulsions; extremities cold; not in anywise collected; suppression of urine. On the sixteenth loss of speech. On the seventeenth, she died. **Phrenitis.** . . .

⚓

Chest Trauma During the Battle of Troy

Ancient Warfare and Chest Trauma

GIL HAUER SANTOS, MD

Some of the earliest descriptions of Greek medical knowledge and practices come from Homer's epic poem about the Trojan War: The Iliad. Homer's writings were surprisingly accurate, given that anatomy and physiology were poorly understood. Homer described more than one hundred different wounds and made remarkably correct prognoses about their outcomes. Whereas wounds to the extremities were painful but rarely lethal, head wounds were universally fatal, as were the majority of torso injuries.

In The Iliad, Homer also mentioned healers on the battlefield. In fact, Machaon, one of the most famous physicians of the time, was reputedly the son of the legendary demigod Asklepios. Treatments of the wounded tended toward palliative care only: making the soldier as comfortable as possible and, in many cases, removing the damaging spear or arrow. Most remedies were herbal, to try to staunch blood flow or ease pain, but surgical intervention was essentially unknown.

⚓

In *The Iliad,* that fountainhead of Western literature, Homer describes the events related to the battle of Troy and its disastrous aftermath. All that enormous suffering and bloodshed was incurred to bring back a woman, Helen, who had departed with her lover, Paris, to a faraway land.

An expedition made up by her husband Menelaus, his brother Agamemnon, friends, and allies was assembled in a loose association to go to Troy, punish the Trojans, and bring Helen back to Greece.

Throughout the narrative, Homer gives a majestic and unmatched view of the human

Reprinted from *Annals of Thoracic Surgery,* vol. 69, Gil Hauer Santos, "Chest Trauma During the Battle of Troy: Ancient Warfare and Chest Trauma," pp. 1285–87, Copyright 2000, with permission from the Society of Thoracic Surgeons.

condition. Those who are fortunate enough to read this book are filled with awe and profound admiration for the genius of the one who laid the foundations of Western thinking.

Of special interest for surgeons is the description of 130 injuries occurring during the combats, and we are amazed by Homer's meticulous account of the wounds inflicted to the combatants in that historic and allegory-laden war.

To go from Greece to Troy across the Aegean Sea, the Homeric boats were equipped with a single midship sail and built with decks at the prow and the stern with a single layer of rowers in between. They had no underdeck and the sailors alternated rowing with sleeping on the deck. Rowers and wind moved the craft away from Greece towards the city of Troy. A large flotilla carried 100,000 warriors, most distinguished among them Odysseus, Agamemnon, and Achilles. Most of the warriors were also rowers who alternated at the oars.

On arriving at the proximity of Troy, they camped outside the city walls and on the beaches, staying close to their boats. For 10 years, they attempted to break through the defenses of the city of Priam, until discouraged and exhausted from the long time already passed and their losses in battle, they decided on a stratagem to get inside the walls of the well-defended city, as later described by Homer in *The Odyssey.*

One hundred and thirty battle wounds are described in *The Iliad,* of which, 26 (20%) were in the chest. Other anatomical areas with a large incidence of wounds were the head with 22, the abdomen with 23, and the neck with 19. Only one wound was described in a foot.

For weapons, the combatants used spears, swords, arrows, and stones, protecting themselves with helmets and shields made of leather, wood, and bronze. In a typical clash, the chiefs rode chariots pulled by two horses, while their men ran close to them. Frequently, during the heat of battle, the chiefs were dragged out of their chariots and had to face the other combatants on the same footing.

Apparently, horseback fighting was still an unknown art, possibly because stirrups, which permitted the rider to stay in a steady position to keep his balance and use his weapons, had not yet been invented. The first known rigid stirrups were found in China dating from the fourth century AD. In the Western world, stirrups were found in Avar tombs in Hungary dating from the seventh century AD. It is possible that Avar and other nomadic tribes brought stirrups from the East across the steppes of northern Asia. It was with the help of the cavalry provided with stirrups that Charles Martel, chief of the Franks and grandfather of Charlemagne, consolidated his kingdom, defeating the Moslems at a battle near Poitiers in the year 732.

Looking at the weapons used, we read that 72 of 130 wounds described at the battle of Troy were produced by a spear, some of them specifically described as bronze-tipped spears. Bronze spearheads like the ones described have been recovered on archaeological excavations, notably by Schliemann late in the nineteenth century on excavations conducted by him at the hill of Hissarlik, where ancient Troy is supposed to have stood. Those bronze spearheads measured an average of 65 cm and were likely used as part of a thrusting spear. Its size and weight would have made it difficult to use them as a throwing weapon, yet in several instances they are described as being thrown against the enemy.

Fifty-eight injuries were caused by weapons other than spears. Of those, 12 were inflicted by swords. These were short swords made to be used in close combat. Arrows were responsible for nine other injuries. In nine other instances, wounds were caused by hurled large stones found in abundance where the battle took place. Most of the head injuries were produced by those heavy stones. We find four victims of an initial injury by spear followed by a blow with a sword, and one victim of a combined stone and sword attack. One combatant died as a result of a hand-to-hand fight, while for 22 injured fighters, there is no mention of the weapon used.

Of the 26 chest wounds, the majority, that is 20, were produced by spears. Two chest injuries were inflicted by arrows, one was made by a combination of spear and sword, while in three cases there is no mention of the weapon that was used.

Most of the injuries are succinctly described by naming the weapon and the anatomical area afflicted, but in some cases, a more elaborate description is made, as with the description of the charge of Patroclus against Sarpedon:

> "The spear sped not from his hand in vain, for he hit Sarpedon just where the diaphragm bounds the ever-beating heart. He fell like some oak or silver poplar or tall pine to which woodmen have laid their axes upon the mountain to make timber for ship building. Even so did he lie stretched at full length in front of his chariot and horses moaning and clutching at the blood stained dust. Death closed his eyes as he spoke. Patroclus planted his heel on his breast and drew the spear from his body, whereon the diaphragm came along with it and he drew out both spear point and Sarpedon's soul at the same time."

In the same way, the vivid description of Alcathous's death has some poignant graphic details:

> "Idomeneus struck him with a spear in the middle of his chest. The coat of mail that had hitherto protected his body was now broken and rang harshly as the spear tore through it. He fell heavily to the ground, and the spear stuck to his heart which still beat, and made the butt-end of the spear quiver till dread Ares put an end to his life."

Peirous wounded by Thoas was hit in two areas:

> "Thoas struck him in the chest near the nipple, and the point fixed itself in his lungs. Thoas came close up to him, pulled the spear out of his chest and then drawing his sword, smote him in the middle of the belly so that he died."

A more straightforward encounter was the one when: "King Agamemnon knocked mighty Odius from his chariot. The spear of Agamemnon caught him on the broad of his back, just as [he] was turning in flight; it struck him between the shoulders and went right through his chest, and his armour rang round him as he fell heavily to the ground."

Two physicians attended the Greek forces in battle. One of them was Podalirius and the other Machaon. When Machaon was wounded by Alexandrus with an arrow on his right shoulder, Idomeneus said to Nestor: "Mount your chariot at once and take Machaon with you and drive your horses to the ships as fast as you can. A physician is worth more than several other men put together, for he can cut out arrows and spread healing herbs." However, when soon after Eurypylus was wounded with an arrow in the thigh, he asked help from one of his companions: "Noble Patroclus . . . save me and take me to my ship, cut out the arrow from my thigh, wash the black blood from off it with warm water and lay upon it those gracious herbs . . . for of the physicians Podalirius and Machaon, I hear that the one is lying wounded in his tent and is himself in need of healing, while the other is fighting the Trojans upon the plain." Patroclus clasped him round the middle and led him into the tent, and a servant, when he saw him, spread bullock-skins on the ground for him to lay on. He laid him at full length and cut out the sharp arrow from his thigh; he washed the black blood from the wound with warm water, he then crushed a bitter herb, rubbing it between his hands, and spread it upon the wound; this was a virtuous herb which killed all pain, so the wound presently dried and the blood left off flowing."

Serious injuries bringing suffering and death resulted from this conflict. Yet as a sad part of the human condition, bloody episodes continue, with no interruption, to punctuate our history from distant past to present days, and it always appears that through the centuries no lesson has yet been learned because war continues to be a way to solve disputes among nations. Weapons are getting more formidable and the damage produced by them on the fragile human body equally more horrendous.

Surgeons continue to be dedicated to preserve and restore the integrity of the delicate human body not only by confronting diseases but also repairing injuries caused by civilian and war trauma.

An extra role for the surgeon should certainly include his or her participation as an active voice in the worldwide dialogue searching for a future of peace when disputes will be decided at the negotiating table instead of the battlefield.

⋏

The Parallels Between Asclepian and Hippocratic Medicine on the Island of Kos

Spyros G. Marketos

The Western medical tradition prior to the teachings of Hippocrates was magicoreligious. Earliest Greek medicine followed that model in the form of Asclepian medicine, founded by Asklepios, son of Apollo, god of the sun and patron of all physicians. His temples were scattered all over the eastern Mediterranean and Aegean, places of healing based on prayers for the intervention of the Homeric gods. Supplicants slept in the temples and hoped the gods would cure them in their sleep. If a cure was not achieved, people assumed that, for whatever reasons, the gods chose not to intervene.

Hippocratic medicine offered a complete contrast to the Asclepian model. Hippocrates' teachings focused on a rational approach to health, based on close observation, a variety of natural remedies, few surgical treatments, and a decidedly holistic approach to illness. At first glance, it would appear to be the antithesis of the magicoreligious model, but, in fact, as this selection shows, both traditions existed in a noncompetitive spirit of cooperation. Hippocrates was originally an Asclepian, and although he did not give divine action a primary place in the explanation of disease, neither did he totally reject the idea.

⋏

Introduction

Medicine has existed on earth—either in the form of primitive medicine and/or magicoreligious medicine—from the first day that humans appeared on the planet. Religion and medicine, priest and doctor, worked towards the same end: the defence of the individual against evil forces. Ancient Greece during the pre-Hippocratic period was the time of the priestly Asclepian medicine. To Asclepios—or Aesculapius in Latin—the god of the healing art were dedicated many therapeutic centres-temples around the Mediterranean sea, the so-called Asclepieia. Pre-Hippocratic medicine was based on religious belief, on surgery and on regimen. The physician was closely connected with religion and, predominantly, a herb gatherer. Hippocratic medicine (5th century BC) was based on a right way

of thinking (rationalism) and on a whole, humane approach to the patient. The Hippocratic physician treated the whole patient, not only the organs of the body. It is obvious that when a sick patient was not cured by the rational medicine, then an attempt was made to find healing in religious and/or alternative types of medicine, as occurs even today.

Ancient Greek medicine . . . is based on the coexistence of both the Asclepian art and Hippocratic medicine and comprises a part of the history of general culture. The fact that the priestly Asclepian medicine, which relied on dreams and faith, and rational Hippocratic medicine occurred together from the 5th century BC reveals that alternative medicine is nothing new. Although there is no evidence to support cooperation between the Hippocratic physicians and the priests of Asclepieia, there is no proof of hostility between them.

Reprinted by permission of S. Karger, Basel, Switzerland, from Spyros G. Marketos, "The Parallels Between Asclepian and Hippocratic Medicine on the Island of Kos," *American Journal of Nephrology* 17 (1997): 205–208.

Although the medical work of Hippocrates had little in common with that of the priests of Asclepieia, the parallels between creativity in the Asclepian art and Hippocratic medicine were closer than medical historians usually realise, since the rise of rational medicine did not exclude a parallel rise in religious medicine in Greece. Asclepios' followers respected the tradition, did not reject the old divine status, claimed that they were the descendants of Asclepios and were loyal to the Hippocratic oath.

The Asclepian Medical Art

Ancient Greek medicine had its origins in primitive medicine and took a magicoreligious form. Throughout antiquity, the roles of religion, magic and medicine were confused because they used different methods for the same purpose: the treatment of diseases, supposed to be caused by the supernatural forces of evil divinities, often called spirits or demons. . . .

In ancient Greece, the art of healing and the relief of suffering derived from Asclepios whose oracles are found everywhere around the Mediterranean. In Homeric times (12–8th centuries BC), the period of the famous Minoan and Mycenaean civilisations, the physicians were respected and skilful craftsmen. In the *Iliad,* the greatest epic in any European language, Machaon and Podaleirius, surgeons and noble-warriors, are the sons of the king of Tricca. The two noble Greek physicians gave their attention to the treatment of wounds and treated diseases by dietetics. Both were Asclepiads, in fact sons of Asclepios the blameless physician, as the poet says.

Asclepios was the son of Apollo, the god of the sun, the leader of the muses and the patron of physicians, worshipped at Delphi, a centre for medical advice. Asclepios was taught the art of medicine by the famous centaur Chiron. Chiron was the first to institute the medical art of surgery and then of herbs. The sage Chiron trained physicians, guided musicians and made righteous men.

Asclepios had a large family, all of whose members were connected with health care activities. His wife Epione soothed pain, his daughter Hygeia provided preventive medicine, another daughter, Panacea, represented treatment and cure for everything; his son Telesphorus, always represented as a child, cared for convalescence. It is important to note that every member of Asclepios' family presided over a different form of health care or specific medical services.

During the next ten centuries (6th century BC–5th century AD), temples dedicated to Asclepios, cults of 'temple healing' associated with his name (Asclepieia), developed into therapeutic centres, where, besides his adoration, medical care was given by the priests. The establishment of the Asclepieia in specially selected places took account of the influence of climate, water supply and situation to offer a naturally healthy environment to patients. . . .

Asclepios was worshipped in magnificent temples throughout the Aegean islands, more than 400 temples all over the Greek world and further, from Rome to Asia Minor and from Africa to Scythia. It is important to emphasise that the ancient Greek origins of the Western tradition of medical care rooted in the pattern of the physician-god Asclepios and that in antiquity there was neither competition nor enmity between the physician and the healer god.

Rational Hippocratic Medicine

Hippocrates (460–377 BC) worked on the island of Kos before the founding of the Asclepieion. He came from an old, local, priestly family and travelled extensively before dying in Larissa, Thessaly. His pupils established a centre of healing on Kos after his death, using the old Hippocratic methods (**anamnesis,** diagnosis, therapy), and the Hippocratic oath has become the ethical nucleus of the medical profession.

The Greek 'father of medicine' . . . is connected with the most creative period of scientific medicine in antiquity. He was the one most able to assimilate the accumulated knowledge of the previous centuries for the transition from empiricism to rational medicine. This progress in cosmology and human physiology was acquired by the physical or pre-Socratic philosophers, who played the role of a bridge between the Asclepian and the Hippocratic physician. The latter inaugurates a new approach to all the natural phenomena, attempting to offer scientific explanations.

Early Greek philosophy flourished on the periphery of the Greek world and Hippocratic medicine mirrored this geographical localisation. The intellectual background of Hippocratic medicine was pre-Socratic philosophy. Hippocrates was born on the island of Kos very close to the coast of Asia Minor, and was a contemporary of Pericles and his 'Golden Age'. His name is mentioned in the works of the two greatest philosophers of ancient Greece, Plato and Aristotle. 'Asclepiad', the former called him, and 'leader of the Asclepiads', the latter. He was taught the first principles of medicine by his father Heraclides, a direct descendant of the god Asclepios, according to a widespread legend.

The Hippocratic diagnostic system, based on logical reasoning, observation and belief in the 'healing power of Nature', formed the basis of medical practice. Hippocrates was one of the most significant figures in the history of science because he released the healing art from demons, superstition and magic, and established the ethical and moral rules of the medical profession. Diseases had a logical interpretation, they were no longer a curse of the gods or a punishment due to divine wrath. Sharing the human suffering, he adopted an attitude summarised in the phrase 'the place of a physician is at the bedside of his patient'.

The Hippocratic physician is basically a craftsman, accompanied into his workshop by an audience of pupils and other bystanders, who discusses the diagnosis and treatment of every case. When he goes to the patient's home he has the duty to persuade not only the patient but the relatives as well. He follows the more communal character of life in antiquity, which does not permit any special discretion or intimacy in his behaviour. His authority is related to his education (usually philosophical and medical) and to his therapeutic abilities. If he makes a reputation for himself, then this extends beyond his town and he probably attracts patients from other regions or is invited to visit other cities. If he is called to undertake the treatment of a serious disease, he may refuse or accept, explaining the slight prospects of a cure. Certain situations, with a predictable fatal outcome, where intervention was prohibited, justified the Hippocratic dogma 'to help or at least not to harm'.

The Hippocratic physician must also possess the oratorical skill to express his ideas about human nature and the structure and composition of the body as well as to answer the medical questions of the people, or simply for the better handling of human relations. Some theories can only be proved by dialectics and logical argumentation. This aspect of medical science is accessible only to those educated in philosophy and rhetoric. The healing art, according to Hippocrates, is linked to three conditions: the disease, the patient and the physician; the latter is needed to be, moreover, a servant of the art (the 'techne'). Every patient is a different case and this individuality makes a fixed dogma for curative methods impossible. Hippocrates was, above all things, both a practitioner and philosopher-physician, who took care of his patients from prognosis to treatment.

Hellenic (Asclepian and Hippocratic) Medicine

Ancient Greek medicine combines rationalism and empiricism but it is also influenced by religious ideas. God is a power reckoned into the theories and practice of the physicians. At first glance, the medical texts do not usually mention magic or religious healing. If a miracle occurs, it is accepted because philosophy acknowledges this possibility. Hippocratic writings recognise the divine influence but only as a factor like nature, which is a power of its own. In the treatise *On Sacred Disease,* Hippocrates concludes that there is no need to put the disease in a special class, to consider it more divine than the others: they are all divine and all human. Each has a nature and power of its own. He also attacks those who attribute epilepsy to the direct influence of a god or demon and calls them magicians, faithhealers, quacks and charlatans.

On the other hand, Asclepios, almost throughout antiquity, was the ancient hero of medical care and the main representative of divine healing in his cult centres, a form of medical treatment never opposed by ancient physicians. Moreover, the worship of the God of Medicine, beyond its medical significance, came to play a significant role in the religious life of later centuries, in the final stage of paganism. While Galen's rational and experimental medicine was still preserved in the encyclopaedias, the new and prevailing spirit of medicine was that of religion and magic. A significant historian calls Galen 'the last Greek medical scientist of antiquity', and declares, 'Man's mind had moved from a scientific toward a religious and magical view of the universe'. This explains the survival of Asclepian medicine, because scientific medicine was worsted in the rivalry and gradually degenerated from rational treatment to wild speculation and even quackery.

In the period in which rational and religious medicine coexisted, they had equal value. The latter, performed in the Asclepieia, adopted scientific elements, changing its character. Yet an influence of religious ideas on science is also conceivable. It is possible that the physicians recognised the practice of priests and magicians as an activity parallel to but separate from theirs, an alternative healing method.

Conclusion

From the preceding discussion, we may draw five conclusions. (1) Ancient Greek medicine . . . has a scientific and cultural orientation throughout its history. (2) Asclepian medicine reflects some of the virtues and the duties of contemporary society for providing care to the underserved. (3) Hippocratic medicine developed in close company with philosophy and cannot be separated from that of pre-Socratic philosophy. (4) Hellenic medicine highlights the coexistence of traditional and rational medicine. (5) Alternative medicine may function in a complementary way to conventional primary medical care.

Sport and Medicine in Ancient Greece

THIERRY APPELBOOM, MD, CHRISTINE ROUFFIN, MA,
AND ERIC FIERENS, MA

One of the fastest-growing medical specialties is sports medicine, which has its roots in the practices of ancient Greece. As medicine became increasingly based on Hippocrates' rational model, athletic injuries were considered to be not divine punishment, but the result of specific damage, both treatable and preventable. Early practitioners of sports medicine focused on two aspects: preparation of the athlete so that he could compete at his physical best, and the medical and surgical treatment of the myriad injuries sustained in the competitions. Thus, from the beginning of organized sports in Greece, the doctor closely attended the athlete.

Thierry Appelboom, Christine Rouffin, and Eric Fierens, *American Journal of Sports Medicine* (vol. 16, no. 6), pp. 594–96, copyright © 1988 by Sage Publications, Inc. Reprinted by permission of Sage Publications, Inc.

The civilization of ancient Greece has made a profound and lasting impression on modern culture. Greece's geographic position, at the junction of East and West, and the diffusion of its influence, have given it the reputation of being one of the most brilliant civilizations in history, and with good reason. One is immediately struck by the position of both sport and medicine in ancient Greece. The development of sport was the result of a tradition of increasing spiritual awareness through physical activity; indeed, physical culture not only took high priority in Greek upbringing and daily life, but also in the social organization of the city states. Moreover, the great openness of Greek intellectual life allowed significant progress to be made in the field of medicine. This was to become codified, and thus enriched and perpetuated. The position of sport was therefore to encourage the development of the medical knowledge associated with it. The athlete's preparation was conceived in a new and original way, and medicine was taken out of the hands of the priests and placed in the hands of physicians and surgeons.

Sport in Ancient Greece

Ancient Greece is not only the world of purity that we think of when we see its white temples today, which originally were painted in bright colors. Ancient Greece was also a world of violence and cruelty, fire and blood, often existing in a state of war. Evidence of this is provided by the accounts of Homer, especially by that of the Trojan War as portrayed in the *Iliad*. These accounts bear witness to violent trauma, cranial fractures, dislocations, abdominal wounds, etc., which are described with such accuracy that one could even ask if Homer the poet was not also a military surgeon.

Nevertheless, one must remember that long conflicts like the Trojan War were interrupted by periods of peace. The spirit of rivalry and confrontation inherent in man and previously unleashed in war, in ancient Greece came to be channeled into the practice of competitive sports. Competitions were held during religious festivals or political gatherings and were always placed under the auspices of the gods. For instance, games were organized by Achilles around the funeral pyre of Patroclus. On the other hand, religious ceremonies were intimately involved whenever games were held. The spirit of Agon presided over these competitions. The name in fact lies at the root of the term "agonistics," the nearest synonym we have to "sport." The victor symbolized both physical and moral courage and was the incarnation of the mastery of the balance between corporal and spiritual achievement. He was rewarded with a crown of olive, taken from the tree planted by Heracles himself. Although at the moment of victory he would necessarily be exhausted in body and disheveled in appearance, his depiction by the artist was idealized to immortalize his victory in the public mind. Thus sport influenced Greek civilization through the sculptor's chisel, which so skillfully rendered that harmonious beauty of bodies observed in scenes from the competitions, as evidenced in the "Discobolos" by the sculptor Myron (5th century BC).

The sanctuary of Olympia dedicated to Zeus was renowned for the athletic competitions that took place there. The site was not a city, but an athletic and religious center, focused around a temple dedicated to Zeus. The buildings for the athletes (palaestra, gymnasium, stadium), as well as the lay buildings, were all outside the sacred enclosure. The games reached their peak at the beginning of the 5th century BC, thanks to a period of relative peace between Sparta and the other Greek cities. At this time, Olympia was the landmark of panhellenistic unity. However, the participation of non-Greek citizens . . . corrupted the spirit and the Olympic ideal. Finally, the Roman conquest reduced the contests to the level of an entertainment: certain "tests of nobility" disappeared, and there was an increase in those contests where violence reigned supreme. Gladiator fights, taken over from the Etruscans by the Romans, developed separately and as spectacles for a distinct public. The last blow came from Christianity, which strove vigorously against even the principle of athleticism: Theodosius II (in 426 AD) ordered the destruction of the temple of Olympia because he considered it far too pagan. An earthquake in the 6th century finished the destruction of the lay buildings, and the site was finally covered by alluvium from the Alpheius River, not to be rediscovered until the 19th century.

Medicine in Ancient Greece

The medicine of antiquity was very much of its time, with its good and its bad points. Before Hippocrates, it was a mythological and magical activity; illness resulted from the will of the gods; all therapeutic intervention began with an offering and often stopped at just that. Medicine was thus in the hands of the priests. The god to whom they had recourse was Aesculapius, who was not an Olympian deity, being the result of the union of Apollo (a god) and Coronis (a nymph). The legend persists that after being fed by a goat, Aesculapius was recognized by a shepherd, thanks to the aureole on Aesculapius' forehead. He was initiated into the practice of medicine by the centaur Chiron, who also became associated with medical education. Chiron is, indeed, the only centaur from the mythological tradition who is associated with knowledge and wisdom, his peers always being conceived as brutal and ignorant creatures.

As an extraordinary physician, Aesculapius brought back a person from the dead, thus being likely to upset the natural order of things. Disturbed by this, Zeus struck him down with a thunderbolt, later deifying him. In this way, Aesculapius became the Greek god of medicine. An analogy can be made between him and the image of Christ as the son of God and a mortal, being crucified and resurrected.

Probably inherited from Mesopotamian and Egyptian mythology, Aesculapius is commonly depicted with a snake, a wand, and sometimes a dog. The significance of the snake in mythology is double: good and evil, because it can kill (e.g., The Laocoön) or cure (its venom as a basic component of antivenin). It is also a symbol of immortality, which seems to be conferred on it because of its constant changes of skin. Judeo-Christian iconography took over only the evil concept of the snake, to symbolize the devil. The wand represents the philosopher and the sage as guardians of knowledge. As far as the dog is concerned, it is the image of fidelity. Moreover, aware of things not visible to human eyes, the dog guides mankind, and it is the dog who protects intimacy.

The knowledge of Aesculapius was passed on to his sons, renowned warriors who inherited the special medical understanding of their father. Hence Podalirius became the father of medicine and Machaon that of surgery. From the *Iliad,* we know that both attended to wounds and applied remedies that encouraged healing. Appeals were made to them to deal with the wounded, which took place in the sanctuary of Aesculapius. His two daughters, Panacea and Hygeia, became goddess protectors and were invoked by the Greeks, Panacea for healing and Hygeia for good health. No longer controlled by the priests and often working away from the temples, faced with the need to treat athletes, the disciples of Aesculapius drew together a large number of medical procedures from both esoteric tradition and practical experience. They established links between disease and natural causes, without excluding an overriding supernatural influence. Hippocrates (5th to 4th centuries BC) organized and codified the knowledge resulting from these efforts, and added his own concept of the human body's equilibrium based on the theory of the four **humors:** blood, phlegm, yellow bile, and black bile.

Medicine was being separated from the sphere of the divine in this way and was on the way to becoming a rational activity, even if its foundations were still uncertain. Hippocrates considered himself a link in the chain forged by the disciples of Aesculapius of Cos, who claimed direct descent from Heracles and the god Aesculapius himself. This change in outlook also took place at the level of the individual athlete: disease and athletic injuries were no longer considered to be punishments from the gods. In the same way, the athlete's preparation changed and was undertaken with a modified and balanced diet as its basis. There were certain remedies, still sometimes considered as divinely inspired, which were prepared from over 2,500 medicinal plants. For the athletes' well-being, there were recommended infusions: mead, **oxymel**, purgatives, asses' milk, and extracts of onion and of celery. Beyond these, there were other treatments, such as those recommended by Pythagoras—philosopher and mathematician—who prescribed exercise, music, and meditation, but nothing to excess, as Aristotle was also to insist, later on. The latter was to recommend moderation up to puberty, in order to avoid overexertion.

The training diet and regimens, and initial treatment, were rendered not by physicians but by the paedotribes. These trainers fiercely resisted the appearance of doctors at the Olympic games or in the gymnasiums.

On the other hand, parallel with this gentle or moderate approach to medicine, there arose a number of surgical operations mainly oriented to traumatology, which Hippocrates was also to categorize and complete with his personal contributions. A treatise on surgery was to appear, one of the best of its age, probably written by Hippocrates, with an interest for athletes that was very clear. The Games achieved an extraordinary level of violence: fractures, hemorrhages, and being battered unconscious was the lot, especially of boxers. The following is a report by Homer of a boxing match between the Theban chief Euryalus and the noble warrior Epeius: "They hurled themselves one against the other, throwing their heavy punches, their jaw-bones crunching horribly under the blows, sweat coursing over their whole bodies. When his opponent cast a distraught glance around him, the divine Epeius leapt forward and caught him a blow to the cheek. The other would not last much longer; his glistening legs gave way beneath him. . . . After the blow, Euryalus jerked again. But the magnanimous Epeius took him in his arms and stood him on his feet. His faithful seconds surrounded Euryalus and carried him through the assembled company, legs trailing, head lolling, thick blood flowing. It was a man unconscious that they carried away and sat in their midst."

One can grasp straight away the point of having surgical experience on the battlefield, when a doctor had to treat boxers. Hippocrates himself repeated in his treatise on surgery: "Whoever wants to practice surgery needs to go to war." Thus the Greeks knew how to reduce dislocations, withdraw foreign bodies, clean wounds, cauterize bleeding blood vessels, put compresses into place, perfect superior equipment, etc. To fight pain they had mandragora and poppy at their disposal. It can therefore be seen that under Hippocrates, the treatment of sports injuries reached a high level, at least for the period. However, the treatises of Hippocrates had a series of weak points, notably his basic conception of the balance among the four humors, his tendency to be far too passive therapeutically ("Let nature take charge"), and the inaccuracy of his anatomical knowledge. This latter was remedied from the 4th century BC onward at Alexandria, where dissection was authorized by Ptolemy Soter (367–283 BC). Great progress in anatomy and physiology was also brought about in Asia Minor, thanks to Herophilus and Erasistratus (end of 4th century, beginning of 3rd, BC). It was these two who distinguished between sensory and motor nerves.

Conclusions

One can say that sports medicine in ancient Greece developed for various reasons:

- It was in this period that medicine was taken out of the hands of magi and priests, to be handed on to physicians. . . . The previous corpus of medical knowledge was codified and enriched by Hippocrates.
- Military experience was recycled by the athletes' surgeons, to become a genuine sports medicine, helping the athlete in his training.
- Finally, sport occupied an important place in the upbringing of young people, and in the social and cultural organization of the Greek city states.

Developments in medicine and hygiene, especially in the 5th century BC, encouraged athletic performances of a superior quality, because athletes were better prepared and better looked after.

KEY TERMS

Anamnesis, 78 • Bilious, 68 • Defluxion, 71 • Depuration, 71 • Dyspnea, 73 • Humors, 82 • Oxymel, 83 • Phrenitis, 74 • Quinsy, 73

QUESTIONS TO CONSIDER

1. Because the description of the symptoms of the Plague of Athens does not match that of any modern disease exactly, the identity of the plague remains a mystery. An interesting question is also raised: How much have diseases changed during human history? Can we legitimately label ancient outbreaks on the basis of modern symptomology?

2. Modern medicine is based solely on the logical and rational approach that Hippocrates espoused and downplays the magical interpretation of disease. However, an increasing number of physicians are recognizing the importance of a patient's religious and spiritual beliefs in determining how to treat many medical problems. When you look at the way the Asclepians and the early Hippocratics treated their patients, what parallels do you see in this gradual acceptance of the importance of religion?

3. Hippocrates was adamant about the need to gather information from a patient and then to examine him or her for symptoms, much as a modern physician does during a preliminary office visit. After reading Hippocrates' case studies, what other questions would a modern-day health-care practitioner add in order to diagnose and treat a patient? Why do you think Hippocrates did not ask such questions?

4. Do you agree or disagree with Dr. Appelboom's statement that sports can serve as a less-violent alternative to warfare in the competition between politicogeographical entities? To what degree do the Olympic Games involve nationalism or patriotism today?

RECOMMENDED READINGS

Carella, Michael J. *Matter, Morals, and Medicine: The Ancient Greek Origins of Science, Ethics, and the Medical Profession*. New York: Lang, 1991.

Jouanna, Jacques, and M. B. Devevoise, trans. *Hippocrates: Medicine and Culture*. Baltimore: John Hopkins University Press, 1999.

King, Helen. *Greek and Roman Medicine*. London: Bristol Classical Press, 2001.

———. *Hippocrates' Women: Reading the Female Body in Ancient Greece*. New York: Routledge, 1998.

Lloyd, G. E. R., and Nathan Sivin. *The Way and the Word: Science and Medicine in Early China and Greece*. New Haven, CT: Yale University Press, 2002.

Longrigg, James. *Greek Medicine from the Heroic to the Hellenistic Age: A Sourcebook*. New York: Routledge, 1998.

Prioreschi, Plinio. *History of Medicine*. Vol. 2, *Greek Medicine*. Lewiston, NY: Edwin Mellen Press, 1994.

Salazar, Christine F., ed. *The Treatment of War Wounds in Graeco-Roman Antiquity: Studies in Ancient Medicine*. Vol. 21. London: Brill Academic, 2000.

Chapter Five

Rome and Byzantium

INTRODUCTION

Rome was an empire comprising a blend of many attributes of many cultures. Roman medicine followed this pattern, incorporating much of the Greek tradition, which was heavily based in philosophy and the empirical methods of Hippocrates, and adding a strong element of practicality. The Romans contributed substantial knowledge about hygiene, sanitation, and public health. A number of advances, in particular the development of the hospital, were made in the context of the vitally important Roman army.

Although Rome produced a number of important men in the medical field, most of them allied with one or another of several schools of thoughts, one stands out: Galen. His enormous influence on anatomy and physiology, medical ethics, and therapeutics would be felt by all professional physicians for nearly a thousand years. His philosophy of medicine rested heavily on Hippocratic humoral theory and, based on his numerous animal dissections, on a view of a masterful Nature. Unfortunately, many of his theories were incorrect; nevertheless, they were accepted without challenge in Europe throughout the Middle Ages.

After the decline of the Empire in the West, the Byzantine, or Eastern Roman, Empire became the repository of a great deal of written material on medicine. In fact, the preservation of knowledge from Greece and Rome was one of Byzantium's greatest contributions to the art and practice of medicine. Although relatively few new advances were made, Byzantine society preserved works of Hippocrates, Aristotle, Galen, and many others that were lost in Western Europe.

TIME LINE

300 B.C.E.	Herophilus and Erasistratus are teaching in Alexandria—their anatomical discoveries are based on human vivisection of convicted criminals
90 B.C.E.	Marcus Terentius Varro states that disease is caused by particles too small to see that enter the body
45 B.C.E.	Julius Caesar encourages physicians and men of science to settle in Rome; he also begins draining marshes around Rome—a major source of mosquitoes and malaria
25 B.C.E.–50 C.E.	Approximate lifetime dates of Celsus—his *De Medicina*, written for the nonprofessional, was part of a larger encyclopedia; in it he accurately describes the signs of inflammation and discusses topics such as fevers, ulcers, sexually transmitted diseases, surgical hygiene, insanity, and so forth
40–90 C.E.	Dioscorides lives—a Greek surgeon in Nero's army, he describes the medicinal properties of some six hundred plants and more than one thousand drugs, including the use of willow bark to relieve pain, in his *De Materia Medica*
47 C.E.	Fire destroys about forty thousand volumes in the Great Library at Alexandria, repository of most written medical knowledge; most of the rest of the library was destroyed in a civil war in 272 C.E.
97 C.E.	Julius Frotinus is appointed water commissioner for Rome—he then designs the water-supply system of aqueducts for the city
98–138 C.E.	Soranus practices medicine during the reigns of Trajan and Hadrian; about 100, he writes *On Midwifery and the Diseases of Women,* the ob-gyn textbook most used until the Renaissance
129–201 C.E.	Lifetime dates of Galen of Pergamum, the most influential physician of late antiquity and the Middle Ages
140 C.E.	Aretaeus of Cappadocia writes *Acute and Chronic Diseases,* one of the best descriptions of specific diseases in the ancient world

157 C.E.	Galen is appointed physician to the gladiators—his experiences enable him to make many anatomical inferences
165–180 C.E.	Antonine plague in Rome—brought back by troops returning from Seleucia, this unknown disease kills as much as one-third of the population of the city of Rome and decimates the Roman army
170s C.E.	Galen's sixteen works on pulse lore are published; on the basis of this work, he claims that bloodletting is indicated for nearly every pathological condition
180 C.E.	Galen writes *Method of Physicians*, the medical textbook that becomes an accepted authority in medieval medicine
251–266 C.E.	Aurelian plague in Rome; actual disease unknown
325–400 C.E.	Approximate dates Oribasius, author of *Synagogue Medicine* (a seventy-volume medical encyclopedia), lives
541–543 C.E.	Plague of Justinian in the Eastern Roman Empire—the first time bubonic plague appears in Europe; the plague spreads along trade routes and kills as many as two million people in two years, paving the way for the Islamic invasion of the Byzantine Empire

▲

Soranus' Gynecology

SORANUS

Childbirth in the ancient world was attended by women—midwives—rather than physicians. The branch of medicine known as gynecology *had its beginnings with the Hippocratics, and the Hippocratic Corpus contains a great deal of writing about the subject, much of it now known to be incorrect. Soranus, a Greek physician of the first and second centuries C.E. who practiced in Alexandria and Rome, was a specialist in gynecology and the best-known member of the medical philosophical school known as* Methodism. *His textbook,* Gynecology, *in which he openly disagreed with such early concepts as the "wandering womb" as a cause for hysteria, was the largest early treatment of the specialty and remained a standard reference work until the Renaissance. It was divided into four parts—the first two dealing with normal conception, pregnancy, and labor, and the last*

Temkin, Owsei, trans. *Soranus' Gynecology.* pp. 6–7, 34–35, 40–45, 79–80. © 1991 Owsei Temkin. Reprinted with permission of The Johns Hopkins University Press.

two dealing with difficulties in labor and delivery and other problems of the female reproductive organs. Well organized and expertly reasoned, the work offers not only much advice on such matters as choosing a midwife or wet nurse, but also detailed descriptions of neonatal care.

▲

Who Are the Best Midwives?

It is necessary to tell what makes the best midwives, so that on the one hand the best may recognize themselves, and on the other hand beginners may look upon them as models, and the public in time of need may know whom to summon. Now generally speaking we call a midwife faultless if she merely carries out her medical task; whereas we call her the best midwife if she goes further and in addition to her management of cases is well versed in theory. And more particularly, we call a person the best midwife if she is trained in all branches of therapy (for some cases must be treated by diet, others by surgery, while still others must be cured by drugs); if she is moreover able to prescribe hygienic regulations for her patients, to observe the general and the individual features of the case, and from this to find out what is expedient, not from the causes or from the repeated observations of what usually occurs or something of the kind. Now to go into detail: she will not change her methods when the symptoms change, but will give her advice in accordance with the course of the disease; she will be unperturbed, unafraid in danger, able to state clearly the reasons for her measures, she will bring reassurance to her patients, and be sympathetic. And, it is not absolutely essential for her to have borne children, as some people contend, in order that she may sympathize with the mother, because of her experience with pain; for <to have sympathy> is <not> more characteristic of a person who has given birth to a child. She must be robust on account of her duties but not necessarily young as some people maintain, for sometimes young persons are weak whereas on the contrary older persons may be robust. She will be well disciplined and always sober, since it is uncertain when she may be summoned to those in danger. She will have a

quiet disposition, for she will have to share many secrets of life. She must not be greedy for money, lest she give an abortive wickedly for payment; she will be free from superstition so as not to overlook salutary measures on account of a dream or omen or some customary rite or vulgar superstition. She must also keep her hands soft, abstaining from such woolworking as may make them hard, and she must acquire softness by means of ointments if it is not present naturally. Such persons will be the best midwives. . . .

Whether Conception Is Healthful

Some people believe pregnancy to be healthful, because every natural act is useful, and pregnancy too is a natural action. Second, because some women, menstruating with difficulty and suffering uterine pressure, have been freed of their troubles after pregnancy. Opposed to such arguments, one must say that menstruation too is a natural act, but not a healthful one, as we have recalled. As a matter of fact if a thing is useful it is not in every case healthful as well. Indeed, both menstruation and pregnancy are useful for the propagation of men, but certainly not healthful for the child-bearer. For not by conceiving are they relieved of the preceding uterine troubles, rather, being relieved of the latter, they then conceive. Even granted that they are relieved by conception, conception is not a means of preserving health but an aid against disease; just as **venesection** does not become healthful because used as a treatment it resolves diseases. And according to what has been laid down previously, one has to point out that many inconveniences beset the pregnant woman who is heavily burdened and suffers from pica. Moreover, one must realize that the food sufficient for one organism has to be divided for the nourishment and growth of two organisms, so that it no longer remains sufficient for the gravida; for what is devoted to the fetus is of necessity taken away from the gravida. For it is not possible for her to take more food in proportion to the increase in consumption, since the process of digestion will not bear the management of more food. If, therefore, she takes as much food as she can digest and the part of the digested food offered to the fetus is taken away from the gravida, and if this diminution is not healthful, then conception is not healthful either. And that pregnancies bring about atrophy, atony, and premature old age, is manifest from the obvious facts and furthermore from the similarity with the earth which latter becomes so exhausted from continuous production of fruit as not to be able to yield fruit every year. . . .

What Are the Signs, According to the Ancients, Whether the Fetus Is Male or Female?

Hippocrates says that <the signs> of pregnancy with a male are: the gravida has better color, moves with more ease, her right breast is bigger, firmer, fuller, and in particular the nipple is swollen. Whereas the signs with a female are that together with pallor, the left breast is more enlarged and in particular the nipple. This conclusion he has reached from a false assumption. For he believed a male to be formed if the seed were conceived in the right part of the uterus, a female, on the other hand, if in the left part. But in the physiological commentaries "On Generation" we proved this untrue. Other people say that if the fetus is male, the gravida will feel its movements to be more acute and vehement; if, however, it is female, the movements will be both slower and more sluggish, while the gravida too moves with less ease and has a stronger inclination to vomiting. For they say that the good color in women with a male child results from the exercise caused by the movement of the fetus; while the bad color in women with a female child is due to the inac-

tivity of the fetus. But these things are more plausible than true, in as much as on the evidence we see that sometimes one thing, sometimes the opposite, has resulted. . . .

What Is the Best Time for Fruitful Intercourse?

Just as every season is not propitious for sowing extraneous seed upon the land for the purpose of bringing forth fruit, so in humans too not every time is suitable for conception of the seed discharged during intercourse. Now so that the desired end may be attained through the well-timed practice of intercourse, it will be useful to state the proper time. The best time for fruitful intercourse is when menstruation is ending and abating, when urge and appetite for coitus are present, when the body is neither in want nor too congested and heavy from drunkenness and indigestion, and after the body has been rubbed down and a little food [has] been eaten and when a pleasant state exists in every respect. "When menstruation is ending and abating," for the time before menstruation is not suitable, the uterus already being overburdened and in an unresponsive state because of the ingress of material and incapable of carrying on two motions contrary to each other, one for the excretion of material, the other for receiving. Just as the stomach when overburdened with some kind of material and turned by nausea is disposed to vomit what oppresses it and is averse to receiving food, so according to the same principle, the uterus, being congested at the time of menstruation, is well adapted for the evacuation of the blood which has flowed into it, but is unfitted for the reception and retention of the seed. And the time when menstruation starts is to be dismissed because of the general tension, as we have said; likewise the time when menstruation is increasing and at its height because the seed becomes very moist and gushes forth together with the great quantity of excreted blood. Just as a wound does not unite if accompanied by a hemorrhage, and even if united temporarily opens again when the hemorrhage sets in, neither can the seed unite with and grow into the fundus of the uterus when it is repelled by the bloody substance excreted therefrom. Consequently, the only suitable time is at the waning of the menses, for the uterus has been lightened and warmth and moisture are imparted in right measure. For again, it is not possible for the seed to adhere unless the uterus has first been roughened and scraped <as it were> in its fundus. . . .

How to Recognize the Newborn That Is Worth Rearing

Now the midwife, having received the newborn, should first put it upon the earth, having examined beforehand whether the infant is male or female, and should make an announcement by signs as is the custom of women. She should also consider whether it is worth rearing or not. And the infant which is suited by nature for rearing will be distinguished by the fact that its mother has spent the period of pregnancy in good health, for con-

ditions which require medical care, especially those of the body, also harm the fetus and enfeeble the foundations of its life. Second, by the fact that it has been born at the due time, best at the end of nine months, and if it so happens, later; but also after only seven months. Furthermore by the fact that when put on the earth it immediately cries with proper vigor; for one that lives for some length of time without crying, or cries but weakly, is suspected of behaving so on account of some unfavorable condition. Also by the fact that it is perfect in all its parts, members and senses; that its ducts, namely of the ears, nose, pharynx, urethra, anus are free from obstruction; that the natural functions of every <member> are neither sluggish nor weak; that the joints bend and stretch; that it has due size and shape and is properly sensitive in every respect. This we may recognize from pressing the fingers against the surface of the body, for it is natural to suffer pain from everything that pricks or squeezes. And by conditions contrary to those mentioned, the infant not worth rearing is recognized. . . .

▲

Galen on Food and Diet

GALEN

Because of the Hippocratic emphasis on maintaining a proper diet for good health, doctors were expected to know the properties of a wide variety of foods. Each food, as Galen pointed out, had heating and cooling, and moistening and drying attributes, and each affected digestion and the balance of the four humors. Much often depended on whether the food was eaten raw, or the manner in which it was cooked. In these selections, Galen clarified, in his rhetorical and often brash style, which foods he found most healthy and those from which his patients should abstain. The overall diet of Romans wealthy enough to afford such food was healthy by modern nutritional standards; nevertheless, a large percentage of the population may not have eaten all that well.

▲

Reprinted by permission of Taylor & Francis, from Galen, *Galen on Food and Diet*, ed. Mark Grant (London: Routledge, 2000), 78–80, 98–99, 116, 131, 140–41, 169–70, 174–76, 188–89.

. . . The most nourishing wheats are those that are hulled and whose whole substance is dense and compressed, so that they can only be broken by the teeth with difficulty. These wheats furnish the body with a lot of nourishment from just a little volume. The opposite of these wheats can be broken up easily by the teeth, appears loose in texture and spongy after chewing, and furnishes little nourishment from a large volume. If you want to compare an equal volume of each wheat, you will find the compact wheat far heavier. . . .

There is also a type of bread that is precisely halfway between these breads. It carries the name of wholemeal bread, although doctors in the past called it unrefined. It is made from unsifted flour, or in other words from the plain flour from which the bran has yet to be separated. From this derives the name, since every bit of the wheat without any separation is used to make wholemeal loaves, whilst unrefined bread is so called because unrefined flour is gathered together for its manufacture. . . .

The logic of this was clear even without any testing. Since, as I stated earlier, wheat flour when eaten is not easy to digest (unless it has been mixed with salt and yeast, worked and kneaded, and put in the oven), how could anyone not realise that it is the most powerful of indigestible foods? In fact wheats, when eaten like this, possess great power, provided they are digested, and they strongly nourish the body, thereby affording remarkable strength to those who eat them. . . .

. . . The substance of beans is not solid and heavy, but spongy and light. They also possess a cleansing action like barley, for it can be clearly seen that their meal wipes dirt off the skin, something which slave-dealers and women have realised since they use bean meal for washing every day, just as other people use sodium carbonate, which is suitable for washing thoroughly too. . . .

The soup made from beans may be flatulent, but it becomes even more flatulent when the beans are used boiled whole. If they are roasted—

for some people eat them like this in place of sweetmeats—they lose their flatulence, but become difficult to digest and slow to pass through the bowels, whilst for nourishment they distribute a thick juice to the body. Eaten when green, before they have been ripened and dried, they share the same attribute as all other fruits which we serve before their peak has been reached: namely that of supplying nourishment to the body that is moister and consequently more productive of waste, not only in the bowels, but throughout the whole body. So understandably such foods less nourishing and passes through the body faster. . . .

. . . Since all summer fruits afford little nourishment to the body,* ripe figs [in this season] have next to no nutrition; in fact they do not make strong firm flesh, as does bread and pork, but rather spongy flesh, as do broad beans. They fill the stomach with flatulence, and so cause pain, unless on being eaten their passage through the body is swift, and if this is coupled with a prompt evacuation, they cause flatulence of short duration, and so they are usually less harmful than autumn fruit.

Compared to figs that are not ripe, the excellence of ripe figs is considerable, and this excellence is manifest in all other fruits without exception. Figs that are perfectly ripe come close to causing no harm at all, just like dried figs which have many uses, but they are bad for those who eat too many of them. For the blood which they produce is not altogether good, and so the result is a large number of fleas. . . .

. . . It has been shown that kidney stones are produced in those bodies where the thickness of the juices is combined with a fiery heat. You should therefore take special care to avoid ["dry"] cheese, since it is no good for digestion, assimilation, urination, evacuation of the stomach, or for the healthy state of the humours.

. . . Of all the cheeses, the best is freshly produced, such as the sort that is made in my home

---

* Fig trees usually bear two crops a year: The early season (May/June) fruits are inferior and frequently too acidic, and only those of the second, or main, crop (August/September) are of actual value.

town of Pergamum. . . . This is an extremely pleasant cheese for eating and causes no harm to the stomach. It is the least problematic to digest and excrete of all the cheeses. . . .

As regards the differences in variety of the types I have just mentioned, the softer is better than the harder, whilst the loose-textured and porous is better than what is altogether dense and compressed. Cheeses which are very glutinous or are crumbling almost to the point of roughness are bad; those cheeses which are in between are better. . . .

. . . Of all the wines the red and thick are most suited for the production of blood, because they require little change before turning into it, whilst after these come wines that are dark, sweet and thick, then those that are red and dark in colour, but thick in consistency and containing something of an astringent quality. White wines that are at the same time thick and astringent are less able to nourish than these. The least nourishing of all are wines that are white in colour, but thin in consistency and almost resembling the water that is needed for what is called honey-water.

That thick wines are more nutritious than thin wines is revealed by their natural quality and reinforced through experience of them. Sweet wines are digested more easily in the stomach and are better assimilated than harsh wines because they are hotter in power. Thick wines are digested very much more slowly, and the same is true for their assimilation, but if they meet with a stomach strong enough to digest them properly, they furnish the body with plenty of nourishment. It is obvious that their superiority in nutrition over thinner wines is matched by their inferiority in micturition. . . .

Olives generally afford little nourishment for the body, particularly tree-ripened olives. The preferred way of eating these is with bread, but salty olives and pickled in brine olives are eaten without bread before meals with fish-sauce to loosen the bowels. . . .

Chefs prepare olives in many ways. Indeed, I do not consider it right for a doctor to be completely ignorant of the art of cooking, because whatever tastes good is easier to digest than other dishes which may be equally as healthy. . . .

Most people eat [cabbage] as an accompaniment to bread, but doctors use it as a drying medicine. . . . [I]ts juice contains a purgative element, whilst its body contains more that is drying than that is productive for evacuation. So whenever I want whatever is in the stomach to be passed, it is essential to take the cabbage out of the three-legged casserole, in which it has been cooked with water, and put it at once into pots, in which olive oil has been blended together with fish-sauce. It does not make any difference if salt is used instead of fish-sauce.

But whenever I want to dry a moist stomach, I drain off the first lot of water, when the cabbage seems to have been partially cooked, put it in fresh hot water, and then boil the cabbage once again in this water until it is tender, but I do not cook the cabbage in this water when it is taken for clearing the bowels. . . .

Lentils and cabbage dry in almost the same way as each other, and for this reason they affect the eyesight, unless the eye as a whole ever happens to be moister than usual. But for the body, lentils afford considerable nourishment which is thick and full of black bile, whilst cabbage offers meagre nutrition which is wetter than that of lentils, as if this food was not solid but spongy. Cabbage is not a dish full of good juices, like lettuce, but has a wretched juice that smells unpleasant. I have to say that it clearly does nothing good or bad for urination.

Some people, who practise a pathetic form of pseudo-intellectualising, regard 'brassica' as the correct name for this vegetable, as the Athenians did six centuries ago, but not the Greeks of today, who are unanimous in their insistence of applying the term 'cabbage' to only this vegetable. . . .

. . . On the subject of calm and waveless sea, the less fish are exercised, the worse their flesh, so they are inferior when they live in what are called lagoons, and still worse when they are in lakes. . . .

Fish become better and worse according to their diet. Some thrive on weeds and lots of excellent roots which makes them superior, whilst others eat slimy weeds and unwholesome roots. Others again which live in rivers that flow through a big city, feeding off human sewage and similarly unpleasant food, are the worst of all, as I have said, so that, if they are left out dead for a short time, they immediately putrefy and smell disgusting. . . .

Since these are the worst, the best are the complete opposite, their habitat—as I was saying—being the cleanest sea, especially where there are no shores fringed with earth or without any rocks, but rather sandy or rocky coasts. . . .

. . . [White mullet] . . . can be pickled, and the mullet that lives in lakes is far better when prepared like this, because everything that is slimy and smelly in its flavour is removed. Whatever is freshly pickled is better than anything pickled over a long period of time. . . .

▲

Drinkers and Alcoholics in Ancient Rome

E. M. Jellinek

Some sort of intoxicating drink can be found in nearly every culture, and Rome was no exception. Wine was widely drunk by rich and poor alike, although of varying quality, and the wine industry was a vital part of the Roman economy. However, this selection reveals that the stereotype of debauchery and drunkenness often associated with Roman society was untrue during most of Roman history. Not until the first century B.C.E. did true alcoholism begin to appear, and it was in decline within about two hundred years.

▲

The Drinking History of the Romans

The Early Temperate Period (c. 600–200 BC)

The Romans were probably acquainted with wine at the time of the foundation of their city, but one can agree with Ferrero that they were water drinkers during the earliest period of their history. There is not the least indication that they ever practiced brewing and they never acquired a taste for beer. The contempt with which Tacitus and the Emperor Julian spoke of beer is typical of the Roman attitude toward this beverage. . . .

But if the early Romans had no horror of wine, they did not take its use lightly. While there

is no contemporary evidence of women not being permitted to drink wine, and while some of the instances of men killing their wives on account of their drinking, as recounted by Pliny, must be regarded as legendary, it is quite probable that a law against drinking by women existed during the early Period of the Kings. . . .

While we must give credence to the existence of an early law against drinking by women, the claim that the Roman woman had to kiss her male relatives and kin down to the children of cousins to give proof that she had not been drinking is highly questionable. . . .

Even in the times of the first Roman authors known to us the taboo on drinking by women was not in force. It is hard to say when the women of Rome began using wine, but there is a hint in a

Reprinted with permission from *Journal of Studies on Alcohol,* vol. 37, pp. 1718–41, 1976. Copyright by Journal of Studies on Alcohol, Inc., Rutgers Center of Alcohol Studies, Piscataway, NJ 08854.

legend told by Ovid. According to it, the son of King Tarquinius Superbus and some of his friends, during the siege of Ardea, on the spur of the moment ride home to see their wives and "find the King's daughters-in-law, their necks draped with garlands, keeping their vigils over the wine." As Tarquinius Superbus was of Etruscan origin, and as among the Etruscans, according to the fourth-century historian Theopompus, women drank as freely as men, it may be surmised that the use of wine by women was introduced to Rome by Tarquinius Superbus (traditionally King from 534 to 510 BC). If this was indeed the case, the drinking by Roman women must have been as moderate as, or even more moderate than, that by the men over the next 300 years.

There are also allusions to a law of King Numa on age limits for the use of wine by men. Athenaeus, citing Polybius, gives the age limit as 30 years, and adds that neither free-born women nor slaves were permitted to drink. While none of the Roman or Greek authors saw this law in effect, it is quite in agreement with historical facts from other cultures, for instance Sparta. Athenaeus, citing Poseidonius, says that even the wealthy taught their sons to drink water.

The conclusions of McKinlay that in the early period the Romans practiced great moderation in drinking cannot be questioned. Neither did their way of living permit of excess, nor was there a sufficient supply of wine to make excessive use possible. Nevertheless, even in the most temperate societies some intoxication is experienced. The ancient festival of Anna Perenna must have given some occasion to drinking, but it was perhaps not as bibulous as in Ovid's time. . . . [W]e cannot assume that in the early Republic no Roman ever got drunk, but it is safe to say that drunkenness was by no means a common occurrence.

Period of Increasing Use of Wine (c. 200–100 BC)

That the Romans knew by the end of the third century BC . . . such institutions as the *pantopolium,* a drinking place, and the *thermopolium,* where hot drinks were served, is evident from some of Plautus' plays. It is also evident from Plautus that there were expressions for drinking to one's health. . . . And he gives a number of expressions for different degrees of drunkenness, such as *adoptus* which seems to be a more intoxicated state than *ebrius,* and *madidus* which means "soaked." . . .

Some idea of the quantity that upper-class Romans drank in those times may be gained from Justinus on Trogus Pompeius who contrasts Hannibal (c. 247–182) with his Roman adversaries and says that he neither reclined at a meal nor did he indulge in more than one sextarius (a little over half a liter) of wine. . . . The implication of this statement is that the consumption of half a liter of wine with a meal . . . was considered unusually moderate.

Ennius (c. 239–169) in his *Annals* speaks of a victory celebrated with wine . . . ; the victors sleep "conquered by wine." . . . He also speaks of himself as never poetizing unless in a state of gout, i.e., when drunk. . . .

For the second century BC we also have the contemporary evidence of Lucilius (c. 180–103) on the existence of "infamous and shameful eating houses" . . . and *popinones,* the frequenters of such places; and he also has a phrase for winebibbing women, *vini buae.*

Moreover, by the beginning of the second century BC Bacchanalian orgies apparently had spread in Italy. That the Senate was alarmed by this may be seen from a bronze tablet found at Tiriolo . . . inform[ing] [the people] of a Senate resolution respecting the Bacchanalian orgies.

Such concern does not necessarily imply the spread of drunkenness, but rather an increase in the incidence of unbridled ecstatic rituals with sexual excesses which were often indulged without any drinking or only token drinking. Nevertheless the resolution is of significance as an indication of a decline in moral values at the time in question, or even earlier.

The resolution states, among other things, that no one should keep a lodge of Bacchus unless he obtains the permission of the Senate through the praetor of Rome. No man, whether Roman citizen "or person of the Latin name or one of the allies," should attend a meeting of the Bacchant women, but here again an exception is made for those who obtain Senatorial approval through the praetor of the City. The resolution is thus not an absolute prohibition but rather aims at government control of these rituals and at the prevention of their spread to Rome.

To this period belongs of course Cato (234–149) . . . , whose *De Agri Cultura* has come down to us. From th[is] . . . work it is apparent that wine was also the due of the farm hands, although it was inferior even to the ordinary second squeezing. It was made by taking some husks—which after treading had been put in a jar for cattle feed—and soaking them for a while. The alcohol content of this beverage must have been very low, but it is evidence that in Cato's time the laborer too had his wine, even if it was of inferior quality. The boatmen likewise had their wine rations and perhaps of a little better quality than that of the farm hands. According to Pliny, Cato drank the same wine as his crew on his expedition to Spain. This stern upholder of ancient Roman frugality had no contempt for the use of wine but he frowned on those who made a luxury of it and fancied Greek wines.

Cato also mentions medicated wines against snake bite, as a laxative, as a remedy for anuria, for gout, for indigestion, for loose bowels, and other ills. In all these instances some flower, juniper, myrtle, hellebore or pomegranates were macerated in the wine which served as a vehicle for the medicine rather than as the medicine itself.

All this goes to show the common use of wine in the first half of the second century. The most important aspect, however, is the replacement of grain culture by viticulture in the beginning of the century, so clearly reflected in Cato's ranking of the farm land, mentioned earlier. The greater abundance of wine does not of itself make for more abundant drinking, but it does imply a readiness for the acceptance of the product. . . .

By the end of the third or the beginning of the second century the great period of Roman sobriety had come to an end. Probably one cannot speak of widespread drunkenness at this time, but

wine had become a common beverage and intoxication was no longer a rarity. Certainly the situation was still far from one of habitual drunkenness on a large scale, not to speak of alcoholism in the modern sense of the word. However, some instances of true alcoholism must have existed even then.

The Rise of Alcoholism and Drunkenness (First Century BC)

Widespread drunkenness and true alcoholism among the Romans began in the first century BC and reached its height in the first century AD.

In his great poem on the "Nature of Things," Lucretius (99–50) has a few lines which describe the discordance, restlessness and boredom of upper-class Romans of his time. This prevailing mood is the breeding ground of alcoholism and the lines of Lucretius are reminiscent of Cimbal's clinical description of the "decadent boredom drinker." . . .

Among the earliest of the prominent drinkers of the first century BC was the eminent general and statesman, Sulla (138–78), who always worked under high tension. Sallust, who held Sulla's abilities in high esteem, said that he had an avidity for pleasure, and in his leisure time was given to voluptuousness, but that he did not let this interfere with his duties. From Valerius Maximus it appears that this "voluptuousness" included heavy drinking.

The great alcoholic of the century was Antony, of whom Pliny said that he eagerly vied for the palm in this field by publishing a book on his own drunkenness. Unfortunately this book, which would be the first "I'm an alcoholic" story, has not survived. Antony's alcoholism was so notorious that many ancient authors made reference to it. . . .

Seneca . . . cites Cossus who was prefect of Rome in the same period and was "steeped and soaked in wine," came to the Senate drunk, fell asleep and had to be carried home. . . .

By the time of Horace (65–8), there must have been quite a number of drinkers so habituated to wine that it became a physical necessity for them. Thus, Horace mentions wine among those things "which, if denied, would cause pain to human nature," just as would the lack of bread.

. . . [T]he ability to drink large quantities of wine already had become a matter of prestige and there were expressions corresponding to the American phrase, "to hold one's liquor" well or poorly. For example, Seneca mentions that Cimber, one of the conspirators against Caesar, admitted that he could not carry his wine . . . , and elsewhere he asks, "What glory is there in being able to hold much?" . . . The wine-loving nature of the period is reflected in the glorification of wine which runs through the poetry of Horace. . . .

The century also gave rise to the *Satyricon* of Petronius with its famous description of Trimalchio's bibulous banquet. The *Satyricon* refers largely to one class of Roman society, namely, the newly rich freedmen and their hangers-on. As to the drinking by the common folk in that period, there is relatively little information, because Roman authors wrote nearly exclusively of the upper class. Nevertheless we know that wine was a common drink among the lower classes, since there is frequent mention of the distribution of wine to soldiers and the general population. And perhaps more than in Cato's time, wine was the due of farm hands and workmen in general, even though the wine may have been of rather low quality.

Horace mentions a boatman soaked in sour wine (*vappa*) and he also mentions a drunken slave. Tibullus mentions the rustic youth celebrating with wine, and we have a description by Ovid . . . of the festival of Anna Perenna, which he witnessed. The common folk gathered near the banks of the Tiber, the lads lay on the grass beside their lassies and, just as in our days, they sang the songs which they had heard in the theatre. . . . They prayed for as many years as they drank cups, which meant a lot of cups for, as Ovid says, one man drinks as many cups as Nestor numbered years, and a woman would live to Sybil's age if the cups would really accomplish the purpose. They go home reeling, and Ovid saw a drunken old woman dragging her drunken old husband home.

It is safe to assume that the common folk, although in general . . . not . . . habitually hard

drinkers, were given to occasional excess at various celebrations. A wedding, for instance, was an occasion for drinking and it was followed the next day by . . . renewed drinking.

Widespread Alcoholism (First Century AD)

The first century AD outdid the preceding century in drinking. Pliny says that in no aspect of life was more labor spent than on wine. There were many customs which fostered heavy drinking. Pliny mentions wine-drinking contests, drinking as many cups as demanded by a throw of dice, and the fashion set by the Emperor Tiberius . . . to drink on an empty stomach. Of the custom of drinking wine immediately before a meal he says that it was the result of the physicians seeking to advance their interests by introducing some novelty.

To these excessive customs belonged also the custom of frequent toasts which were drunk in as many measures as the honored person had letters to his or her name. "Let Laevia be drunk in six measures, Justina in seven, Lycas in five, Lyde in four, Ida in three"—so runs one of the epigrams of Martial. . . . The measure used was the *cyathus* which contained about 45 ml, so that it would have required almost one-third of a liter to drink Justina's health; but this would be only one of many toasts in the course of a banquet. Of course, long names were a good excuse for a large cup and Martial mentions the name of Caius Julius Proculus whose health was drunk with five, six and eight *cyathi,* that is, more than four-fifths of a liter for one toast. . . .

We get an idea of the quantities drunk by heavy drinkers of the upper classes, but we know little, if anything, about the average for these strata of Roman society, not to speak of the lower classes. . . .

Whatever the annual consumption may have been, it is evident that in Rome of the first century not only excessive drinkers but true alcoholics as well were frequent among the wealthy freedmen, the upper-middle and upper classes.

Seneca, one of the great observers of the morals of the period, says that "the drunkard is often free from drunkenness." . . . As in our day, such drinkers tried to hide their alcoholic breath: aromatic leaves and herbs were chewed, and there were some pills for the purpose on the market.

Pliny describes many features which are well known to us from modern clinical descriptions of alcoholics. He speaks of the drinker who, after his bath, while still naked, grabs a cup and drinks, for he cannot wait until he gets to the meal. These drinkers "never see the rising sun," and they show what we designate today as a withdrawal symptom, namely, the shaky hand. Pliny recognized even alcoholic amnesia or the "blackout": "Next day the breath smells of the barrel, there is oblivion of all things and memory is dead."

Among these alcoholics is the great soldier, the Emperor Tiberius Claudius Nero, whom the army nicknamed *"Biberius Caldius Mero,"* i.e., the tippler who drinks hot pure wine. Suetonius alleged that Tiberius retired to Capri to indulge in drink and perversions. . . . [S]ince Tiberius was undoubtedly a heavy drinker, and his brooding nature, touchiness, and the many frustrations he suffered before his accession to the throne are frequently the making of the pathological drinker, it is quite probable that he was an alcoholic in the modern sense of the term. His retirement to Capri is in keeping with the alcoholic's tendency to withdraw from his customary social milieu to prevent interference with his drinking.

In spite of the foregoing, we should not picture the whole Roman nation of that period as a population of drunkards. There are certain nations at the present time who have tremendous medical, social and economic problems through drunkenness, yet not more than 3 to 7% of the adult population suffers from alcoholism. Such proportions make themselves seriously felt in the life of a nation, and we need not assume that Rome of the first century exceeded the highest incidence of alcoholism known today.

Even during this period of very heavy drinking the rule was to mix water with wine, and the use of undiluted wine was taken as a sign of excess. Not only did the wine have to be diluted, but there had to be more water than wine in the cup.

To mix water and wine half-and-half was regarded as immoderate. . . .

One of the outstanding features of the Roman drinking pattern was that while wine was taken with meals, there followed after the dinner a session of many hours in which drinking was the central activity. This custom of the wine table may have lasted throughout the Empire but apparently it became less and less connected with excess.

Decline of Alcoholism (c. AD 100–400)

After the first century AD and up to the fall of Rome there is a long list of historical figures who are known either for their temperance or for their drunkenness. . . .

In a thoughtful analysis of Roman society of the late Empire Period, Dill has weighed the evidence with great care. One may agree with him that the contentions of St. Jerome and Salvianus—two characteristically ascetic writers—about the prevalence of drunkenness in this period are entirely outweighed by the evidence of the writings of Symmachus, Ausonius, Apolinarius Sidonius—Bishop of Auvergne—and Macrobius. . . .

Dill's conclusion was that the real canker in the late Empire Period was not gross vice but class pride, want of public spirit, absorption in the varieties of a sterile culture, and cultivated selfishness. This is not to imply that in the last years of the Empire there was no drunkenness or alcoholism, but rather that these had decreased to proportions which today would be regarded as a medium-sized alcohol problem. Even the medium-sized problem is a serious matter calling for public action, and it would surely be sufficient to cause the indignation of ascetic writers.

Summary

The grape vine . . . is indigenous to all the great wine-producing countries of Europe and the Near East. But the art of viticulture may have developed first in Asia Minor, and was probably introduced to other parts of the ancient world by the

Armenians. This must have occurred in very early times since viticulture and the preparation of wine in Italy appear to pre-date the first Greek settlers.

During the earliest period of Roman history wine was relatively scarce, very costly and probably of inferior quality. By the beginning of the second century BC it had become much more readily available and viticulture had begun to assume considerable economic importance. However, qualitatively, Italian wines did not achieve a first rank in the world for another 200 years. By that time the predominance of vineyards over grain land had increased to such a degree that food shortages were feared and unsuccessful legislative attempts were made in the first century AD to restore a balance. Although wine remained a major source of wealth throughout the Empire Period, its production and export declined, and by the middle of the second century AD perhaps as much as half of Rome's supply was imported.

The drinking history of the Romans falls into five stages as indicated by the literature of the times. In the early temperate period . . . moderation was necessitated by the cost and scarcity of wine. But also, early Roman attitudes toward the use of alcohol seem to have been relatively puritanical, as illustrated in part by the attitude toward drinking by women.

The appearance of certain drinking words and phrases in Latin, and the reports of such authors as Plautus, Justinus, Ennius, Lucilius and Cato, indicate the dawn of the second stage, involving a change in attitudes toward wine use, and an increase in drinking, from about 200 to 100 BC. The first century BC may be distinguished as the third stage, during which drunkenness became widespread and clear instances of alcoholism were recorded. A number of historical figures provide gross examples of the latter—Sulla, Antony, and Cimber, among others—and the works of contemporary authors such as Lucretius, Horace, Ovid and Seneca are replete with descriptions of drunkenness.

The first century AD may be considered the fourth stage, when alcoholism had become a very serious problem, prevalent in every class of society. However, after AD 100—for whatever reason—there seems to have been a decline in alcohol use and alcoholism, and this trend continued through the last centuries of the Empire.

▲

Roman Medicine and the Legions

A Reconsideration

JOHN SCARBOROUGH

At least as far back as Rome, soldiers going into battle were provided some degree of medical care. Just as today, the purpose of battlefront medicine was to rehabilitate the soldier so that he could return to battle. Medical care for officers in the Roman legions was distinctly different from that for troops; high-ranking officers had personal physicians, but ordinary soldiers had to rely on one another and on the folk medicine of the day. As the Empire expanded and legions were billeted at greater distances, military hospitals were built to care for wounded and sick legionnaires. Thus, even though medical care could be somewhat haphazard and performed by non-professionals, the Roman military recognized the need for it.

▲

Although all general histories of medicine make reference to skilled doctors in the Roman legions, the specialized secondary literature on the subject is not plentiful. . . .

Previous discussions generally argue that the legion was supplied with skilled medical care. . . . [However], like all things Roman, the legions must be considered as a part of the general cultural matrix, and they cannot be separated in a historical analysis from the society from which they took their origin. . . .

The sources which relate the early military history of Rome and her arduous conquest of the Italian peninsula have few references to medical matters in the phalanx-legion as it evolved in the Republic. Medical care was minimal and there was little provision for the wounded. The Romans adapted new techniques on an ill-defined scale and some Hellenistic practices became predominant as time went on. The evolution of medical practice in the legions resembled closely the development of medicine in Roman society at large. The crude medicine practised by the soldiery upon themselves was designed to get the warrior back into battle as quickly as possible. Care was taken of the wounded by the commanding general, and the prevailing attitude caused one modern authority to comment that the Roman army had as its major characteristic a sort of 'stoicism' which allowed the soldiers to be unworried about medical aid.

A good general was one who billeted his wounded in a friendly town or fortress. The soldier was dependent upon his fellows for aid and this medicine resembled that used by the Roman civilian who practised a sort of 'folk' medicine. The contention that there was a voluntary medical corps with the legions which treated wounds and diseases has no foundation on the available evidence, especially from the Republic. The problem of the wounded would not be too important if the Roman legion won its battles; those who were victorious in ancient warfare usually did not lose many men, whereas those who lost normally lost everything.

As the Romans came to know the Hellenistic world, the Roman general adopted a practice that was common among Hellenistic commanders. A personal physician often accompanied the general on the battlefield. On the other hand, before a definite reference from Cicero, there is little indication that the common soldier had access to medical care. The soldiers of the higher ranks, who were of aristocratic extraction, had a 'refreshment retreat' in their tents which they could use and to which they could retire when they became tired or wounded. The Romans apparently regarded the 'retreat' as a portable relaxation point rather than a special place to go for the treatment of wounds.

The Roman consul borrowed some of the devices that are seen in Xenophon and he adopted them with Roman forthrightness; some of the troops functioned as a medical staff as the need arose. Roman consuls were often skilled wound dressers in their own right and their knowledge of such matters stemmed from long years in the legions.

Cicero tells us that the experienced soldier was confident of treatment in the field but the novice despaired at the slightest hurt. His use of *medicus* is the first definite reference we have of medical aid for the legionary. The imprecise Latin, however, leaves the modern reader with the impression the *medicus* was just another soldier, but one who had been judged experienced among the legionaries in problems of wound dressing. Usually the term *medicus* was attached almost indiscriminately to anyone who appeared as if he knew something of medicine. . . .

The stereotype of the military physician, as the Roman thought of him, is presented by Virgil, and the figure fits the evidence that we possess for both the military and civilian modes of life in the late Republic and the Early Empire. . . . Virgil gives clues of the common attitude about a soldier's troubles, and the military man was admired for the amount of physical punishment he could take. . . .

Caesar has many passages which allow us to determine whether or not an official medical corps was available to the Roman legionary. His regard for the safety and well-being of his trusted legions is apparent in his writing. . . .

. . . It seems odd, however, that although Caesar reports numbers of the wounded and the condition of some of the wounded, he fails to account for how they might have been treated. Jacob argues that since Caesar does not bother to talk of this matter, the wounded were taken care of by a medical corps that Caesar took for granted. A sounder conclusion would be that there was a kind of *de facto* medical service of soldier-*medici* which obviated notice.

An official medical service was not a part of the Roman consul's planning on the field of battle. The account given by Plutarch of the disaster at Carrhae shows this clearly. With an elaborate expedition such as Crassus prepared against Parthia, a medical staff would have been included if it was customary to have an official service on the battlefield. Again we can note that the generals supplied themselves with physicians who attended to their personal needs. Caesar recognized the value of billeting his wounded in a safe spot so that they might return to battle, and his system of evacuation of his wounded shows considerable foresight. The major characteristic of the references that Caesar gives us about his sick and wounded is one of praise for the endurance of his troops, and great hints of the typical, cold-blooded, 'stoic' attitude of the Roman legionary.

Thus by the end of the Republic, Roman military medicine was modelled to a certain degree upon precedents common in the Greek armies of the Hellenistic period. The consul and the noble elements of the legion supplied themselves with personal medical care, but the legionary was left in the care of the *medici*. The superb discipline of the Roman legion and its winning record kept the usual incidence of wounded low, but the legionary, like his enemies, suffered from the devastations of disease until the use of the **valetudinarium,** and sanitary measures became common-place in the Empire.

Inscriptions from the Empire, as well as further literary references, indicate the unofficial basis of medical care in the legions. In speaking of the *primorum ordinum* as being a select group of century commanders whom he used as an informal consultation committee, Caesar provides a key to explain the often occurring inscriptional *medicus ordinarius.* Since Caesar's council was one of men taken from the ranks and distinctly one of an informal nature, the *medicus ordinarius, medicus cohortis,* and the *medicus legionis* functioned on the same basis. The inscriptions show that this position was one of great respect, but that the individual so named was first a soldier in his duties, not a physician. It is to the Romans' credit that they recognized the need for such a service, but the solution was not a medical corps whereby trained physicians became a part of the army. The response to the problem of proper care for the sick and the wounded in the legions took the form that the Roman would understand and he thought that it was effective for the need as it was demonstrated. The wounded were cared for, as far as possible on the field, and the transportable sick were placed in *valetudinaria* along with the more severely wounded. The Romans clearly distinguished in the legions between the treatment of the 'sick' and the 'wounded'.

. . . An inscription found in the vicinity of Hadrian's Wall tells in terse terms of the gratitude felt by the soldiers of the first Tungrian Cohort for one Ancius Ingenuus, who had died at the age of twenty-five. His memorial tablet was embellished to an extent that might not be expected, and he is styled *medicus ordinarius.* This indicates his status as one of the ranks, but his status of great respect among his fellow soldiers. Compassion was as highly prized among the Roman legionaries as it is in any age. Titus Claudius Hymnus, *medicus legionis* to the XXI Claudia, is commemorated in a similar fashion. The Cohors IV Praetoria gives us an interesting example of a *medicus cohortis* who erected a memorial to himself and to his dependents. The tone of the inscription allows the modern viewer to observe what could be called 'scientific magic' in the taking of vows in connection with the function of the *medicus* in the legions. The Roman navy had its own variety of 'doctor', termed the *medicus duplicarius,* and his skill was limited.

The great number of inscriptions indicate the *medicus* to be very common, particularly in the frontier posts. We can assume that the *medici* were on hand at most points to render what aid they could, and probably the newer *medici* learned their medicine from the 'senior' *medici* present in the legion.

As the Roman legion developed efficiency and learned to deal with isolated locations which made it impossible for the wounded to be evacuated to a safe Roman fort or allied town, it began to build *valetudinaria* which would serve this function. These structures were the Roman answer to isolation and proved to be an integral part of the *castra,* especially on the frontier. Here the *medici,* experienced as they were in the wounds of war, treated their comrades. The legionary hospitals were carefully planned and show insight into drainage problems with regard to sanitary conditions. Roman engineering skill is apparent and one must admire these islands of hope placed at the edge of the civilized world. Again it should be emphasized that the *valetudinaria* argue for the medical care of the sick as the Roman thought of them in contradistinction from the wounded. They indicate that the Roman army was following good military practice by providing a place for the sick and the transportable wounded near to the source of manpower need. In an age where geographical distances were fantastic, this points to the element of genius inherent in Roman military organization.

Literary evidence spanning the entire course of the Roman Empire points firmly to the lack of an organization of an official medical service which would administer to the common soldier. In his praise of Tiberius, Velleius Paterculus reveals the presence of medical care for the officers of the legions, but not for the common soldier. . . . Even the aristocrat was grateful for good medical care. [Velleius Paterculus] indicates that trained physicians available for the legion at large were rare and that Tiberius followed the practice of the best Roman generals. Such care was not usual and the soldiers received the ministrations of the *medici* in their own ranks. In another context Tacitus crisply notes the thankfulness of the soldiers when Agrippina went among the wounded and acted as a nurse, dressing the wounds and giving clothing to those who needed it. At another point Tacitus states bluntly that the soldiers took care of their own wounds and doctored one another. The image of medicine in the legions shows no trained physician in attendance, and that the training of the

medici consisted of experience with a common knowledge of anatomy and medicine in the day-to-day needs of the legion.

Celsus remarks that anatomy can be learned from the wounds of a soldier in battle and Galen says that the medical attendants in the German Wars were like untrained empirics not to dissect the bodies of the dead German warriors to learn something more than they knew. Celsus gives us a detailed account of missile injuries and this may show the level of skill attained by the best of the military *medici.* From the evidence that we have of the *medicus,* he gathered his craft within the legion and was not a trained physician in either the Hellenistic fashion of Galen or in the Latinized manner that Celsus suggested.

The often-cited reliefs of a *medicus* treating the wounded, as depicted on Trajan's Column, reinforce the conclusions that the inscriptions and literary evidence give us. The *medici* treating the wounded on Trajan's Column are dressing superficial wounds and their dress is identical with that of the soldiers they are aiding. Trajan's Column would thus bear out the general picture: the *medici* were those soldiers of a legion or of an auxiliary detachment who had demonstrated their capabilities for wound dressing and a primitive surgery, but who were not trained physicians. This tradition reached back many centuries in Roman warfare. Whether or not the best of the Roman legionary *medici* consulted medical handbooks such as Celsus must remain theoretical.

Returning to further references from the literary sources, one notes the unofficial basis admitted in many cases. As time passed the soldiers seemed to have received less attention of the quality noted in the Early Empire, and the camp *praefect* was put in charge of what medical care they got. . . . If trained physicians were present among the legions in the Later Empire, the type of medicine they practised seems to remind us of the repute of certain doctors often noted in authors of the Early Empire. Galen tells us that he was summoned to give proper medical treatment at the front where little apparently existed—as he saw it. Galen notes that many doctors 'talk' medicine without proving their skill.

A

Four Different Ways of Philanthropic Aid to the Blind in Medieval Eastern Christendom

A. H. DIAMANDOPOULOU-DRUMMOND,

A. A. DIAMANDOPOULOS, AND

S. G. MARKETOS

Caring for the blind is one of the oldest forms of medical attention, having roots at least as ancient as the Old Testament. The Byzantines carried the concept considerably further, not only because doing so was an integral part of their culture and Christian faith, but also because blindness was a major problem throughout the area. The Byzantine leadership and government were well known for their philanthropy, and a significant portion of the care for the less fortunate was devoted to persons without sight. Legislation supported the growth of institutions for individuals who were sight impaired and demonstrated the Byzantines' particular concern for the welfare of people in need.

A

Until recently, the provision of health care and welfare by the Byzantine State has been a neglected and misunderstood subject. Papers dealing with this topic have been presented rarely to the International Society for the History of Medicine, usually by Greek authors such as Rozos and Eftychiadis.

In particular, the provision of aid for the blind has attracted even less attention. As a consequence, erroneous beliefs have entered the literature. For example, according to W. H. Levy writing at the end of the nineteenth century, the first organized institution for the care of the blind was the asylum of the Quinze-vingts in Paris. It was established in 1260 AD by Louis IX (or St Louis) of France, in order to deal with the epidemic of ophthalmia which occurred on the return of the Crusaders from the East. The same information, surprisingly, is given in a Greek encyclopaedic dictionary of the 1950s.

In this paper we will demonstrate that several types of provision for the blind had been made earlier by the Byzantine State. . . .

. . . Blindness was a common and serious problem throughout the Middle East. From ancient times there are indications of the existence of eye disease in the area. The Stele of Hammurabi (*c.* 1700 BC) mentions the surgical treatment of an eye tumour. The ancient Egyptians are known to have recognized several eye diseases leading to blindness, and trachoma was recognized from Pharaonic times. Homer, according to ancient biographers, is reported to have become blind after contracting an eye disease on his travels. More importantly, from a Byzantine point of view, is that of all the miracles performed by Christ, incidences of the Healing of the Blind represent 16% of the total, and constitute the greatest number concerned with the treatment of a particular

Reprinted by permission of Blackwell Publishing, from A. H. Diamandopoulou-Drummond, A. A. Diamandopoulos, and S. G. Marketos, "Four Different Ways of Philanthropic Aid to the Blind in Medieval Eastern Christendom," *Ophthalmic and Physiological Optics* 15, no. 6 (1995): 609–13.

sense. At the time of the Byzantine Empire, blindness continued to be a widespread problem in the area, as is evidenced by the frequent references to the blind in Byzantine texts.

. . . The seriousness with which the handicap of blindness was regarded by the Byzantine State can be appreciated first from the fact that it was used as a punishment for crimes such as treason, attempts on the throne and for prisoners of war. . . . Strange as it may seem to us, the Byzantines regarded this punishment as a philanthropic act since the alternative was the death penalty. Belisarius, a general of the sixth century, is reported to have begged in the streets of Constantinople after he had been subjected to the penalty of blinding for treason. The use of blinding as a punishment had been known of course since antiquity, particularly as retribution from the gods. We are all familiar with the *'lex talionis'* and the expression 'an eye for an eye'. Blinding was also a popular form of punishment in the Roman Empire. . . . [U]nder Byzantine law a man could not become emperor if he was blind, since the emperor was expected to embody the worldly and spiritual perfection appropriate to God's representative on Earth.

Second, the large number of 'miraculous' shrines which were to be found throughout the length and breadth of the Byzantine Empire emphasize the importance with which the restoration of sight was regarded. From the shrine of the Virgin at Sozopolis (Pisidia) in western Asia Minor to the shrine of the doctor-saints Cyrus and John at Menouthis in northern Egypt, miracle cures of eye disease and blindness were recorded at innumerable shrines. Characteristically, one of the oldest holy-water shrines (or agiasmata), Zoodohos Pege in Constantinople is famous for the cure of a congenitally blind man by the use of the clay from the spring. This cure occurred in the presence of the man who later became Emperor Leon the Great (fifth century). This tradition continues. Even today, the agiasmata shrines of St Paraskevi (the patron saint of the Blind), which exist in Constantinople, far outnumber those of the other saints. From a total of 470 shrines for 70 different saints we have an average number of approximately 6.9 shrines per

saint. It is quite striking that St Paraskevi had ten times this average, i.e. 69 shrines. . . .

. . . There was great interest in optical, astronomical and ophthalmological subjects. The Byzantines inherited much of the knowledge amassed on these topics by the ancient Babylonians, Egyptians and Greeks. From the Roman period there is evidence that doctors who specialized in eye diseases used both drug remedies and surgery. Doctors such as the Greek Rufus of Ephesus (*c.* 100 AD) helped to lay anatomical foundations for later advancement of ocular and ophthalmic knowledge. The Byzantines, while playing a major role in the transfer of ancient knowledge to the post-medieval world, also made important additions. From Oribasius and Eustathios of Antiochia in the fourth century AD to Andreiomenos in the fifteenth, there was continual interest and progress in ophthalmology and related subjects. Of particular interest are the following.

Around 500 AD Anthemios of Tralles, mathematician, engineer and also one of the architects of St Sophia, experimented with parabolic mirrors. His brother Alexander was a doctor and his two books *Peri Ophthalmon* [on Eyes] were translated into Latin, Arabic, Hebrew and Syriac during the medieval period. The seventh chapter of the *Tetravivlos* [Four Books] of Aetius Amidenus (sixth century) contains virtually all the ophthalmological knowledge of his time. He recognizes 61 eye diseases including trachoma. In the seventh century Paul of Aegina mentions the treatment of pterygium and trachoma. Meletius the Monk, who is considered to have lived in the ninth century, wrote a treatise *On the Constitution of Man* of which the longest chapter is that on the eyes. . . .

. . . Society as a whole, that is the emperor and his court plus the Church and its lay members, realized that it had a responsibility to provide care and welfare for those with loss or impairment of vision. The Byzantine State built upon and extended the ancient Greek idea of philanthropy. There were no exceptions made on the basis of sex, age, race, creed or social status.

While the Byzantine concept of philanthropy included philosophical, religious and political elements, its greatest expression was by actively providing for the needs of all types of weak members of society. It achieved this by personal involvement in the service of the needy. This could take the form of contributions of money or goods, but most important of all was actual 'hands-on' service. Hence, emperors and empresses are known to have tended the sick. Philanthropy was considered one of the best qualities an emperor could have, since it brought him closer to his role model, Christ the 'Philanthropic Saviour'. All Christians, however, were expected to contribute to aiding the poor, the sick and the infirm. In return, they could hope that their chances of a place in Heaven would be improved. Philanthropy as far as the Byzantines were concerned was a way of life. The most impressive aspect of this was the establishment of special philanthropic institutions throughout the empire. Many of these made particular provision for the care of those afflicted by ophthalmic disease.

For these four reasons, a steady and continuing system of health care and social welfare for the blind developed. . . .

. . . From the very beginning, under Constantine the Great, the Byzantine State began to make legal provision which would emphasize its philanthropic character. . . . Measures such as tax concessions for philanthropic institutions and for doctors facilitated these improvements. In parallel with the State Laws many of the Canon Laws of the Church encouraged the establishment of philanthropic institutions and the provision of care and welfare for the needy. . . .

The fifty-seventh of the Apostolic Canons, which predate the first Synod of Nicaea and were observed even before the fourth century declares:

> If a clergyman or a layman shall ridicule a lame, or deaf, or blind person, he shall be excommunicated.

This is a remarkably progressive statement for its time, and it demonstrates that blindness was not considered to be some kind of Divine Justice, and also that the sufferer was to be treated with respect. Later comments by the twelfth century canonists Zonaras, Balsamon and Aristenus make clear the Church's continued stance that the blind are to be aided and guided, but not patronized or

ridiculed, since to do so is to mock God. This is an attitude in keeping with modern ideas on the provision of help for the blind, and all those with special needs, which does not interfere with their self-respect.

. . . The first sources referring to any kind of charitable foundations date from the fourth century AD, and deal with provisions made for the care of the poor and of strangers. These first institutions seem to have been of a general nature. . . . Slightly later, Bishop Basil of Caeserea (370–379 AD) built several other establishments or *katagogia* for the use of both hale and ill strangers. He hired doctors and nurses for the care of the latter. At the end of the fourth century Bishop John Chrysostom (398–404 AD) opened similar institutions in Constantinople, which were referred to as *nosokomeia,* that is hospitals. By the end of the sixth century more specialized medical care was being offered throughout the empire.

The *Miracula Sanctii Artemii* of the mid-seventh century refers to a deacon of St Sophia (Constantinople), suffering from a groin complaint, who was assigned a bed in the hospital (or Xenon) of Sampson, next to the section for ophthalmic patients. This indicates that as early as the seventh century separate medical care was provided for those afflicted by eye diseases. The problem of eye disease was not confined to the capital. Of the same period is the *Typhlokomeion,* or home for the blind in Jerusalem, which is referred to in the *Miracula S. Anastasii Persae.* In the early twelfth century the Emperor Alexios Komnenos (1081–1118 AD) rebuilt many philanthropic institutions. According to his daughter Anna, he built a second town near the area of the ancient Greek Acropolis in Constantinople to house the poor, both men and women. Anna emphasizes the charitable nature of this establishment by relating that many of the inhabitants of what today would be called 'sheltered housing' were blind or otherwise infirm. Later in the same century, the famous Pantocrator Xenon founded by John II Komnenos had five wards, one of which was solely for ophthalmic cases. Hence, we note a steady interest and progress in the care of those with eye disease.

. . . At the end of the eighth century the Patriarch of Constantinople Tarasios who was lauded for his philanthropic good works, distributed allowances to the blind on important religious occasions, such as during Lent and at Easter.

At least initially, philanthropic institutions were associated with monastic communities, or churches. It is characteristic that those 'men of God' who became saints are often described as 'the light of the blind' and 'the doctor of the ill'. Monks at the Monastery and Baths of Panagia Odegetria (The Guiding Virgin) in the Mangana district of Constantinople, acted as guides for the blind who had gone there seeking a cure. Similarly, Anna Komnene in praising her father's good works describes that he arranged for sighted people to lead the blind.

. . . When all else failed, the blind were not left to despair. The hope of a miraculous cure remained. Throughout the empire from early Byzantine times, centres for the miraculous cure of eye diseases were well known. Sophronius of Jerusalem (seventh century) consulted Alexandrian medical professors for an ocular problem but was not cured by them. In his 'Miracles of Cyrus and John' he describes a votive plaque at the entrance to their healing shrine at Menuthis, which concerns the cure of a man who had been blind for eight years. The later 'Vita' of St. Luke the Younger (or Steiriotes) describes the immediate healing at his tomb of a Boeotian woman suffering from an eye ailment, again after the doctors had failed to effect a cure. Votive eyes of gold, silver or wood were left at the healing shrines in thanks for successful cures.

All the previously mentioned factors influenced both Western and Eastern countries outside the boundaries of the Byzantine Empire. After the Crusades, hospitals and hospices were founded in Western countries such as the aforementioned asylum of the Quinze-vingts. Also, in the Islamic/Jewish world of the same period reference is made both to hospitals and to oculists' treatments.

. . . From the examples above it is evident that a very progressive policy of health care and welfare was followed throughout the Byzantine State in order to cope with the problem of blindness. . . .

KEY TERMS

Valetudinarium, 100 • Venesection, 88

QUESTIONS TO CONSIDER

1. What kinds of questions does an expectant mother ask when she is selecting her obstetrician or midwife? What attributes is she most apt to be concerned about? How are they similar to or different from the criteria Soranus suggested for selecting a midwife? How have priorities changed?

2. The foods that Galen discussed are still considered healthful, and he clearly stated how the properties of each affect the body. Because nutrition science is no longer based on Galen's humoral theories, on what basis do we consider these foods to be healthy? Why is barley good for us, or beans, cheese, or eggs? Are any of Galen's observations still valid?

3. During the Roman Empire, and later the Byzantine Empire, institutions such as legionnaires' hospitals for the sick and facilities for the sight impaired began to appear. Why

do you think they appeared at this point in history? What needs did they satisfy? How well do you think these needs were met?

4. According to modern addiction experts, certain behaviors indicate alcoholism, such as drinking excessively, losing control, denying the existence of the problem, having blackouts, and experiencing withdrawal upon not drinking. On the basis of such criteria, does alcoholism appear to have been as common in Rome as it is in modern-day society? Or, are such criteria specific to the current-day experience? Can we apply them to an ancient society such as Rome? Why or why not?

RECOMMENDED READINGS

Barzel, Uriel S., ed. and trans. *The Art of Cure: Extracts from Galen.* Haifa, Israel: Maimonides Research Institute, 1992.

Grant, Mark. *Dieting for an Emperor: A Translation of Books 1 and 4 of Oribasius' Medical Compilations with an Introduction and Commentary.* Leiden, the Netherlands: Brill, 1997.

Jackson, Ralph. *Doctors and Disease in the Roman Empire.* Norman: University of Oklahoma Press, 1988.

Kottek, Samuel S. *Medicine and Hygiene in the Works of Flavius Josephus.* Leiden, the Netherlands: Brill, 1994.

May, Margaret T., trans. *Galen—On the Usefulness of the Parts of the Body.* 2 vols. Ithaca, NY: Cornell University Press, 1968.

Rocca, Julius. *Galen on the Brain: Anatomical Knowledge and Physiological Speculation in the Second Century AD.* Leiden, the Netherlands: Brill, 2003.

Salazar, Christine F. *The Treatment of War Wounds in Graeco-Roman Antiquity.* Leiden, the Netherlands: Brill, 2000.

Scheidel, Walter. *Death on the Nile: Disease and the Demography of Roman Egypt.* Leiden, the Netherlands: Brill, 2001.

Smutny, Robert J., ed. *Latin Readings in the History of Medicine.* Lanham, MD: University Press of America, 1995.

von Staden, Heinrich, ed. *Herophilus: The Art of Medicine in Early Alexandria.* Cambridge: Cambridge University Press, 1989.

Chapter Six

Europe, 500–1500

INTRODUCTION

The period in European history between the fall of the western part of the Roman Empire and the fifteenth-century Renaissance is often referred to as the *Middle Ages*. It was the age of feudalism, courtly love, and chivalry, but it was also a time of significant urban growth, the rise of trade, population growth (until the Black Death), and the beginnings of such modern nations as Great Britain, France, Russia, and Spain. This time frame is often portrayed as a period of decay and stagnation of knowledge, but it was also a "staging period" for the medical developments of the sixteenth and seventeenth centuries.

From a medical viewpoint, the Middle Ages was generally a dormant period for learning except for the works of Greece and Rome. Even much of that ancient knowledge was lost in the West until the gradual reintroduction of the works of Galen, Hippocrates, and others through the newly established universities and their medical schools beginning about 1200. Oxford, Padua, Bologna, and above all Salerno, all became the pipeline through which the classic works that had been preserved in the East, and the new writings of a number of Islamic physicians, began to infiltrate Western medicine. Additional East-West contacts also occurred during the Crusades, bringing both medical knowledge and new diseases to Europe.

Most doctors were not men of letters, and surgery was conducted mainly by barber surgeons, who learned their craft through apprenticeship. Licensing was generally unknown and where found was nearly impossible to enforce, the result of which was surgeons with a wide range of abilities. Further, few doctors of any kind existed, and most Europeans had no medical assistance beyond the services of midwives and herbalists. Neither cleanliness nor balanced nutrition was known, which resulted in a population at high risk for infectious disease and nutritional deficiencies, if not outright starvation on occasion. Infant and child mortality rates were high even in years when no epidemics or plagues were raging, women routinely died in childbirth, and any accident that broke the skin raised the terrible danger of tetanus and gangrene. In general, for most Europeans, the Middle Ages were decidedly unhealthy.

TIME LINE

625–690 C.E.	Paul of Aegina writes *Epitomae medicae libri septem (Seven Books of Medicine),* his only work to survive
794	St. Albans Hospital is built in London
829	Dame Trotula is teaching at the Salerno medical school, which becomes the most important teaching facility of the entire period
1095–1099	First Crusade—crusaders return home bringing new diseases such as leprosy
1127	Stephen of Pisa writes *Liber regius (The Royal Book),* translating the works of Persian physician Ali ibn al-Abbas and introducing Arabic and Greek medicine to the West
1131	Council at Rheims forbids monks to practice medicine for money
1161	Jewish physicians in Prague are burned for "poisoning wells"—such persecutions for "causing" disease outbreaks are common during the Middle Ages
1179	Church requires authorities to identify and isolate lepers
1214	Maurus of Salerno writes *Anatomia mauri (Anatomy of a Moor),* one of the earliest Latin texts on anatomy
1247	St. Mary of Bethlehem Hospital is founded in London; later becomes known as Bedlam, an infamous insane asylum
1249	Roger Bacon writes his treatise on convex lens use for farsightedness; by the end of the century, spectacles are in common use
1267	Council of Venice prohibits Jewish physicians from practicing among Christians
1315–1322	The Great Famine occurs in northern Europe and the British Isles
1347–1351	The Black Death sweeps across Europe, killing millions
1363	Guy de Chauliac writes *Chirurgia magna (The Great Surgery),* describing treatments for wounds, fractures, and other ailments

1400s	In this century, anatomical teaching using demonstrations with human cadavers becomes common in universities and surgeons' guilds
1403	Venice, Italy—a quarantine (forty-day isolation period) is instituted for people suspected of having plague
1414	Influenza breaks out in Paris
1452	First professional association of midwives is formed, in Germany
1478	Galen's *De medicina (On Medicine)* is produced in print for the first time
1485	Outbreak of English Sweating Sickness (etiology unknown) occurs in London
1489	Spanish soldiers returning from Crete introduce typhus to Europe
1493	First European outbreak of a disease named the *Great Pox,* or *syphilis;* concurrently, severe smallpox and malaria epidemics occur throughout Europe

Medieval Compendium of Women's Medicine

DAME TROTULA

Dame Trotula became known in the twelfth century as an outstanding female physician, a distinct rarity in the Middle Ages. As a professor at the prestigious School of Medicine at Salerno, she authored a number of writings, only a few of which have survived. Her Medieval Compendium of Women's Health *is the most famous, even though she was probably not the sole author. Written from a uniquely feminine perspective, it became the authoritative text on obstetrics for centuries. While it depended heavily on Galen's teachings, strong elements of local Italian midwifery practices, as well as remedies then slowly making their way from the Muslim world into the West, can also be seen in it. Some of Trotula's ideas sound familiar to the modern ear: the benefits of a balanced diet, regular exercise, cleanliness, and reduced stress, and the use of the birthing chair, which is again becoming popular in some obstetrical suites.*

Reprinted by permission of the University of Pennsylvania Press, from Monica H. Green, ed. and trans., *The Trotula: An English Translation of the Medieval Compendium of Women's Medicine* (Philadelphia: University of Pennsylvania Press, 2001), 83–84. Copyright © 2001, 2002, University of Pennsylvania Press. All rights reserved.

On the Regimen for the Infant

The ears of the infant ought to be pressed immediately, and this ought to be done over and over again. Then, attention needs to be paid that the milk does not enter the ears and the nose when [the child] is nursing. And let the umbilical cord be tied at a distance of three fingers from the belly, because according to the retention of the umbilical cord the male member will be greater or smaller. And so that it might talk all the more quickly, anoint the palate with honey and the nose with warm water, and let it always be cleaned with unctions, and let the mucous secretions always be wiped off and cleaned. And so the child ought always to be massaged and every part of its limbs ought to be restrained and joined by bandages, and its features ought to be straightened, that is, its head, forehead, nose. The belly and loins should be tempered, lest much oiliness or humidity exit from them. If either of these appears, for a time try to abstain from the accustomed bandaging and let it sleep for a while. Then let it be bathed in warm water and let it be restored to the accustomed practice [of binding]. A little bit of soporific medicine should be given so that it sleeps. Its skin ought equally to be massaged, which also is customary to be done after taking the breast. Right after birth its eyes ought to be covered, and especially it ought to be protected from strong light. There should be different kinds of pictures, cloths of diverse colors, and pearls placed in front of the child, and one should use nursery songs and simple words; neither rough nor harsh words (such as those of Lombards) should be used in singing in front of the child. After the hour of speech has approached, let the child's nurse anoint its tongue frequently with honey and butter, and this ought to be done especially when speech is delayed. One ought to talk in the child's presence frequently and easy words ought to be said. When the time for the extrusion of its teeth comes, the gums ought always to be rubbed each day with butter and goose grease, and they ought to be smeared with barley water. The throat and the vertebrae ought to be anointed. If its belly becomes lax, let a plaster which is made from cumin and vinegar and mixed with sugar be placed over it; gum arabic, Armenian bole, and similar things ought to be mixed together and given to the child. But if its belly is constricted, let a suppository be made for it from honey and cotton and mouse dung, which should then be inserted. When the time comes when it begins to eat [solid foods], let lozenges be made from sugar and similar things and milk in the amount of an acorn and let them be given to the infant so that it can hold them in its hand and play with them and suck on them and swallow a little bit of them. The meat of the breast of hens and pheasants and partridges ought to be given because after it begins to take these things well, you will begin to change reliance upon the breasts and you should not permit the child to suck them at night, as was said above. Thus, it ought to be drawn away [from the breast] day by day and in an orderly way, and care should be taken that it not be weaned during a hot season.

If one limb of any child is larger than another, it can be reduced to its customary size if the affliction is recent. If it is old, there is no way it can be reduced. For a recent affliction, we aid in this manner. First, let the limb be fomented with a decoction of these herbs, that is, bear's breech with root of marsh mallow and with leaves of wild celery, parsley, and fennel, and all diuretic herbs. Boil these in water. And let the limb of the patient be placed above the vessel, and let it be covered with a linen cloth so that it sweats. Then let chamomile and marsh mallow be cooked in water, and in this thick mixture let wax be melted, and let the whole limb then be covered with this. Afterward, let it be tied tightly with linen bandages, and thus let the limb of the patient sweat through one night; in the morning, let it be rubbed so that the spirits are aroused and flow to the painful part. This having been done, let the limb be rubbed with *dialtea,* thus composed: two parts *dialtea* and a third of laurel oil mixed together; and let the limb be anointed in the above-mentioned manner three or four times a day. Now take *diaceraseos, ceroneum,* and *oxicroceum,* and let them be powdered in turn. Then let marsh mallow be cooked and let the powder be softened with this viscous liquid until it adheres well, and let the whole limb of the patient be covered and tied with bandages, and thus it will be able to be ameliorated with fomenting and the application of plasters. These things having been done, let rest and leisure be ordered; let the patient have a warm and moist diet, with good quality, moderately red wine, which s/he should drink until s/he is cured. Let the patient use baths of fresh water.

▲

Disease of the Soul

Leprosy in Medieval Literature

SAUL N. BRODY

The diagnosis of leprosy was one of the most dreaded pieces of news any medieval person could hear. Nobility, guild member, or peasant, it meant forced exile from all human society, including church and even family. Such a radical reaction was due to two principal factors: the Biblical teachings about the disease and the fear that it was contagious (which it generally is not). As a result, when the examination and diagnosis was made, by a priest rather than a physician, the victim was forced to leave behind everything of his or her former life and to live on the fringes of society—his or her only company being other lepers. As a visible act to demonstrate cutting all social bonds, the leper was officially declared dead in a ceremony that must have been utterly devastating to the unfortunate person, was promised redemption in the afterlife, and was sent away.

▲

. . . The physical examination of a suspected leper could come to one of four conclusions. The suspect could be declared healthy and given attestation that he was not leprous. Or, if the examiners thought that because of poor regimen the suspect might become leprous, he would be so admonished. If, however, the subject suffered a skin disease which could not be confirmed as leprosy, he would be confined to his home and strongly warned that he might have to enter a leper asylum if a later examination indicated the presence of leprosy. Finally, if the leprosy was confirmed, the victim would be told that he would have to be separated from the healthy population.

In 1179, the Third Lateran Council issued a decree which urged that the segregation of lepers from society be accompanied by appropriate ceremony. The decree provided a number of specimen rituals, and the *separatio leprosorum* in time came to be accepted widely, though not universally, for lepers continued to be treated with varying rigor. For instance, in England, where segregation was perhaps more lax than elsewhere, the ceremony of the symbolic burial service was not in force. . . .

The sequestration of lepers was carried out with appropriate solemnity. Jeanselme outlines a representative office of separation by synthesizing rituals followed in seventeen dioceses. During the ceremony, the leper knelt before the altar, beneath a black cloth supported by two trestles. (However, at Amiens and elsewhere, he was required to stand in a grave in a cemetery.) His face was covered by a black veil as he heard the mass. The officiating priest threw a spadeful of earth from the cemetery on the head of the leper three times, explaining that the ritual symbolizes the death of the leper to the world. The priest said: "Be dead to the world, be reborn to God," and the leper replied, "O Jesus, my redeemer, you formed me out of earth, you dressed me in a body; let me be reborn in the final day." Then, using the vernacular, the priest read the prohibitions that made the alienation of the victim explicit:

> I forbid you to ever enter the church or monastery, fair, mill, marketplace, or company of persons. I forbid you to ever leave your house without your leper's costume, in order that one recognize you and that you never go barefoot. I forbid you to wash your hands or any thing about you in the stream or in the fountain and to ever drink; and if you wish water to drink, fetch it in your cask or porringer. I forbid you to touch anything you bargain for or buy, until it is yours. I forbid you to enter a tavern. If you want wine, whether you buy it or someone gives it to you, have it put in your cask. I forbid you to live with any woman other than your own. I forbid you, if you go on the road and you meet some person who speaks to you, to fail to put yourself downwind before you answer. I forbid you to go in a narrow lane, so that should you meet any person, he should not be able to catch the affliction from you. I forbid you, if you go along any thoroughfare, to ever touch a well or the cord unless you have put on your gloves. I forbid you to ever touch children or to give them anything. I forbid you to eat or drink from any dishes other than your own. I forbid you drinking or eating in company, unless with lepers.

Following the reading of the proscriptions, the leper put on his costume and was given the signal with which he was to warn the healthy of his approach. Both signal and costume varied with locality. The instrument for warning the popu-

lace of the leper's approach was usually a rattle or castanet, but it was sometimes a bell, either carried or worn on the shoes. At Lille, the leper carried a small horn, and at Arles he sang the "De Profundis" to warn the healthy of his presence. As for his clothing, he usually wore gloves and long robes. In certain areas, the costumes were distinguished by cut or color . . . , though in England there was little uniformity. . . .

Equipped with his clothing and various utensils, the leper would be led to his place of retreat, often a hut situated in an open field outside of the town. At the threshhold of his hut, the leper had to say, "This retreat is mine, I will live here always because I have chosen it." The priest would bless the outcast's utensils and encourage him to be patient. The ritual of St. Albin d'Angers directs the cleric to say:

> Because of greatly having to suffer sadness, tribulation, disease, leprosy, and other worldly adversity, one reaches the kingdom of paradise, where there is neither disease nor adversity, but all are pure and spotless, without filth and without any stain of filth, more resplendent than the sun, where you will go, if it please God. But so that you be a good Christian and so that you bear this adversity patiently, God gives you grace.

In the ritual of separation used at Reims, the priest consoles the leper that even if he is separated from the healthy,

> this separation is only corporeal; as for the spirit, which is uppermost, you will always be as much as you ever were and will have part and portion of all the prayers of our mother Holy Church, as if every day you were a spectator at the divine service with others. And concerning your small necessities, people of means will provide them, and God will never forsake you. Only take care and have patience. God be with you.

The priest would next place a cross before the leper's door, hang a box for alms on the cross, and place an offering in it, at the same time admonishing those gathered for the ceremony not to injure the leper by word or action, but rather—having a remembrance of the human condition and the formidable judgment of God—to provide liberally for all his needs. The congregation would presumably follow the priest's example and place alms in the leper's cup. Finally, the priest advised parents, or whoever was

in guardianship of the leper, to remain close to him for at least thirty-two hours in order to provide comfort and assistance if the leper were to enter a physical or spiritual crisis. The leper was now separated from the world. . . .

▲

Fracture Trauma in a Medieval British Farming Village

Margaret A. Judd and Charlotte A. Roberts

Farming has always been a dangerous occupation, even before the advent of modern machinery. Falls, gashes from tools, and blows from unruly livestock have been common injuries to farmers since ancient times, and the medieval peasant was no exception. Rural activities were simply far more apt to produce injury, especially fractures, among both men and women than were urban jobs. In this selection, the author looks specifically at the incidence of broken bones in a farming village and compares it with that of a medieval urban population and that of modern farmers. The results clearly show that farming has always been, and remains, one of the most dangerous human activities.

▲

Agriculture ranks among the top three most dangerous occupations in industrialized nations, accompanied by construction and mining. In many regions it is the leading cause of fatal and nonfatal injuries and therefore, the identification of physical hazards is an essential topic in clinical research. Epidemiological study of farming-related trauma identifies the etiology of injury, designs preventative strategies, creates safer equipment, and disseminates knowledge to reduce high trauma statistics. While these modern investigations of occupational trauma strive to prevent injury in present-day populations, they also provide insight with which to assess trauma among archaeological populations.

Fracture traumas are common pathological lesions observed in archaeological skeletal material and represent the accumulation of physically traumatic events in an individual's life that resulted in broken bones. While observations of trauma are conscientiously reported during a skeletal analysis, tabled in skeletal reports, and adeptly described, there remains a paucity of systematic investigations at the populational and etiological levels.

Early studies of archaeological trauma were either case studies of violence or summaries covering an immense time span with equally diverse recording methods. Since then, studies of trauma have emerged as investigations that integrate physical and cultural factors within a specific

Reprinted by permission of Margaret A. Judd, Dept. of Anthropology, University of Pittsburgh, from Margaret A. Judd and Charlotte A. Roberts, "Fracture Trauma in a Medieval British Farming Village," *American Journal of Physical Anthropology* 109 (1999): 229–31, 234, 236–42.

environmental context into the interpretation of the trauma pattern observed. The report by Lovejoy and Heiple of Late Woodland hunter-gatherer longbone fractures at the Libben site in Northern Ohio was perhaps the earliest in-depth methodical trauma study conducted at the populational level, and it ushered in a new standard for paleotrauma research. Numerous methodical and interpretive issues were addressed: a systematic data collection, the expression of frequency of fractured bones per bone type in addition to fractures per individual, accidental vs. intentional trauma, and years at risk of trauma. . . . Larsen reviewed more current research areas in populational investigations of ancient trauma, e.g., the role of elemental patterning in determining whether a lesion was due to violence or accident, the effects of immigration, subsistence strategy, industrialization, ritualized violence, and child abuse. Paleotrauma research has advanced significantly, although much of the focus remains directed towards violence, i.e., both domestic and external warfare. Other areas such as occupational trauma, however, remain neglected.

Stirland previously cautioned about attempts to associate specific occupations with paleopathology, especially when the activities are known only through artifacts, but stressed the need for rigorous similarity studies between temporally and/or geographically contemporary groups so that group activity or general occupation could be assessed. However, the greatest obstacle for such intersite comparisons of paleotrauma that seek to examine variables such as age and sex variation, environment, subsistence strategy, or lifestyle is the lack of use of standard recording procedures that facilitate comparison, although various protocols and recommendations exist. This investigation will address this potential by examining fracture trauma as a product of daily living in a specific environment, in this case, rural medieval Britain.

Farming is a unique "occupation" as it is a lifestyle composed of multiple activities, rather than one specific occupation, performed in a simple setting that serves as both a residence and

workplace, and allows for only intermittent escape to different surroundings, a situation amplified in the isolated medieval village. This study will assess the longbone fracture patterns and frequencies from a rural medieval British skeletal sample and compare the results to those of four other British samples, one rural and three urban, dated to the medieval period, from which data were similarly recorded. With the temporal and geographic components constant, the role of the living and working environment of these sites can be explored as an injury risk factor. By comparing longbone fracture patterns and frequencies of rural medieval British samples to those of their contemporary urban samples, it is possible to determine whether the activity complex associated with farming posed an occupational hazard in antiquity as it does in the present day.

. . . Raunds Furnells . . . was a small agricultural community located in the Nene Valley of the English East Midlands just northwest of the present village. The site was occupied from the late 6th–15th centuries AD, and consisted of approximately 40 villagers at any one time. The Christian Saxon cemetery from which this skeletal sample derived was established during the 10th century and used for about 200 years. A total of 363 burials was excavated by the Northamptonshire Archaeology Unit from 1977–1980, and the remains are currently stored at the Department of Archaeological Sciences at the University of Bradford. Only adults of known sex as determined by the skeletal analysis of Powell were included in this investigation.

. . . The longbones (clavicle, humerus, radius, ulna, femur, tibia, and fibula) of each individual were identified as present (90%+bone present), incomplete (50–90% bone present), fragmentary (<50% bone present), or absent. Each bone was examined for evidence of antemortem or perimortem fracture. Incomplete bones with fractures and all complete bones formed the observable corpus.

The side affected and the position of fracture (proximal, middle, or distal third of the shaft) were recorded for each bone. The fracture type was assigned as transverse, oblique, spiral, comminuted, incomplete, impacted, compressed, crush, or avulsion, following the definitions . . . summarized by Lovell. This information assists in determining the type of energy that caused the fracture, such as a direct force resulting from a blow, an indirect force due to fall, or repetitive stress. . . . Each fractured bone and its opposite were measured for length. . . .

Most fractures heal successfully, but problems may arise that affect the function of the bone, joint, or soft tissue, or threaten the survival of the individual. General complications develop rapidly after the injury occurs and are not visible in skeletal paleopathology due to their acute and fatal nature. Such developments include **crush syndrome** and tetanus that may both result in death, gangrene that may lead to limb amputation, and fat embolism, the catalyst for cardiovascular accident. Local complications may occur shortly after the injury or years later and are visible in skeletal remains. Fractured bones were examined for periosteal lesions and osteomyelitis. The presence of osteoarthritis, mal-union, post-traumatic **ossification**, atrophy, and **avascular necrosis** determined joint alterations due to bone fracture. . . .

Rural vs. Urban Sites

. . . Both males and females from the rural sites suffered a higher prevalence of longbone fractures than persons from the contemporary urban settings. Females were predisposed to upper body fractures in both environments, although the rural females were particularly vulnerable to forearm fractures. These results suggest that there was a distinct difference in fracture frequencies between both males and females in rural and urban environments in medieval Britain.

. . . In order to evaluate the role of the medieval rural environment in fracture etiology, it is necessary to briefly review the daily activity and lifestyles of the medieval peasant. Daily subsistence activities included routine chores such as those illustrated by the "Labors of the Months," a recurrent medieval theme in sculpture, painting, stained glass, architecture, and manuscripts. These scenes depict farming activities as functions of the season, such as plowing in March, threshing in September, and killing hogs in December. In addition to recording activity and the associated perishable ecofacts, these icons also provide visual evidence of information not detectable from the archaeological record alone, such as the posture and actions required to perform the activity, the type of equipment used, who usually performed the task, and the role of animals in the local economy.

Milk, eggs, cheese, and vegetables made up a large portion of the peasant diet and were less frequently traded. Butter and cheese were particularly valued, as they could be stored for longer periods of time than the 2-day life span of fresh milk. Chicken and geese were relatively cheap to maintain since they did not require a special diet. They were therefore plentiful and provided a continuous source of eggs. Crops such as barley, wheat, oats, and rye were common and the labor required for a successful bounty was part of the annual routine: plowing, sowing, harvesting, threshing, winnowing, and milling. Apple, pear, and nut trees comprised the orchard, while wild nuts and berries were also gathered to enhance the diet. Peasants living near woodlands hunted or poached rabbit, deer, boar, birds, and squirrel, especially during the harsh winter months. Husbandry was practiced along with agriculture, rendering each family unit self-sufficient. Pigs were kept strictly for meat, cattle provided milk, and sheep produced milk and wool. Horses, bulls, and oxen were used primarily for labor, although their meat was eaten out of necessity. Some households supplemented their income with dairying, brewing, butchering, baking, thatching, milling, timber production, and carpentry, or by selling agricultural produce to neighboring towns.

Men were responsible for heavier labor and work located at a distance from the homestead, such as fieldwork, plowing, transporting, fishing, tree felling, and herding. Females assisted in field chores such as planting, weeding, and gleaning, but the majority of their work focused on the *croft* (garden) at home. Here, activities included gardening, fowling, brewing, baking, tending the orchards, milking cows, making butter and cheese, spinning, and weaving. The close proximity to the house allowed women to provide vigilant child care, while attending to food preparation for the family and workers. It was essential for females to remain flexible during the peak seasons of harvest and planting to assist in the fields. Men reciprocated by performing tasks closer to home during the winter months, such as butchering and dairying. Both sexes in poorer households hired themselves out when additional workers were in demand, especially during the harvest.

Medieval farming, therefore, was not a distinct occupation with specific tasks, but rather a way of life composed of a medley of activities required to maintain the household throughout the year. The actions involved in accomplishing these tasks and the surroundings in which they were performed provided the arena for potential injury.

. . . Clinical investigations of [modern] farm living reveal that residents and hired laborers are exposed to greater occupational and environmental hazards than any other occupation, but was this also true in antiquity? It may be argued that the high incidence of modern farm injury is due to increased mechanization and heavy equipment such as tractors, combines, and harvesters, but current epidemiological research finds that fractures due to nonmechanized causes still account for a substantial majority (about 40%) of nonfatal farming injuries. For example, an extensive 12-year investigation of agricultural trauma in rural Wisconsin, Minnesota, and Iowa discovered that of 739 cases of farm-related injuries, 225 (30%) were attributed to falls, kicks, or assaults by farm animals, while 77 individuals (10%) fell from the hayloft, hay wagon, or silo. The study by Jones of trauma in an American Amish community in Ohio described fracture patterns in a "traditional" farming community and thus provides a source of injury mechanisms that may also have been present in a medieval British farming

village such as Raunds. The Amish practice a frugal, preindustrial agricultural lifestyle and avoid modern technological innovations such as electricity, telephones, engines, and automobiles. The division of labor is clearly defined: males are employed predominantly as farmers although some now work in the community as carpenters, blacksmiths, carriage makers, and butchers, while women tend the garden, process and prepare food, provide child care, and create handicrafts. In Jones, 60 cases of trauma were observed in 272 hospital admissions over a 3-year period. Injuries that occurred during chore performance accounted for 58.3% of fractures and were attributed to the following etiologies: throws from a buggy or saddle (18.3%), horse kicks (5%), falls predominantly from a ladder or hayloft (28.3%), and encounters with horse-drawn equipment (6.7%).

The dominance of animal-related injuries is echoed in clinical studies of automated farming sectors. While a portion of injuries are attributed to falls over the family pet that usually result in fractures to the upper extremities, more aggressive damage is associated with falls from horses, bovine assaults, and falls from animal-drawn vehicles. An association with beef and dairy farms presents an increased hazard for all agricultural workers, where injury may occur from close contact with the animal during feeding, milking, dehorning, calving, and foot treatment.

Virtually everyone residing on a farm, including children and the elderly, is involved with daily chores and therefore vulnerable to injuries unique to a farm setting. When women are active in farm chores, males generally exhibit a greater proportion of injuries, such as 2.8:1 and 3:1, although Zhou and Roseman found that females incurred more injuries than males. The greater propensity for male trauma has been attributed to the riskiness of male labor, the number of hours worked, and being the owner/operator. The majority of all female farm injuries, even in a modernized operation, are attributed to animals, especially dairy cows, with short falls in the barn being second; the arms are the most frequent injury location. During peak harvest seasons, a work reciprocity exists, and all able bodies may be recruited to perform essential tasks, thereby exposing everyone to the hazards of the activity. It is during these intense periods that more injuries occur and may be attributed to the inexperience of temporary workers or exhaustion.

Small farm operation is unregulated and therefore mandatory retirement is not essential. As a result, many older adults continue to perform tasks that physically challenge their aging bodies. Physiological deterioration such as failing eyesight and hearing, slow reaction time, impaired [movement] of the lower limbs, vertigo, and impaired coordination in the dark increases with advanced age and therefore is an added factor to farm injury susceptibility. Bone loss due to **osteoporosis** in older males and females creates a more fragile, brittle bone that breaks easily, especially during low-energy traumatic impacts caused by falling and tripping. Longbone sites that are particularly vulnerable include the proximal humerus, distal radius, proximal femur, and proximal tibia. However, while rural activities produce an increased general injury risk, a rural lifestyle results in a decreased incidence of osteoporotic fracture in modern populations and is credited to the higher activity levels of the farm residents that creates a greater maximum bone mass.

Children are overlooked as members of the agricultural workforce, even though they constitute a large majority of the injuries reported. Common sources of fatal injury to children include drowning in irrigation ditches, suffocation in grain bins, animals, and farm machinery, while nonfatal injuries are ascribed to falls and animals. A child may not necessarily be working when an accident occurs, but because they often accompany the parent during chores, they are also exposed to similar workplace dangers.

It is clear that a substantial number of agricultural injuries on modernized farms are related to nonmechanical factors such as farm animals and falls. It would seem reasonable that the longbone fracture pattern at Raunds may reflect the complex of activities associated with the "traditional" farming lifestyle.

. . . Several common injury sources exist between the nonmechanized aspects of modern farming and the medieval farming environment, such as the role of animals in the economy, animal-drawn vehicles and equipment, structures such as haylofts and silos, the use of ladders, harvesting, and butchering. Nonmechanical equipment used in antiquity has not changed functionally or morphologically over time and is similar to that used in traditional farming communities. Langdon compiled a list of hand tools available on a well-equipped medieval farm with their associated activities; tools such as axes, mallets, sickles, forks, ladders, and wheelbarrows were used much as they are today. Therefore, the injury etiology, pattern, and frequency sustained by ancient peoples while using this equipment or performing manual farm chores should also be similar.

Injuries sustained by rural females from Raunds . . . are characterized by distal, oblique fractures to the forearm, which are associated with indirect forces due to tripping or short falls caused by a shift in body weight and loss of center of gravity. When upright balance is lost due to a slip, the individual falls backward and instinctively extends the arms to break the fall, thereby placing additional stress on the forearm's shaft. During a trip, the step is obstructed and the body falls forward; the head and trunk resist by arching back while the arms abduct to regain balance to absorb the impact force. Likewise during a stumble, due to erratic or unstable foot movement, the body attempts to regain its center of gravity by arm abduction and by doing so, the arms are again unprotected. In any case, should balance be recovered, stress is placed on the lower leg in the process, predisposing it to fracture or sprain. Women and children were likely prone to tripping, slipping, or stumbling while procuring, transporting, and processing items such as fuel, water, milk, eggs, grains, fowl, and produce. Dairying, a task relegated to medieval women, would have exposed females to tibia injury, which is frequently encountered during the course of milking the animal.

In this northern region of England, ox-pulled carts predominated during the early medieval period. The heavier ox-drawn carts were much larger than the horse-drawn vehicles and had spoked rather than solid wheels, a sinister web for an unguarded leg. By the eleventh century, plough technology allowed for more efficient breaking of the ground and ridging. Teams of 6–8 horses or oxen were required to power this equipment. While men were alleviated of some injury from maneuvering the human-powered push-plough, they now worked intimately with large draft animals and faced a different occupational hazard. Falls from wagons or horses, or being caught under overturned vehicles, most probably happened in antiquity, with males the more frequent victim, since they habitually traveled to the fields and worked with the animal teams. Injuries received in these situations are identified clinically by lesions typical of direct blows, such as clavicular or midshaft transverse breaks, especially when the more robust humerus or femur [is] involved. Falls from heights are commonly associated with lower limb and clavicle fractures, as individuals typically land on their shoulder or lower leg. These types of injuries are typical of the diverse fractures observed among the Raunds males.

Living conditions, combined with the deterioration of the senses and motor skills, were a particular bane to the elderly. Small . . . , low-ceilinged houses afforded shelter to both humans and animals in one long room before separating the living area from the barn in later periods. A central hearth provided the internal heating and light source, but left the perimeter and entrance in darkness, although candles, ceramic lamps, and lanterns generated additional lighting sources. The cohabiting smaller animals such as dogs, cats, rats, and fowl also functioned as mobile or sedentary obstacles, and chances of stumbling were heightened by inadequate lighting even during the day-time, since there were few windows. While this living environment would challenge the physical dexterity of any individual, when combined with the sensory impairments of aging, a rugged terrestrial environment, and daily farming activity, a considerable number of daily hazards confronted older adults.

Fractures sustained by Raunds adults over 45 years of age accounted for 25% of all longbone lesions. Three of 15 (20%) females presented injuries: one had a clavicular fracture, one exhibited a midshaft break to the forearm while pronated, and the third had a Colles' and distal ulna fracture, all typical of injuries received during a short fall. Injuries displayed by 7 older males were also typical outcomes of falls (4 clavicles, 2 distal fibulae, and 1 radius) and accounted for 28% of the male fractures. However, these injuries did not necessarily occur in old age and represent the accumulation of trauma at the time of death. These data also contradict the clinical evidence for increased older female trauma due to osteoporosis, but endorse the advantages of a physically active farm life.

Five incomplete fractures on shafts of the ulnae or clavicles, the characteristic results of falls, were observed in the Raunds sample. The incomplete or "greenstick" fracture is associated with childhood trauma as children are especially resilient to fractures, but the lesion is often difficult to verify without X-ray and even then may be indiscernible. Although children were not examined in this study, the incomplete lesions etched in the adult longbones did not reflect abuse, but more likely a childhood fall, as the injuries were discrete incidents that did not exhibit localized multiple healing, an indicator of abuse in adults and children. This observation, combined with the lack of metaphyseal and spiral shaft fractures, especially to the humerus and tibia caused by yanking and twisting the unfused longbone, would have served as a possible indicator of earlier abuse.

. . . The urban males sustained a greater number of fractures to a variety of anatomical locations, possibly reflecting riskier and more diverse activities when compared to females. The fracture frequency of urban females was also significantly lower than that of the rural group, although the fracture locations were similar. This disparity suggests a difference in general activity and/or environmental conditions, especially between urban females and other groups. Documentary evidence for urban occupations can be determined from a variety of medieval sources such as poll taxes, assessment rolls, court records, registered wills, depositions due to debt, defamation, and marriage records. Urban male professions included cook, baker, butcher, miller, tailor, carpenter, armorer, and dyer. Women were frequently involved in the sale of produce rather than the actual production, i.e., they were the vendors of bread, but rarely the bakers. In addition to retail trade, traditional female professions included spinster, brewer, seamstress, and laundress, all of which were more sedentary and less dangerous than the farm chores performed by the rural females or the activities of the urban males.

Fracture trauma among townspeople was minimal, as previously suggested by Grauer and Roberts. They proposed that the trauma pattern of St. Helen-on-the-Walls was comparable to that of other medieval urban sites, in that longbone fractures were uncommon; the radius and/or humerus were the most frequently fractured bones; and males displayed a higher percentage of trauma. Grauer and Roberts concluded that the hazards of medieval urban centers were minor. The results obtained in the present investigation

support this argument, and show no significant difference between the individual fracture frequencies among the urban groups, although a significant difference exists between the fracture frequencies of the urban and rural samples.

. . . Fractures at rural medieval British sites were indiscriminately distributed between males and females. The locations and types of fractures, however, do reflect a segregation in activity. This activity, probably associated with labor, was recorded historically and iconographically and provides a possible explanation for some of the injuries observed in this sample. Rural activity has changed little over time, especially when compared to modern "traditional" farming and small-scale operations where some chores are still performed manually. As in the present, all individuals were expected to help out on the medieval farm and therefore were susceptible to farm-related dangers. A high individual fracture frequency is significantly associated with farming in medieval Britain, and suggests that this type of environment was more hazardous than that of urban neighbors, just as it is today.

⋏

The Great Surgery

GUY DE CHAULIAC

During the Middle Ages, most surgeons were referred to as barber surgeons, *men who trained through apprenticeship and military service rather than formal education. Barber surgeons set bones, performed phlebotomies, and shaved and cut hair; the symbol of the barber pole with its red spirals portrays the flow of blood from bloodletting. Most physicians considered barber surgeons to be inferior technicians.*

The fourteenth-century French surgeon Guy de Chauliac was unusual: First and foremost, he was a physician, university educated, but he was also a surgeon, with training in anatomy. In service to the Avignon popes, he wrote one of the great classics of early surgical texts: his Chirurgia magnus, *or The Great Surgery, dated 1363. Widely copied and translated into several languages, his* Chirurgia *became the principal surgical treatise until the eighteenth century. His work relies heavily on Galenic principles as well as those of a number of the best-known Islamic physicians.*

Reprinted from W. A. Brennan, trans., *Guy de Chauliac On Wounds and Fractures* (Chicago: W. A. Brennan, 1923), 1, 84–86, 147, 151–52.

The selections included here from the Chirurgia *cover several topics. The first is a broad statement describing what a surgeon ought to be in manners, training, and attitudes, whereas the second lists the nine basic principles of the treatment of head wounds. The final two selections deal with fractures of the arm and leg, common injuries in battle and everyday life, as indicated in the previous reading.*

⋏

What the Surgeon Ought to Be According to Guy de Chauliac

The conditions necessary for the surgeon are four: first, he should be learned; second, he should be expert; third, he must be ingenious; and fourth, he should be able to adapt himself. It is required for the first that the surgeon should know not only the principles of surgery, but also those of medicine in theory and practice; for the second, that he should have seen others operate; for the third, that he should be ingenious, of good judgment and memory to recognize conditions; and for the fourth, that he be adaptable and able to accommodate himself to circumstances. Let the surgeon be bold in all sure things, and fearful in dangerous things; let him avoid all faulty treatments and practices. He ought to be gracious to the sick, considerate to his associates, cautious in his prognostications. Let him be modest, dignified, gentle, pitiful, and merciful; not covetous nor an extortionist of money; but rather let his reward be according to his work, to the means of the patient, to the quality of the issue, and to his own dignity. . . .

Nine Teachings Which Must Be Observed in the Treatment of Wounds of the Head

The *first teaching* to be known is that wounds of the head the same as a fracture of the limb have many peculiarities and differences from wounds of the other organs, as much by reason of the vicinity and nobility of the meninges of the brain as that on account of the rotundity of its form, it cannot be either united or held by bandage, as the other organs.

The *second teaching* is that in wounds of the head you must observe with particular note the common intentions . . . concerning bleeding, purgation and care of the bowels; that at least once a day the patient should go to the stool of his own accord or by help of a suppository or clyster or some laxative. Of the manner of living it should be very spare. The extraction of infixed things should be the least noxious. Flowing of blood should be restricted, and of the correction and preservation of the wound from complications, as it has been and will be said.

The *third teaching* is that in wounds of the head before all things the hair should be removed and the head shaved, softening it with water and oil, as William says, taking care that neither hairs, water nor oil should enter into the wound, because these things hinder the consolidation. . . . From the commencement let discharge of matter be restricted and pain appeased by putting egg albumin over and in the wound. After the commencement let the other suitable steps be taken, let the surrounding parts always be kept anointed with unguent of bol armenian or red oil, so that pain and fever may be appeased and aposthemation prevented.

The *fourth teaching* is: Let one guard the wound from cold, because as you have often heard from Hippocrates, cold is an enemy of nerves and of the bones and meninges; and air is also offensive to these organs. For this William counseled that in winter, when such wounds are being dressed, it should be done near a brazier with hot coals; the windows should be closed and light can be obtained from candles. After the bandage of the head it should be covered with a sheepskin cap.

The *fifth teaching* is that if sanious matter is discharged from the place it should be cleaned away once a day in winter and twice in summer; and that the changing and cleaning may be made with cotton, lint and soft cloths gently and without pain.

The *sixth teaching* is that above the meshes a piece of soft sponge should be placed in order that by it the sanious discharge may be soaked up and prevented from descending to the brain.

The *seventh teaching* concerns: That convenient bandage may be accommodated to it; thus when we wish to incarnate, let there be made a bandage with two ends which at least is half incarnative. It is made thus: that one may take a band more than a yard long and four fingers wide and let it all be rolled up except two spans. Then, commencing along the forehead, proceed toward the ear which is opposite the wound, and the other rolled part unrolled toward the ear of the side of the wound (not, however, covering the ears) is brought back to the other end of the bandage and there, near the ear, let it be twisted and tightened and let the free end of the bandage be turned downward and the rolled part let upward toward the head, winding it by the side behind the head toward the end of the spans; and then as before twisting it with the other and returning it on the head. Let that be done so many times that all may be covered and well bandaged. That being done, the Bolognese tie the two ends under the chin and the Parisians suture them in the middle of the forehead.

If we only wish to retain the medicaments we will make a bandage with several ends, which is made for the head by this means: That one may have a large piece of linen about three spans long and two spans wide. Let it be cut from each end at about three fingers' widths of the breadth until there only remains one span in the center. Then one of its end may be tied with the other behind, tightening it around the head. The other two ends being passed over each other by the neck, let them be bound under the chin in front.

The *eighth teaching* is that if by chance any fragment of bone may have remained in the wound, let it be treated by wine abundantly (if there is no fever) and with the capital powder of pimpinella, betoyne, gariophylata, valeriana, and osmius in equal parts of each, and as much of pilosella as of all the others together.

The *ninth teaching* is that the patient be placed in bed in the beginning on that part in which it will be least painful, and after on the side wounded as soon as sanious discharge appears in order that the sanious matter may discharge better. . . .

Concerning Fracture of the Forearm and Its Bones

It happens sometimes in the forearm that the two bones are fractured and sometimes one of the two only. The fracture of the inferior and greater bone is of greater vehemence and severity than that of the superior smaller bone, as Avicenna says and Albucasis the same. All agree that in this fracture, whether one or both bones be broken, that it should be extended by two assistants, the one pulling toward the elbow, the other softly toward the hand. Let them be gently equalized and bandaged and do the other things necessary. . . . In the arm when one of the bones is broken, little splinting is necessary, but when the two bones are broken it requires five or six splints. It is placed over the abdomen hanging from the neck. It is consolidated in thirty days. . . .

Concerning the Thigh

When the thigh is broken, strong extension is necessary for it, as Avicenna says. Now for this fracture . . . of the thigh it is scarcely exempt from lameness, as Avicenna says. Still it is necessary to know especially that almost all agree that one must proceed the same in its regimen as in the fracture of the adjutory bone; save that it is necessary that one use stronger extension. And for this it is also necessary that there should be two attendants to tie the ligaments above and below the fracture. They also order that the limb may be very strongly bound and splinted with six or seven splints, and William wishes that the external splints may be long and strong.

Three suffice for Albucasis. Because it is commanded that the leg be bound to the thigh in place of using splints in such a manner that the calcaneum reaches to the buttocks, which does not please me. With regard to the position of the patient, there are different modes; some (such as Roger, Albucasis and William) put the patient in a plain bed and apply cloths and poultices about and beyond the fracture, which I do not praise. Others (as Master Peter) support it with long straw supports reaching to the feet and covered with a cloth, which is sutured and held from above with three or four bands. Others (as Avicenna and Brunus, to which Roger agrees) apply two splints which reach to the feet, similarly tied with bands. Some, as Lanfranc and several modern practitioners, put the limb in a cradle as far as the feet. Yet, however divergent they may be, all endeavor to so situate the reduced broken thigh that it may repose without trouble and does not budge nor decline to either side. For this Roger warns the operator that the injured thigh may be kept alongside the healthy limb. For greater caution Roger situated the patient in a narrow perforated bed in order that he might go to stool without getting up from the place and tied the thigh and the leg in three or four places to the edges of the bed and the foot to a post so that the patient cannot drag it of his own accord, as Theodorus does.

With regard to myself, the thigh being bound with long splints to the feet, I sometimes sustain it with the above-mentioned means with straw or some other thing; and I attach to the foot a leaden weight, passing the cord over a little pulley so that it will keep the leg in its proper length; and if there is some defect in the equalization, by pulling little by little it will be rectified. The dressings are removed every nine days or more and the fracture is consolidated in fifty days.

▲

Biological Warfare at the 1346 Siege of Caffa

Mark Wheelis

The Black Death of 1347–1351 is probably the most famous epidemic in history, killing about a third of the affected populations in Europe and Asia. Although modern researchers are not sure that the actual disease was bubonic plague, and most indications are that it was not, no one can doubt the intensity and far-reaching effects of the pandemic. The Black Death was a history-altering event. Although its origins are still unclear, historians know that the disease first manifested during a siege by the Mongols against the Italian trading enclave on the Black Sea at Caffa in 1346. Gabriele de' Mussi's account, written after the fact, is the principal source for the outbreak at Caffa, and it is supported by most known facts.

In this selection, the use of disease by the besiegers of Caffa reveals a clear-cut case of biological warfare. The method was simple and effective, and the results were devastating. However, the author also points out that the plague spread to Eurasia by several routes, only one of which was the diaspora of survivors of Caffa. In any case, following is one of the earliest recorded cases of biowarfare, a subject much on the minds of modern-day people.

▲

Reprinted from Wheelis M. Biological warfare at the 1346 siege of Caffa. Emerg Infect Dis [serial online] 2002 Sep [2/25/03];8. Available from: URL: http://www.cdc.gov/ncidod/EID/vol8no9/01-0536.htm

The Black Death, which swept through Europe, the Near East, and North Africa in the mid-14th century, was probably the greatest public health disaster in recorded history and one of the most dramatic examples ever of emerging or reemerging disease. Europe lost an estimated one quarter to one third of its population, and the mortality in North Africa and the Near East was comparable. China, India, and the rest of the Far East are commonly believed to have also been severely affected, but little evidence supports that belief.

A principal source on the origin of the Black Death is a memoir by the Italian Gabriele de' Mussi. This memoir has been published several times in its original Latin and has . . . been translated into English (although brief passages have been previously published in translation). This narrative contains some startling assertions: that the Mongol army hurled plague-infected cadavers into the besieged Crimean city of Caffa, thereby transmitting the disease to the inhabitants; and that fleeing survivors of the siege spread plague from Caffa to the Mediterranean Basin. If this account is correct, Caffa should be recognized as the site of the most spectacular incident of biological warfare ever, with the Black Death as its disastrous consequence. After analyzing these claims, I have concluded that it is plausible that the biological attack took place as described and was responsible for infecting the inhabitants of Caffa; however, the event was unimportant in the spread of the plague pandemic.

. . . The disease that caused this catastrophic pandemic has, since Hecker, generally been considered to have been plague, a zoonotic disease caused by the gram-negative bacterium *Yersinia pestis,* the principal reservoir for which is wild rodents. The ultimate origin of the Black Death is uncertain—China, Mongolia, India, central Asia, and southern Russia have all been suggested. . . . Known 14th-century sources are of little help; they refer repeatedly to an eastern origin, but none of the reports is firsthand. Historians generally agree that the outbreak moved west out of the steppes north of the Black and Caspian Seas, and

its spread through Europe and the Middle East is fairly well documented. However, despite more than a century of speculation about an ultimate origin further east, the requisite scholarship using Chinese and central Asian sources has yet to be done. In any event, the Crimea clearly played a pivotal role as the proximal source from which the Mediterranean Basin was infected.

. . . Caffa (now Feodosija, Ukraine) was established by Genoa in 1266 by agreement with the Kahn of the Golden Horde. It was the main port for the great Genoese merchant ships, which connected there to a coastal shipping industry to Tana (now Azov, Russia) on the Don River. Trade along the Don connected Tana to Central Russia, and overland caravan routes linked it to Sarai and thence to the Far East.

Relations between Italian traders and their Mongol hosts were uneasy, and in 1307 Toqtai, Kahn of the Golden Horde, arrested the Italian residents of Sarai, and besieged Caffa. The cause was apparently Toqtai's displeasure at the Italian trade in Turkic slaves (sold for soldiers to the Mameluke Sultanate). The Genoese resisted for a year, but in 1308 set fire to their city and abandoned it. Relations between the Italians and the Golden Horde remained tense until Toqtai's death in 1312.

Toqtai's successor, Özbeg, welcomed the Genoese back, and also ceded land at Tana to the Italians for the expansion of their trading enterprise. By the 1340s, Caffa was again a thriving city, heavily fortified within two concentric walls. The inner wall enclosed 6,000 houses, the outer 11,000. The city's population was highly cosmopolitan, including Genoese, Venetian, Greeks, Armenians, Jews, Mongols, and Turkic peoples.

In 1343 the Mongols under Janibeg (who succeeded Özbeg in 1340) besieged Caffa and the Italian enclave at Tana following a brawl between Italians and Muslims in Tana. The Italian merchants in Tana fled to Caffa (which, by virtue of its location directly on the coast, maintained maritime access despite the siege). The siege of Caffa lasted until February 1344, when it was lifted after an Italian relief force killed 15,000 Mongol troops and destroyed their siege machines. Janibeg renewed the siege in 1345 but was again forced to lift it after a year, this time by an epidemic of plague that devastated his forces. The Italians blockaded Mongol ports, forcing Janibeg to negotiate, and in 1347 the Italians were allowed to reestablish their colony in Tana.

. . . Gabriele de' Mussi, born circa 1280, practiced as a notary in the town of Piacenza, over the mountains just north of Genoa. Tononi summarizes the little we know of him. His practice was active in the years 1300–1349. He is thought to have died in approximately 1356.

Although Henschel thought de' Mussi was present at the siege of Caffa, Tononi asserts that the Piacenza archives contain deeds signed by de' Mussi spanning the period 1344 through the first half of 1346. While this does not rule out travel to Caffa in late 1346, textual evidence suggests that he did not. He does not claim to have witnessed any of the Asian events he describes and often uses a passive voice for descriptions. After describing the siege of Caffa, de' Mussi goes on to say, "Now it is time that we passed from east to west to discuss all the things which we ourselves have seen. . . ."

. . . The de' Mussi account is presumed to have been written in 1348 or early 1349 because of its immediacy and the narrow time period described. The original is lost, but a copy is included in a compilation of historical and geographic accounts by various authors, dating from approximately 1367. The account begins with an introductory comment by the scribe who copied the documents: "In the name of God, Amen. Here begins an account of the disease or mortality which occurred in 1348, put together by Gabrielem de Mussis of Piacenza."

The narrative begins with an apocalyptic speech by God, lamenting the depravity into which humanity has fallen and describing the retribution intended. It goes on:[*]

. . . In 1346, in the countries of the East, countless numbers of Tartars and Saracens were struck down by a mysterious illness which brought sudden death. Within these countries broad regions, far-spreading provinces, magnificent kingdoms, cities, towns and settlements, ground down by illness and devoured by dreadful death, were soon stripped of their inhabitants. An eastern settlement under the rule of the Tartars called Tana, which lay to the north of Constantinople and was much frequented by Italian merchants, was totally abandoned after an incident there which led to its being besieged and attacked by hordes of Tartars who gathered in a short space of time. The Christian merchants, who had been driven out by force, were so terrified of the power of the Tartars that, to save themselves and their belongings, they fled in an armed ship to Caffa, a settlement in the same part of the world which had been founded long ago by the Genoese.

Oh God! See how the heathen Tartar races, pouring together from all sides, suddenly invested the city of Caffa and besieged the trapped Christians there for almost three years. There, hemmed in by an immense army, they could hardly draw breath, although food could be shipped in, which offered them some hope. But behold, the whole army was affected by a disease which overran the Tartars and killed thousands upon thousands every day. It was as though arrows were raining down from heaven to strike and crush the Tartars' arrogance. All medical advice and attention was useless; the Tartars died as soon as the signs of disease appeared on their bodies: swellings in the armpit or groin caused by coagulating humours, followed by a putrid fever.

The dying Tartars, stunned and stupefied by the immensity of the disaster brought about by the disease, and realizing that they had no hope of escape, lost interest in the siege. But they ordered corpses to be placed in catapults and lobbed into the city in the hope that the intolerable stench

---

* Reprinted by permission of Rosemary Horrox and Manchester University Press, from Rosemary Horrox, trans. and ed., *The Black Death* (Manchester, UK: Manchester University Press, 1994), 16–20.

would kill everyone inside. What seemed like mountains of dead were thrown into the city, and the Christians could not hide or flee or escape from them, although they dumped as many of the bodies as they could in the sea. And soon the rotting corpses tainted the air and poisoned the water supply, and the stench was so overwhelming that hardly one in several thousand was in a position to flee the remains of the Tartar army. Moreover one infected man could carry the poison to others, and infect people and places with the disease by look alone. No one knew, or could discover, a means of defense.

Thus almost everyone who had been in the East, or in the regions to the south and north, fell victim to sudden death after contracting this pestilential disease, as if struck by a lethal arrow which raised a tumor on their bodies. The scale of the mortality and the form which it took persuaded those who lived, weeping and lamenting, through the bitter events of 1346 to 1348—the Chinese, Indians, Persians, Medes, Kurds, Armenians, Cilicians, Georgians, Mesopotamians, Nubians, Ethiopians, Turks, Egyptians, Arabs, Saracens and Greeks (for almost all the East has been affected)—that the last judgement had come.

. . . As it happened, among those who escaped from Caffa by boat were a few sailors who had been infected with the poisonous disease. Some boats were bound for Genoa, others went to Venice and to other Christian areas. When the sailors reached these places and mixed with the people there, it was as if they had brought evil spirits with them: every city, every settlement, every place was poisoned by the contagious pestilence, and their inhabitants, both men and women, died suddenly. And when one person had contracted the illness, he poisoned his whole family even as he fell and died, so that those preparing to bury his body were seized by death in the same way. Thus death entered through the windows, and as cities and towns were depopulated their inhabitants mourned their dead neighbours.

The account closes with an extended description of the plague in Piacenza, and a reprise of the apocalyptic vision with which it begins.

. . . In this narrative, de' Mussi makes two important claims about the siege of Caffa and the Black Death: that plague was transmitted to Europeans by the hurling of diseased cadavers into the besieged city of Caffa and that Italians fleeing from Caffa brought it to the Mediterranean ports.

. . . de' Mussi's account is probably second-hand and is uncorroborated; however, he seems, in general, to be a reliable source, and as a Piacenzian he would have had access to eyewitnesses of the siege. Several considerations incline me to trust his account: this was probably not the only, nor the first, instance of apparent attempts to transmit disease by hurling biological material into besieged cities; it was within the technical capabilities of besieging armies of the time; and it is consistent with medieval notions of disease causality.

Tentatively accepting that the attack took place as described, we can consider two principal hypotheses for the entry of plague into the city: it might, as de' Mussi asserts, have been transmitted by the hurling of plague cadavers; or it might have entered by rodent-to-rodent transmission from the Mongol encampments into the city.

Diseased cadavers hurled into the city could easily have transmitted plague, as defenders handled the cadavers during disposal. Contact with infected material is a known mechanism of transmission; for instance, among 284 cases of plague in the United States in 1970–1995 for which a mechanism of transmission could be reasonably inferred, 20% were thought to be by direct contact. Such transmission would have been especially likely at Caffa, where cadavers would have been badly mangled by being hurled, and many of the defenders probably had cut or abraded hands from coping with the bombardment. Very large numbers of cadavers were possibly involved, greatly increasing the opportunity for disease transmission. Since disposal of the bodies of victims in a major outbreak of lethal disease is always a problem, the Mongol forces may have used their hurling machines as a solution to their mortuary problem, in which case many thousands of cadavers could have been involved. de' Mussi's description of "mountains of dead" might have been quite literally true.

Thus it seems plausible that the events recounted by de' Mussi could have been an effective means of transmission of plague into the city. The alternative, rodent-to-rodent transmission from the Mongol encampments into the city, is less likely. Besieging forces must have camped at least a kilometer away from the city walls. This distance is necessary to have a healthy margin of safety from arrows and artillery and to provide space for logistical support and other military activities between the encampments and the front lines. Front-line location must have been approximately 250–300 m from the walls; trebuchets are known from modern reconstruction to be capable of hurling 100 kg more than 200 m, and historical sources claim 300 m as the working range of large machines. Thus, the bulk of rodent nests associated with the besieging armies would have been located a kilometer or more away from the cities, and none would have likely been closer than 250 m. Rats are quite sedentary and rarely venture more than a few tens of meters from their nest. It is thus unlikely that there was any contact between the rat populations within and outside the walls.

Given the many uncertainties, any conclusion must remain tentative. However, the considerations above suggest that the hurling of plague cadavers might well have occurred as de' Mussi claimed, and if so, that this biological attack was probably responsible for the transmission of the disease from the besiegers to the besieged. Thus, this early act of biological warfare, if such it were, appears to have been spectacularly successful in producing casualties, although of no strategic importance (the city remained in Italian hands, and the Mongols abandoned the siege).

. . . There has never been any doubt that plague entered the Mediterranean from the Crimea, following established maritime trade routes. Rat infestations in the holds of cargo ships would have been highly susceptible to the rapid spread of plague, and even if most rats died during the voyage, they would have left abundant hungry fleas that would infect humans unpacking the holds. Shore rats foraging on board recently arrived ships would also become infected, transmitting plague to city rat populations.

Plague appears to have been spread in a stepwise fashion, on many ships rather than on a few, taking over a year to reach Europe from the Crimea. This conclusion seems fairly firm, as the dates for the arrival of plague in Constantinople and more westerly cities are reasonably certain. Thus de' Mussi was probably mistaken in attributing the Black Death to fleeing survivors of Caffa, who should not have needed more than a few months to return to Italy.

Furthermore, a number of other Crimean ports were under Mongol control, making it unlikely that Caffa was the only source of infected ships heading west. And the overland caravan routes to the Middle East from Serai and Astrakhan insured that plague was also spreading south, whence it would have entered Europe in any case. The siege of Caffa, and its gruesome finale, thus are unlikely to have been seriously implicated in the transmission of plague from the Black Sea to Europe.

. . . Gabriele de' Mussi's account of the origin and spread of plague appears to be consistent with most known facts, although mistaken in its claim that plague arrived in Italy directly from the Crimea. His account of biological attack is plausible, consistent with the technology of the time, and it provides the best explanation of disease transmission into besieged Caffa. This thus appears to be one of the first biological attacks recorded and among the most successful of all time.

However, it is unlikely that the attack had a decisive role in the spread of plague to Europe. Much maritime commerce probably continued throughout this period, from other Crimean ports. Overland caravan routes to the Middle East were also unaffected. Thus, refugees from Caffa would most likely have constituted only one of several streams of infected ships and caravans leaving the region. The siege of Caffa, for all of its dramatic appeal, probably had no more than anecdotal importance in the spread of plague, a macabre incident in terrifying times.

Despite its historical unimportance, the siege of Caffa is a powerful reminder of the horrific consequences when disease is successfully used as a weapon. The Japanese use of plague as a weapon in World War II and the huge Soviet stockpiles of *Y. pestis* prepared for use in an all-out war further remind us that plague remains a very real problem for modern arms control, [more than] six and a half centuries later.

The Black Death

John Clynn

Regardless of the origins of the Black Death, its sweep across Europe was unstoppable. From Italy, it moved north to France, the British Isles, and Scandinavia, eastward into central Europe and Russia, westward to Spain and Portugal, and south across the Middle East and into Asia. It struck nobility and peasant, priest, soldier, and guild member alike; young and old; men, women, and children. No place was immune, whether hamlet, city, castle, or monastery. The plague experience was nearly universal.

Among the eyewitness accounts of the Black Death, the most famous is Boccaccio's Decameron, *but one of the most poignant is that of a Franciscan monk in Ireland. Writing in 1348, John Clynn described the horrors of the plague in Kilkenny from his deathbed, fully anticipating his own death. Not at all sure whether the human race would survive, he nevertheless tried to record the events in case some people might live to read his account in the future.*

In 1348, particularly during the months of September and October, bishops and prelates, ecclesiastics and members of religious orders, nobles and others, everybody in fact, women as well as men, gathered in droves from all over Ireland to make the pilgrimage to Tech-Moling and wade in the water, with the result that on many days you might have seen thousands of people assembled. Some came out of devotion; others, the majority in fact, came because of their fear of the plague which was then raging. It first began near Dublin, at Howth, and at Drogheda, and virtually wiped out those cities, emptying them of inhabitants. In Dublin alone 14,000 people died between the beginning of August and Christmas. This pestilence was said to have arisen in the east and to have killed some forty million people as it swept through the Saracens and unbelievers. In Avignon in Provence, where the Roman Curia was then based, it began in the previous January, in the pontificate of Clement VI. There were not enough churches and burial grounds in the city to hold all the dead bodies, and the pope himself ordered a new burial

From Richard Butler, ed., *Annalium Hiberniae Chronicon* (Dublin: Irish Archaeological Society, 1849), 35–37, as translated and edited by Rosemary Horrox, *The Black Death* (Manchester, UK: Manchester University Press, 1994), 82–84. Reprinted by permission of Manchester University Press and Rosemary Horrox.

ground to be consecrated for the burial of those killed by the pestilence. From May to the Translation of St Thomas [3 July] more than 50,000 bodies were buried there. . . .

Since the beginning of the world it has been unheard of for so many people to die of pestilence, famine or other infirmity in such a short time. Earthquakes, which extended for many miles, threw down cities, towns and castles and swallowed them up. Plague stripped villages, cities, castles and towns of their inhabitants so thoroughly that there was scarcely anyone left alive in them. This pestilence was so contagious that those who touched the dead or the sick were immediately infected themselves and died, so that penitent and confessor were carried together to the grave. Because of their fear and horror men could hardly bring themselves to perform the pious and charitable acts of visiting the sick and burying the dead. Many died of boils, abscesses and pustules which erupted on the legs and in the armpits. Others died in frenzy, brought on by an affliction of the head, or vomiting blood. This amazing year was outside the usual order of things, exceptional in quite contradictory ways—

abundantly fertile and yet at the same time sickly and deadly. Among the Franciscans at Drogheda 25 brothers died before Christmas, and 29 died at Dublin. . . . At Kilkenny the pestilence was strong during Lent, and eight Dominicans died between Christmas and 6 March. It was very rare for just one person to die in a house, usually husband, wife, children and servants went the same way, the way of death.

And I, Brother John Clynn, of the Friars Minor of Kilkenny, have written in this book the notable events which befell in my time, which I saw for myself or have learnt from men worthy of belief. So that notable deeds should not perish with time, and be lost from the memory of future generations, I, seeing these many ills, and that the whole world is encompassed by evil, waiting among the dead for death to come, have committed to writing what I have truly heard and examined; and so that the writing does not perish with the writer, or the work fail with the workman, I leave parchment for continuing the work, in case anyone should still be alive in the future and any son of Adam can escape this pestilence and continue the work thus begun.

Key Terms

Avascular necrosis, 115 • Crush syndrome, 115 • Ossification, 115 • Osteoporosis, 117

Questions to Consider

1. Consider the various ministrations Dame Trotula recommended for newborns. Regardless of the reasons given, which actions would likely be taken in a modern birthing suite? Which would not? Consider what is done to the newborn today. How do these procedures differ from those performed on the medieval infant, and why are they recommended?

2. In light of Guy de Chauliac's description of the essential traits of a surgeon, which, if any, would apply equally well to current-day surgeons? Which, if any, are seemingly unimportant to the modern surgeon?

3. We tend to look at popular attempts to stop the spread of the Black Death as hopelessly confused and ignorant at best and scapegoating at worst. Prayers, killing dogs and cats, fleeing the cities, using sweet substances to clear the air, even blaming the

plague on the sins of the world, or worse, on the Jews, did nothing to stop the relentless spread. However, would we react any differently today, even with all the diagnostic tools available? How would modern populations react to an unknown disease that spread in an unknown manner, had no cure, and was seemingly unstoppable?

4. The current threat of biowarfare centers on technology, ease of dissemination of information, and the speed of intercontinental travel. Yet, consider how easily the Mongols introduced plague to the city of Caffa, with only the most primitive equipment. Why have bioweapons become such an important threat? What do they offer that traditional methods of warfare do not? What special dangers are involved, as the Mongols discovered?

5. Medieval women were underserved by physicians, a profession dominated by men. Women had to rely on their own remedies and on other women, such as midwives, for help. In modern-day America and Europe, women have much better access to both medical knowledge and care. Yet, throughout the rest of the world, women remain on the fringe of the medical profession both as practitioners and as patients. What parallels can be drawn between women of the European Middle Ages and contemporary women in underdeveloped countries?

6. One issue historians must consider carefully regarding historical evidence is cause and effect. For example, we know that the Mongols hurled plague victims' bodies over the Caffa wall, and we know that shortly thereafter, plague broke out inside the city. Does the first fact explain the second? Or might another explanation be offered as to why plague broke out inside the city walls? What other explanations might be equally valid? (*Hint:* Think about the behavior of rats, the animal vector believed involved in the spread of plague.)

RECOMMENDED READINGS

Boccaccio, Giovanni. *The Decameron.* New York: Signet Classics, 2002.

Cadden, Joan. *The Meaning of Sex Differences in the Middle Ages: Medicine, Natural Philosophy, and Culture.* Cambridge: Cambridge University Press, 1995.

French, Roger. *Medicine Before Science: The Business of Medicine from the Middle Ages to the Enlightenment.* Cambridge: Cambridge University Press, 2003.

Green, Monica H., trans. *The Trotula: A Medieval Compendium of Women's Medicine.* Philadelphia: University of Pennsylvania Press, 2001.

Horrox, Rosemary, trans. and ed. *The Black Death.* Manchester: University of Manchester Press, 1994.

Ogden, Margaret S., ed. *The Cyrurgie of Guy de Chauliac.* London: Oxford University Press, 1971.

Orme, Nicholas. *Medieval Children.* New Haven, CT: Yale University Press, 2001.

Rowland, Beryl, trans. *Medieval Woman's Guide to Health.* Kent, OH: Kent State University Press, 1981.

Siraisi, Nancy. *Medieval and Early Renaissance Medicine: An Introduction to Knowledge and Practice.* Chicago: Chicago University Press, 1990.

Strehlow, Wighand, and Gottfried Hertzka. *Hildegard of Bingen's Medicine.* Santa Fe, NM: Bear and Company, 1988.

Ziegler, Philip. *The Black Death.* New York: John Day, 1969.

Chapter Seven

Medicine in the Muslim World and the Americas, 700–1500

INTRODUCTION

While the state of medical knowledge in Europe languished, and even regressed, during the early Middle Ages, the practice of professional medicine flourished in other regions of the world, most notably in the Muslim Empire. Arabic medical practices and writings were firmly grounded in the principles of Hippocrates and Galen and the other scientific and medical writers of classic Greece and Rome. In fact, one of the greatest contributions of the Muslim world to modern medicine was the preservation of many of the original works of such philosophers, poets, and physicians, without which the entire Greco-Roman tradition could have vanished.

In addition to simple preservation, however, the great scholar-physicians of the Muslim Empire (which stretched from Spain to India) produced many new works on topics ranging from the use of hot-iron cautery for battle wounds to the humoral foundations of disease. These individuals were also responsible for a number of advances in surgery and ophthamology and added an enormous number of substances to the study of pharmacology. One of the clearest definitions of the practice of medicine came from Ibn Sina, who began his famous *Canon on Medicine* by saying that medicine "is the art whereby health is conserved and the art whereby it is restored, after being lost" (*Canon*, Book 1, Part 1, Thesis 1).

Halfway around the world, the great urban civilizations of Mexico and the Andean countries developed their own medical traditions. The Mayan and Aztec cultures of Mexico, which reached an advanced stage of sophistication by 1500, depended on a combination of a natural ingredient–based pharmacoepia and a firm belief in the supernatural cause and cure of disease. Further south, centering around the Peruvian capital of Cuzco, the Incan Empire placed a high value on its citizens' health. With an extremely broad range of ecosystems available to the Incas, their materia medica was at least as developed as that of their European conquerors, and their surgical methods included even the successful opening of the skull. The complex responses to death and disease in the Americas reflected a strong cultural commitment to relieving the discomfort and anxiety of the ill and wounded.

However, the development of these medical systems was abruptly truncated, beginning in 1492, not by the military might of the Spanish and other Europeans, but by the arrival of their traveling companions: a host of infectious diseases such as smallpox and measles, to which the native peoples had no immunity. The arrival of Old World epidemics and the catastrophic die-off they caused permitted the European conquest of the New World and the successful imposition of European control over an entire hemisphere. It also abruptly halted the further development of some sophisticated medical systems.

TIME LINE

600–900 c.e.	The Mayan Empire reaches its height in southern Mexico and Guatemala
ca. 700	The Maya begin using the concept of *zero,* which reflects their considerable achievements in both mathematics and astronomy
707	Teaching hospital is built in Damascus; many such hospitals are built throughout the Muslim Empire, the most famous of which is Jundi-Shapur, founded about 530
711–778	Spain is conquered by the Muslims; the Western Caliphate reaches its fullest extension
ca. 860–ca. 932	Al-Razi (name Latinized to *Rhazes*), a highly prolific Muslim alchemist and physician-scholar, lives—writes more than two hundred books during his career
936–1013	Al-Zahrawi (Latinized to *Albucasis*), a great Islamic physician and surgeon, lives—writes *On Surgery,* the first illustrated comprehensive surgical text
980–1037	Ibn Sina (Latinized to *Avicenna*) lives—probably the most influential Arabic physician-scholar; writes his *Canon on Medicine* about 1010
ca. 1091–1162	Ibn Zuhr (Latinized to *Avenzoar*), an eminent physician-scholar of Seville, lives—writes primarily on clinical medicine
1095–1258	The Crusades, a series of religious conflicts between Christians and Muslims, take place—crusaders returning home bring new diseases to Europe
1126–1198	Ibn Roschd (Latinized to *Averroes*), a scholar-physician-jurist of the Western Caliphate, lives—writes

	extensively on medicine, law, and mathematics, but most of his works are later burned
1135–1204	Moisés Maimónides lives—a Jewish physician of the Western Caliphate
1200	Incan Empire is founded in Peru; at its peak in the 1530s, it will extend from Colombia to Chile
ca. 1250	First Islamic medical school in Turkey is founded
1284	Mansari Hospital is built in Cairo
1325	Aztec capital city of Tenochtitlán is founded; site of modern-day Mexico City
1347–1348	Black Death sweeps throughout the Muslim Empire
1409	Insane asylum is built in Seville
1430s	Portuguese voyages begin the Age of Discovery
1492	"Discovery" and permanent occupation of the New World by Europeans begins; Muslims are finally expelled from Spain
1493	First Old World epidemic breaks out in the Caribbean; exact disease is unknown
1493	Syphilis epidemic in Europe gives rise to the Columbian theory that the disease was imported from the New World, the only infectious disease to have done so; this theory has been widely disputed
1498	Portuguese reach India, the first European contact by sea
1503	Sailors on Columbus's fourth voyage probably introduce malaria to the New World
1520	Smallpox arrives in Mexico with the Spanish, causing catastrophic mortality
1521	Hernán Cortés defeats the Aztec Empire, beginning the destruction of Aztec learning and culture and establishing Spanish hegemony in Mexico and Central America
1524	Cortés builds the first hospital in Mexico City
1532	Francisco Pizarro conquers the Incan Empire, aided by the smallpox epidemic that preceded his arrival
1542	By this date, Amerindians are virtually extinct in the Caribbean
1614	Less than one hundred years after first contact with Europeans, the population of Central Mexico has decreased from twenty-three million to about two million, primarily as a result of the introduction of Old World diseases

⋏

The Canon on Medicine

Ibn Sina

The Canon on Medicine, *written about 1010 by the great Islamic physician-scholar Ibn Sina, is one of the most famous and influential textbooks on medicine throughout history. Written in Arabic, it was translated into Latin in the twelfth century and immediately became a standard reference in European schools of medicine. The Canon is divided into five sections: general principles, simple drugs and remedies, diseases of specific organs, diseases that affect the entire body, and compound medicines. It clearly demonstrates the influence of Greek medicine; Ibn Sina's theories are solidly founded on Hippocratic humoral theory and reflect considerable reading and research on his part.*

For the physician of his day, few diagnostic tests were available to aid in identification of specific diseases. Ibn Sina stated that symptoms denote the location and cause of the disease, and that the physician must use all his senses to observe symptomology. The best example of Ibn Sina's thinking is his lengthy analysis of urine, a practice known as uroscopy.

Uroscopy was extremely popular among medieval European physicians, and the specially marked flask was as symbolic of medical practice then as the stethoscope is now. As this reading shows, a physician was supposed to examine the urine with regard to color, clarity, density, and sediment, and, on the basis of his findings, he could pinpoint both cause and location of the presenting malady.

⋏

Urinoscopy

The Urine

Precautions Necessary in Collecting the Urine, Before Forming an Opinion as to Its Character

It must be collected in the early morning; it must not have been kept over from the night before.

The person must not have taken either food or drink before passing it.

The previous food must have been free from colouring agents like crocus and cassia fistula (these render the urine lemon yellow or ruddy), and from potherbs (which make the urine a greenish tint), and from salted fish (which renders the urine dark), and from intoxicating wines (which tend to render the colour of the urine similar to themselves).

The patient should not have been given an agent which expels some humour . . . by the urine.

Physiological state. The patient should not have undertaken severe exercise or toil, or be in a praeternatural mental state; for in each case the colour of the urine may alter. . . .

The whole of the urine should be collected into one single vessel lest anything should be spilt out of it; one should allow it to settle before scrutinizing it. . . .

The vessel used for the specimen must be clean, and the previous sample must have been rinsed out of it.

The material of which the vessel is made should be clear white glass or crystal.

Reprinted by permission of Augustus M. Kelley Publishers, from O. Cameron Gruner, trans., *A Treatise on the Canon on Medicine of Avicenna* (New York: Augustus M. Kelley, 1970), 323–27, 331–33, 336–39, 341–48.

The urine must not be exposed to the sun or wind or freezing cold, until the sediment has separated out and the various characters have properly developed. . . .

The sample must be inspected in a light place where the rays do not fall directly upon it, as otherwise the brilliant light would interfere with the colours and give rise to erroneous deductions.

The nearer one holds the sample to the eye, the denser does it appear. The further away it is, the clearer does it seem. In this way one can distinguish urine from other fluids brought to the doctor in a falsified state. . . .

The first and foremost object of observing the urine is to form an opinion about the state of the liver, the urinary passages and the blood-vessels. The various disorders of these organs are revealed by it. But the most precise information to be obtained is that concerning the functional capacity of the liver.

. . . The following are the points to observe in a sample of urine:

quantity

odour

colour

foam

texture

clearness

sediment

. . . By *colour* we understand the various shades of colour perceived by the sense of sight—whiteness, darkness, intermediate shades.

By *texture* we refer to the coarseness or fineness.

By *clearness* or turbidity we refer to the ease or otherwise with which light traverses it. . . .

There is a difference between texture and translucence, for a urine may be coarse and yet as clear as egg-white or liquid fish-glue; and a rarefied urine may be turbid. . . .

Turbidity depends on the presence of certain variously coloured particles—opaque or dark, or tinted with other colours which are imperceptible to the sense of sight and yet are impervious. . . .

The Significance of the Colour of the Urine

The Degrees of Yellowness. Among the shades of yellow colour are: (1) straw-yellow; (2) lemon-yellow; (3) orange-yellow; (4) flame-yellow, or saffron-yellow; that is, a very deep yellow; (5) clear reddish-yellow. All except the first two denote a hot intemperament, in degrees varying with the amount of exercise, pain, fasting, and abstinence from water. The fourth variety denotes predominance of the bilious humour.

The Degrees of Redness. (1) Rose-red or roseate; (2) very dark red; (3) purple red, which has a brilliance about it like a certain rose; (4) smoky red or dull red. All these denote dominance of the sanguineous humour, for dullness of colour points that way. A flame-yellow shows the presence of more "heat" than dull red because it shows there is bilious humour in it, and this is hotter than sanguineous humour. . . .

The Degrees of Green Colour. (1) A colour approaching that of pistachios; (2) the colour of verdigris; (3) rainbow green; (4) emerald green; (5) leek-green. The first denotes a cold intemperament, as do all things the shade of whose green is not (2) or (5). These (2, 5) denote extreme combustion, but (5) is not as unhealthy as (2). If it should be met with after physical labour it denotes "spasm." A green-coloured urine in adolescence points to the same condition. . . .

The Degrees of Blackness. (1) Dark urine approaching blackness, through a saffron colour. This occurs in jaundice, for instance. It denotes (*a*) denseness and oxidation of the bilious humour; (*b*) **atrabilious** humour derived from bilious humour; (*c*) jaundice. (2) Deep-brown-black. This shows the presence of sanguineous atrabilious humour. (3) Greenish-black. This shows the dominance of pure atrabilious humour. . . .

The Compound Colours of the Urine *Like raw meat washings* (i.e. blood-stained water). This means hepatic insufficiency due to plethora of blood or to any form of intemperament, resulting in deficient digestive power and dispersal of the vitality. Were the vital power adequate, it would show that there is plenty of blood, even to great excess; and in such a case, the secretory power would be hardly adequate for dealing with it.

Oleaginous. Oily. The fat of the body is being destroyed. The appearance is like a lemon-yellow tinged with the greenness of the mistletoe growing on larches. It is called oleaginous because it is viscid and translucent, and also has the lustre of fat, and shows a certain brilliance or refulgence in spite of a certain opacity. It is not a good sign in many states, not to say it is bad. For it shows there is neither maturation, nor a change for the better. In rare cases it indicates the critical evacuation of unctuous matter, but for it to mean this, alleviation must follow. . . .

Purple (-black). This is a very bad sign. It means oxidation of both bilious and atrabilious humour.

Ruddy colour admixed with a tinge of blackness. This occurs in composite fevers and in fevers arising from gross superfluities. If it clarifies, and the darkness settles down from the surface, it denotes an inflammatory mass in the lung.

The Signs Afforded by the Density, Quality, Clearness or Turbidity of the Urine

Urine may be transparent or opaque, or intermediate in density.

Transparent (Limpid) Urine Whatever be the state, a urine of limpid consistence denotes: (*a*) deficient digestion (lack of maturation); (*b*) venous congestion; (*c*) renal insufficiency (for the kidneys only separate out fine matter, or if they attract other matter, they fail to discharge it until it has been rarefied or rendered capable of excretion); (*d*) excessive fluid-intake; (*e*) a very cold or a dry intemperament.

When it occurs in the course of an acute illness, it denotes deficient digestive power, and inability to complete digestion (absence of maturation: cf. above). It may indicate that the weakness

of the other faculties is so marked that they cannot influence water at all, and hence it passes through the body unchanged.

Prognosis. It is worse for urine to be very transparent at puberty than in adolescence, because during the former period of life urine is naturally more opaque than in adolescence. Being more moist in their temperament, their bodies attract moisture more readily, and, in addition, moisture is essential for their growth. Hence, if acute fevers arise during the age of puberty, the urine is decidedly abnormal if it is transparent; and, should it continue of that character, it would be a very ominous sign. Should it continue and favourable symptoms should not appear, and should the vitality not be maintained, it would be a sign that an abscess is forming below the liver. . . .

Opaque (Thick) Urine If the urine is very opaque, it shows that maturation has failed to take place; or, more rarely, it denotes the maturation of "gross" humours, such as occur at the height (status) of humoral fevers, or after the opening of abscesses. In acute fevers, the appearance of opaque urine is usually a bad sign, though not as bad as a persistently transparent urine. The fact that urine is opaque shows that there is a certain degree of digestion proceeding, because digestion adds to the opacity of urine to a certain extent, and shows that there is some power of expulsion (of effete matter). But it is a bad sign in so far as it denotes the breakdown of, and abundance of, humours, and that the evacuation of the separated materials is hindered. . . .

Good signs Opaque urine easily voided, whose sediment falls easily: when occurring in palsy, etc. . . .

Limpid plentiful urine following upon thick turbid urine or thick and scanty urine. . . .

Diagnostic points. Opaque urine, with a sandy sediment, denotes **calculus**. Opaque urine, with pus, a bad odour, and scaly particles separating out, denotes rupture of an abscess. A thick urine, with the clinical evidences of an inflammatory mass or of an ulcer in the bladder, kidney, liver or chest, shows that there is an abscess about to burst.

If the urine prior to that were like the washings of raw meat, it would show that there is unhealthy blood flowing from the liver; and if the faeces were also similar, it would show there is an inflammatory mass in the interior of the liver. If prior to this there was shortness of breath, with a dry cough, and a stabbing pain in the chest, then one knows that an abscess has ruptured which arose in the chest or (round the) aorta. If the pus is "mature," it is satisfactory.

Discharge of urine resembling pus may benefit a person who takes no exercise and lives in an unhygienic manner. . . . Such "matter" is not "pus." It is only pus if it appears in the urine after the bursting of an abscess; the urine is then not only thick but dark. . . .

Turbid urine of the appearance of poor wine, or of chick-pea-water, may occur during pregnancy, and may be met with in persons with long-standing internal "hot" inflammatory masses. . . .

If the urine resembles the colour of some member for some time, it forewarns that disease is about to arise there. . . .

The Signs Derived from the Odour of the Urine

Fetid Odour. A fetid odour, with signs of maturation in the urine indicates ulcers in the urinary passages, or "scabies." . . .

Such a urine, in acute fevers, without disease in the urinary organs, is a bad sign. . . .

If such a urine appears in acute diseases, it forewarns of death by extinction of the innate heat and predominance of the extraneous cold.

Sweetish Odour. This denotes predominance of the sanguineous humour. If also very fetid, a predominance of the bilious humour. . . .

The Indications Afforded by the Foam on Urine

Foam arises from the moisture and the gases forced into the urine as it is passed into the urinal. The vapour which leaves the body with the urine doubtless adds to the consistence of the urine, especially if gases predominate in it, as occurs in cases of obstructions. The urine then shows many bubbles.

One notices the following points in regard to the foam:

Colour: it is dark or reddish in jaundice.

Size of bubbles: large ones indicate viscidity.

Number of bubbles: if numerous it denotes viscidity and much gas.

Rate of bursting of the bubbles: if slow, it indicates viscidity, and coarse glutinous humour.

Prognosis. Hence if small bubbles persist in a specimen, in cases of kidney disease, it shows that the illness will be of long duration. . . .

The Indications Derived from the Divers Kinds of Sediment

. . . In the first place one must specify the meaning of the term "sediment." It is not "that which sinks to the bottom of the vessel." It is "that whole substance (denser in essence than wateriness) which separates out from the wateriness—regardless of whether it settles down or not, floats or not, sinks or not."

Therefore we may say that there are various characters pertaining to the sediment—its "structure," its quantity and quality, the arrangement of its components, its position, duration, and mode of permixture.

. . . A sediment is natural, laudable, evidence of normal digestion and maturation, when it is white, sinks to the bottom of the vessel, when its particles are in continuity . . . , uniform, and all alike. In contour it is rounded. It is light, homogeneous, delicate, like the deposit which forms in rosewater. . . .

Abnormal Sediments *Flaky or squamous.* This is composed of large red or large white particles. . . . They suggest the shedding of mucous linings. Particles from the bladder or kidneys may not be of moment; in fact, if **vesical** they are a sign of recovery. . . .

Another form resembles the scrapings from intestines; . . . this indicates the presence of oxidized particles which are derived from (*a*) the liver, (*b*) the kidney, or (*c*) blood. . . .

Another form, more strictly scaly, consists of small bodies like the husks or hulls of grain. Such a sediment denotes (i) bladder trouble, or (ii) grave colliquative disorder of the system as a whole. . . .

Fleshy sediments. These, as you already know, are usually of renal origin. They are not so if the flesh is healthy and there is no breakdown in the body. . . .

Fatty sediment. This, like the preceding, denotes colliquative processes in the body. It is more serious if it resembles "gold water" in appearance. . . .

Mucoid sediment. This denotes an unnatural humour, which is too plentiful within the body and passes out either by the urinary tract, or a critical hip-gout, or joint pains. . . .

Ichorous sediment. This differs from a crude sediment in being fetid. It is preceded by the evidences of abscess. . . .

Hair-like sediment. This is produced by the coagulation of any internal humour, which has been exposed to the innate heat on its way from the kidney to the bladder. . . .

A sediment having the *appearance of yeast soaked in water,* is evidence of gastric and intestinal weakness and of depraved digestion (often due to milk and cheese having been taken).

Sandy or gritty sediment ("Gravel"). This is always a sign of calculus whether in process of formation or actually formed, or in process of solution. . . .

Cineritial sediment. This is a sign that serous humour or pus has altered in colour through long stagnation and breaking up of its particles. . . .

Hirudiniform. The sediment is of the (appearance and) colour of leeches. If well mingled with the urine, this denotes hepatic insufficiency. If less closely intermingled with the urine, it denotes a trauma in the urinary passages which breaks their continuity. . . .

The appearance of bodies like red leeches in the urine, associated with evidences of disease in the spleen, denotes a destructive disease in that organ. . . .

Position A laudable sediment may swim like a cloud or nubecula; may float on the surface; or be suspended in the middle layers. . . .

Time Occupied in Sedimentation If the sediment settles rapidly, it is a good sign, showing that maturation is correct. If it settles slowly, it is not good, for it shows deficient or absent maturation, according to its amount. . . .

Signs Relative to the Daily Quantity of Urine

Generally speaking, **oliguria** means weakness of vitality. If the amount is less than the fluid consumed, it points to great loss by diarrhoea or to a tendency to dropsy. . . .

Variation of quantity. It is a bad sign if the urine is at one time abundant, at another scanty, at another suppressed. It shows that there is a hard conflict between the vitality and the disease. A plentiful urine in an acute illness, occurring without any abatement of symptoms, and associated with copious sweats, shows hectic fever and may be followed by convulsions. . . .

A scanty urine, passed involuntarily, drop-by-drop in acute diseases, indicates cerebral disease, affecting nerves and muscles.

If a fever subside and there are other signs of recovery, one may predict **epistaxis.** Otherwise delirium will ensue and death is likely. . . .

Variations According to Age

Infancy. The urine tends to the characters of milk, considering the food and their moist temperament. Hence it is nearly colourless.

Childhood. The urine is thicker and coarser than in adolescents, and more turbid. This has already been mentioned.

Adolescence. The urine tends to **igneity,** and homogeneity.

Later life. The urine tends to be white and tenuous, but it may be coarse ("thick") because of the effete matters which are now being evacuated to a greater extent by way of the urine.

Decrepit age. The urine is whiter and still more tenuous. A similar coarseness to that of the preceding may occur, but this is rare. If the urine becomes very thick, it intimates liability to develop calculus.

Variations According to Sex

Women. The urine is always thicker, whiter and less pellucid than in males. The reason is fourfold: In women there is feebleness of digestion; abundance of effete matters; width of **emunctory** channels; material discharged by way of the uterus, which draws similar material down the urinary passages also.

Men. When the urine is shaken, it becomes turbid and the turbidity ascends to the surface,

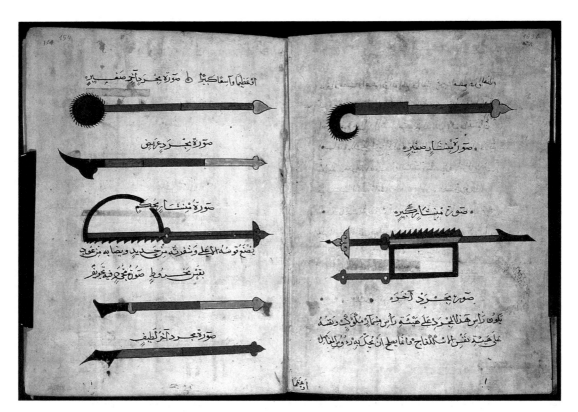

FIGURE 7–1 Albucasis's Surgical Instruments
In addition to contributing the work of such men as Ibn Sina and preserving the ancient writings, the Muslim physician–philosophers devised a number of surgical advances. The most influential surgeon, Al-Zahrawi of Cordoba (Latinized to *Albucasis*) wrote the first detailed illustrated surgical text, some fifteen hundred pages long and completed about 1000 c.e. In this treatise, titled *Al-Tasrif (On Surgery),* he wrote about a number of new developments, including the use of cautery, as well as new surgical and orthopedic procedures and the use of various new instruments. This book became the single most important surgical text in European medical schools until the Renaissance.

though occasionally it remains throughout the whole bulk of the urine. When the urine in women is shaken, it does not become turbid because the particles are barely discrete, and there is usually a circular foam on top. Even if such urine becomes turbid, it does so only to a light extent.

If male and female urine be mingled, a filamentous network forms at once. (Filaments also appear in male urine if passed immediately after intercourse.) . . .

The Urine of Animals and Its Difference from Human Urine

It is often desirable for a doctor to know some thing about the urine of animals, so that when he is tricked by a patient, he can quickly and truly discern it, difficult though it be to do so. . . .

Dentistry in the Bible, Talmud and Writings of Moses Maimonides

FRED ROSNER, M.D., F.A.C.P.

Care of the teeth was minimal throughout early history. Teeth wore down quickly because of sand and gravel in grain, abscesses were common, and the only certain way to stop a toothache was to pull the offending tooth. Bad breath was nearly universal, and dental floss and the toothbrush were virtually unknown.

The great Jewish physician Maimónides served the Sultan and wrote several important medical texts, the most famous of which was his Medical Aphorisms. *The twenty-five chapters of this work focus on medical subspecialties, including dentistry, and his comments reflect both the religiophilosophical authority of the Bible and the Talmud and the popular remedies available for toothache. Thus, as is evident in this selection, vinegar was a good remedy for toothache, but it could not be used as a remedy on the Sabbath; however, if it was simply used in the food eaten on that day, and the toothache stopped, the sufferer had not violated the Sabbath.*

The medieval giant of Judaism, Moses ben Maimon (1138–1204), known to the world as Maimonides was a rabbi, physician, philosopher, astronomer and codifier of Jewish law. His best known works are his philosophical masterpiece, the *Guide of the Perplexed,* and his Code of Jewish Law known as *Mishneh Torah.* The latter is a monumental compilation of all biblical and talmudic law and remains a classic to this day. His *Guide of the Perplexed* is one of the most influential philosophical works of any time and is full of original thinking in law, theology and ethics.

Maimonides also wrote a variety of other books, essays, treatises, and commentaries as well as a voluminous correspondence. Some of his ten authentic medical works are cited later in this article as they pertain to dentistry. His works cover a gamut of disciplines including theology, mathematics, law, philosophy, astronomy, ethics and medicine. His contributions to these fields

Reprinted by permission of the American Academy of the History of Dentistry (www.histden.org), from Fred Rosner, "Dentistry in the Bible, Talmud and Writings of Moses Maimonides," *Bulletin of the History of Dentistry* 42, no. 3 (1994): 109–112.

have been described in innumerable books and essays.

Among the many things about which Maimonides wrote is the subject of dentistry with a variety of references to the teeth. These are part of the subject of this essay.

The *Regimen of Health* is one of the most renowned of Maimonides' medical writings. It was written in response to a letter requesting medical advice from Al-Malik Al-Afdhal, eldest son of Saladin the Great of Egypt. The Sultan was a frivolous and pleasure-seeking man of thirty, subject to fits of melancholy or depression due to his excessive indulgences in wine and women, and his warlike adventures against his own relatives and in the Crusades. He complained to his physician of constipation, dejection, bad thoughts and indigestion. Maimonides answered his royal patient in four chapters. The first chapter is a brief abstract on diet taken mostly from Hippocrates and Galen. The second chapter gives advice on hygiene, diet and drugs in the absence of a physician. The third extremely important chapter contains Maimonides' concept of "a healthy mind in a healthy body," perhaps an early description of psychosomatic medicine. He indicates that the physical well being of a person is dependent on his mental well being and vice versa. The final chapter summarizes his prescriptions relating to climate, domicile, occupation, bathing, sex, wine, drinking, diet and respiratory infections. The *Regimen of Health* was originally written in Arabic and several Arabic manuscripts are extant. . . .

This . . . essay presents a review of dentistry as found in the Bible and Talmud as well as a description of vignettes and authentic statements about dentistry in the medical and rabbinic writings of Maimonides.

Dentistry in the Bible and the Talmud

. . . The prophet Jeremiah laments that G-d broke his teeth with gravel stones. Homiletically, a broken tooth is said to be "like confidence in an unfaithful man in time of trouble." Esau wept at his encounter with Jacob because his teeth were loose and painful. A priest lacking teeth is not fit for temple service because of his unsightly appearance.

Vinegar is harmful to the teeth, as is smoke to the eyes. Vinegar loosens healthy teeth but heals a toothache or gum wound. On the other hand, sour fruit juice is efficacious for toothache and does not harm healthy teeth. In case of need, one may even use vinegar produced during the Sabbatical yean when fields must lie fallow; such fruits are otherwise only permitted "for nourishment." Vapors of a bathhouse are also harmful to the teeth. Prolonged fasting causes the teeth to become black.

Rabbi Judah, the Prince, was liberated from a severe toothache by the Prophet Elijah touching his tooth. A special remedy for the teeth is to place a garlic root ground with oil and salt on the side where the tooth aches. A rim of dough should be placed around the tooth taking care that the medication not touch the flesh, as it may cause leprosy.

Tooth extraction in antiquity was a serious operation. Rab told his son not to have a tooth extracted. The Talmudic commentator there explains that if one extracts a molar tooth, one's eyesight may be affected. Great emphasis was placed on beautiful teeth. A person who whitens his neighbor's teeth is better than one who gives him milk to drink. Lovers extol one another by saying that their teeth are like a flock of sheep which came up from the washing. Jacob promised his son Judah "teeth whiter than milk."

Spleen is considered in the Talmud to be good for the teeth whereas leek is considered harmful. However, the spleen should be chewed and spit out because if it is swallowed, it harms digestion. Sour grapes set teeth on edge.

Artificial teeth of silver and gold are described in the Talmud as is a wonder toothpick. A reed should not be used for this purpose because it may injure the gums. A gold tooth prepared for a young maiden rendered her beautiful so she was able to be married. Artificial teeth were prepared by craftsmen. Wood chips or toothpicks were constantly carried between the teeth, perhaps to achieve proper alignment of misaligned teeth. The expression "take the chip out from between your teeth" was often followed by the retort "take the beam out from your eyes."

The teeth also play an important and specific role in the Jewish legal sphere. The phrase, "an eye for an eye, and a tooth for a tooth" is not interpreted literally in Jewish law. Rather it refers to financial compensation to which the injured party is entitled. The Code of Hammurabi, however, interprets the "tooth for a tooth" literally so that a man who knocks out the teeth of another man must have his teeth knocked out. Not so in Jewish law which rules that if someone knocks out the tooth of his servant, the servant is given his freedom as a substitute for the tooth. This rule applies even if the tooth is already loose but still usable, and also if the tooth was only loosened but became unusable as a result of the blow by the master. Even a physician who drills his servant's tooth and causes it to fall out must give his servant his freedom.

Various remedies are cited for scurvy of the gums. This ailment is defined as bleeding from the gums if one places anything between the teeth. The cause of this illness is said to be the chill of cold wheat-food and the heat of hot barley-food, as well as the remnant of fish hash and flour. The remedies are leaven water with olive oil and salt or goose fat smeared with a goose quill or ashes from burned unripe seeds of an olive.

Dentistry in the Writings of Moses Maimonides

The most voluminous of Maimonides' ten authentic medical treatises is his *Medical Aphorisms of Moses* which is comprised of twenty-five chapters, each dealing with a subspecialty of medicine. Most of the approximately 1500 aphorisms in this work are based on the writings of Galen including the latter's commentaries on the works of Hippocrates. In the first chapter, quoting Galen, Maimonides states that nerves do not insert into the cartilage, ligament or adipose tissue of bone except in one organ, the penis. Teeth are the ex-

ception among bones because fine nerves are found in their roots.

In the seventh chapter, again quoting Galen, Maimonides states:

> The reason which necessitates the tranquilization of pain following extraction of a painful tooth is that the nerve which attaches to the root of the painful tooth heals through the severance of this connection and attachment to the bone through which thus stretching was originally produced. Thus, place is formed therein through which dissolved liquids which have gathered there can exit. The cause for breaking of teeth and their corrosion lies in their softening. Therefore, it is important to harden them and strengthen them with astringent medications. The same is true for changes in their appearance to yellow and the like which occurs due to bad liquids which descend to them. Heal them with remedies which produce an intermediate degree of dryness and [believe] not, as some physicians think, that the more powerful the drying agent, the more beneficial it is [to the teeth].

In the ninth chapter of his *Medical Aphorisms* Maimonides points out that a warm cataplasm or compress applied on the teeth either externally or directly inside the mouth should be applied before meals on an empty stomach or after a long period following a meal.

In his *Treatise on Poisons and their Antidotes* Maimonides discusses the treatment of someone bitten by a poisonous snake or other animal. He recommends that one immediately tie a ligature above the site of the bite to prevent the poison from spreading throughout the body. An incision should be made at the site of the bite and the wound sucked. The person sucking on the wound should spit out all that he sucks. He should first rinse his mouth with olive oil or wine and oil. He should not have any oral illness nor any decayed teeth.

In the Arabic version of his *Regimen of Health* . . . Maimonides cites the following remedy for toothache and tooth extraction.

> The remedy is that the sufferer should take two grains of mountain raisins and wrap them in cotton

wool and wet them in water and crush them between two stones and apply to the affected tooth for it will soothe the pain locally; or take one *qirat* [1/16 of a drachm] of *Colotropis procera* and wrap it in cotton wool and apply to the tooth for it alleviates pain. He [the sufferer] may also use alkali, tar, cautery or betel leaves and others. For tooth extraction without using steel [instruments] take pyrethra and leave it [immersed] in vinegar for a month until it becomes soft as dough; then apply it to the [affected] tooth which should be removed instantly; or take the root of the mulberry, let it solidify in the sun in a glass and apply it to the tooth which will drop out immediately.

Another remedy for the teeth is the following:

Take one ounce of *kabuli* [myrobolan of Kabul] and an ounce of *Phyllanthus embelica,* and half an ounce each of cinnamon bark and coriander, two drachms of Indian nard and one drachm of mastic. Each is pounded alone and then the whole is crushed together and rubbed against the teeth, then rinse in the bath.

In his famous compilation of all Biblical and Talmudic law known as *Mishneh Torah,* Maimonides describes therapeutic and hygienic rules on the Sabbath. He rules that

If one has a toothache, he may take sips of vinegar, but may not spit it out—he must swallow it. If one has a sore throat, he may not gargle with oil, but may drink it in large quantities, and if this cures his soreness it does not matter. One may not chew mastic or rub his teeth, with a medicament on the Sabbath if his purpose is medicinal, but if the intention is to remove mouth odors he may do so.

Maimonides is alluding to the Talmudic discussion about the efficacy of vinegar for a toothache. One should not sip vinegar or rinse one's teeth with it on the Sabbath since healing, except in the case of danger, is ordinarily prohibited, lest he crush the ingredients on the Sabbath. One may, however, dip one's food in vinegar and eat it in the usual manner, and if the toothache is cured, he has not broken the law.

Also in the laws pertaining to the Sabbath, Maimonides rules that a woman may not go out on the Sabbath into a public domain wearing:

an artificial tooth worn in the mouth to replace a missing tooth, or a gold tooth worn over one of her own teeth that has turned black or red. A silver tooth, however, is permissible, because it is not noticeable. The reason she is forbidden to go out wearing any of these articles is that it might fall off and she would then be tempted to carry it home in her hand, or else she might take it off to show it to her friends.

Maimonides bases his ruling on the Talmudic discussion as to whether or not a woman is allowed to go out on the Sabbath with an artificial or gold tooth. Rabbi Judah, the Prince, permits it but the Sages forbid it. Rabbi Zera states that this prohibition only applies to a gold tooth but that all Rabbis agree that a silver tooth is permitted. The Talmudic commentator, *Rashi,* explains that a gold tooth, being valuable, is likely to be removed by a woman from her mouth and displayed to her friends. Meanwhile, she may carry it on the street, an act forbidden on the Sabbath. Maimonides explains the permissive ruling of Rabbi Judah, the Prince, in that the gold tooth is covering one of the woman's own diseased teeth; therefore, she will not take it out to show to her friends because that would uncover her blemish.

Summary and Conclusion

The art of dentistry in ancient times was closely related to that of its mother science, medicine. Ancient and medieval Jewish sources such as the Bible and Talmud are replete with references to both dentistry and medicine. Those relating to dentistry are briefly reviewed in this essay.

The greatest Jewish scholar of the Middle Ages was twelfth century Moses Maimonides. A few limited references to dentistry are found in his medical and rabbinic writings. Maimonides is an important figure in the history of dentistry primarily as part of his stature and renown as a physician. His medical legacy is found in his ten medical treatises.

⋀

Insanity and Its Treatment in Islamic Society

Michael W. Dols

In the history of the Christian world, care of individuals who were mentally ill was regarded on an entirely different level from that for the care of persons who were physically ill. With the philosophical and religious linkage of insanity and sin, medieval Christians regarded mental illness as the "fault" of the patient-sinner. In the Islamic world, however, such a linkage did not exist, which meant care was generally much more benevolent than that in the Christian West. Most patients were kept at home under family care, but institutions were available for persons who presented a danger to themselves or others. Physical restraints were used, but so were medications, baths, and diets, all designed to lessen symptoms and make the patient both comfortable and manageable. In general, the patient with mental illness was treated with care and gentleness in an Islamic hospital.

⋀

A description of the actual treatment of the insane in medieval Islamic society is a difficult task for three major reasons. First, the medical texts, especially the well-known treatise on insanity by Isḥāq ibn 'Imrān, give descriptions of various mental disturbances and their therapies; these accounts are, however, usually restricted to the Galenic tradition, are generally nonclinical, and do not emphasize psychoses or florid conditions. Like Islamic law, these accounts are prescriptive rather than descriptive, so that any historical survey of the medical treatment of the insane can rely on them only as supportive evidence or as the rationale for the practice of professional physicians. Second, historical descriptions of disturbed men and women are rare, and one must resort to a wide variety of sources, such as *adab* (belles-lettres), biographical dictionaries, geographers' and travellers' accounts. These depictions of unusual behaviour are, in fact, evaluative. Thus, the third issue is the serious methodological problem of what is meant by

"insanity" or "mental illness". For convenience, insanity may be defined as any behaviour that is judged to be abnormal or extraordinary by a social group at a specific time and place. Within the wide spectrum of human behaviour, members of any society set boundaries to what they believe to be acceptable or permissible. This judgement or consensus depends on the degree to which an individual's behaviour is disturbed as well as on the attitudes of his or her social group toward those actions. Mental illness is, then, more intimately dependent on social attitudes and beliefs than physical illness, and this social context largely determines the care and treatment of the insane. . . .

The development of the early Islamic hospital had coincided with the massive translation of early, primarily Greek, scientific works into Arabic. The translators as well as their translations surely reinforced an orientation to Galenic medicine that was practised by Christian and Jewish doctors in the Hellenistic Near East. Both the hospital and the translations were the direct result of princely patronage that allowed these projects to be carried out on a grand scale. It also allowed medicine to develop as a discipline largely beyond religious constraints. Compared to the transference of Greek scientific knowledge to Rome in antiquity, there appears to have been a conscious effort by the ʿAbbāsid élite to promote medicine especially, making it accessible to Arabic-speaking practitioners and patients. Thus, an adherence to Galenic principles became the criteria for professional medical status in Islamic society and was closely associated with training in the hospital.

Galenic medicine emphasized the physical causation of illness. Insanity was a disturbance or dysfunction of the brain, which controlled mental activity and emotions. The functioning of the brain, and the body in general, depended upon the proper mixture of the humours and their qualities, so that the treatment of any illness was aimed at the restoration of the balance of these humours. It may be said that this somatic approach created the concept of "mental illness". The physiological approach was further developed in late antiquity and was directly inherited by Islamic doctors. For example, even passionate love, *ʿishq,* was commonly considered by Islamic physicians as a mundane illness. Whereas madness was interpreted in various ways in antiquity, for Galen, it was an illness like all other illnesses; logically, madness should come to be treatable, like all other illnesses, in the hospital. . . .

[A] glimpse of the mental patients in the hospital through the eyes of a prominent doctor leads to the question of the *actual* treatment of the mentally ill in the medieval period. Most conspicuous in the historical accounts, as in that of Ibn Jubayr, is the frequent mention of the various forms of restraint that were placed on the violently insane. Good evidence of the institutional care of the insane is furnished by Leo Africanus (AD 1465–*c.* 1550), who was secretary at the hospital for the insane in Fez for two years. He said that the insane were bound in strong iron chains in the hospital. The walls of their rooms were

strengthened with heavy beams of wood and iron. The person who was in charge of feeding them constantly carried a whip, and when he saw an agitated patient, he administered a good thrashing. Sometimes strangers approached these chambers. The insane called out to them and complained how unjustly they were detained and how cruelly they were handled everyday by the officers, although they were cured of their insanity. Having persuaded the passersby to come closer, the insane would greatly abuse them. Despite the unpleasantness of these conditions of confinement, the asylums were obviously accessible to visitors . . . , and the conditions of the insane appear to have been accepted in the same matter-of-fact way as other disabilities. The asylum is almost a commonplace theme in Arabic literature; for example, a highly entertaining tale in *The thousand and one nights* is about Abūl-Hasan the Eccentric, who was deceived by Hārūn ar-Rashīd into believing that he was the caliph.

The harsh conditions of the asylum should not be misconstrued. The general understanding and treatment of insanity in the Islamic hospital do not fit Michel Foucault's harrowing interpretation of the development of the hospital in seventeenth- and eighteenth-century Europe. The chains and irons in the Islamic hospital were simply necessary devices to prevent harm to the insane or to others; it was not a "great confinement". Despite the apparent cruelty, one can take a benign view. For example, the foreign traveller Jean de Thévenot, who visited Cairo in the mid-seventeenth century, described the Mansūrī Hospital in the following way: "The Hospital and Mosque of Mad People is very near Han Khalil; [the insane] are chained with heavy iron chains, and [they] are led to the Mosque at prayer time. . . . The Hospital is called *Morestan,* and it serves also the sick Poor, who are well entertained and look'd after in it."

Judging by the medieval medical texts, the doctors apparently paid close attention to the patient's regimen; the "**non-naturals**", especially exercise, a restful environment, and ample sleep, should be studied and adjusted, so that the patient's daily life would be conducive to recovery.

Treatment included baths, fomentations (particularly to the head), compresses, bandaging, and massage with various oils. Bloodletting, leeches, cupping, and cautery also appear to have been used. Medication with both simple and compound drugs, usually of vegetable origin, as well as **theriacs,** were given to the mentally ill in every possible form. The drugs included purgatives, emetics, digestives, and sedatives, especially opium. An emphasis on drug therapy may be attributed to Rufus of Ephesus because of his significant influence in this area of Islamic medicine.

The purpose of the diets, baths, and medicines was generally, as Ibn Sīnā said, to increase the moisture of the body in opposition to the presumed drying effect of the black bile. Cold and moist foods were also advised by Isḥāq ibn 'Imrān as a corrective to the burnt yellow bile, the major cause of mania; whey, particularly, was highly recommended on the authority of Galen. The purpose of the bloodletting and purgatives was to evacuate the damaging black bile. And the drugs were obviously intended to calm the excited, stimulate the apathetic, and comfort the depressed.

Ibn Abī Uṣaybi'ah described such drug therapy at the Nūr ad-Dīn Hospital in Damascus: "In the hall [. . .] of the fools [. . .] Muhadhdhab ad-Dīn prescribed for a man who had been stricken by the illness called *māniyā,* that is the bestial madness . . . , an ample amount of opium to be added to the barley water at the time he was given to drink. The man improved and the condition disappeared." . . .

The medical texts also attest to psychotherapeutic techniques that may have been employed. There is clearly a concern in the texts for the personal, educative role of the physician. The psychic healing of the patient's condition can be traced back to antiquity, and anecdotal accounts of the wise physician are often repeated in Islamic garb. In general, however, ancient medicine did not develop a concept of the healing power of words or dialogue. From late antiquity, however, there seems to have developed a "therapy of the word" or a greater belief in the psychogenic causation of mental illness. Professor Bürgel has even suggested that the use of shock or shame therapy, specifically, may have originated with Islamic doctors. In any case, these medieval doctors were apparently sensitive to the psychosomatic aspect of illness, especially some forms of mental disturbance. The treatise of Ibn Bakhtīshū' is a fine expression of this sensitivity. We also get hints of such treatment in the general medical texts. For example, ar-Rāzī sensibly urged the practising doctor to destroy a melancholic's obsession with trifling concerns and to reassure the depressive of his reasonable thoughts.

Following the classical medical texts, especially Rufus of Ephesus, other psychic means of healing were recommended. Music was used in the Islamic hospitals down to Ottoman times. Musical performances were given, for example, at the Mansūrī Hospital in Cairo during the medieval period. Evilyā Çelebi visited the Nūr ad-Dīn Hospital in AD 1648, and he reported that concerts were given three times a day. He also noticed that the treatments of the insane were recorded by the chief physician.

From various sources it appears that other forms of diversion were also employed, such as dancing, theatrical performances, and recitations. Furthermore, Benoit de Maillet, a seventeenth-century Frenchman, recorded that, although most of these features had disappeared at the Mansūrī Hospital in his time, there still existed the custom of announcing the first prayer of the day two hours earlier than in the other mosques of the city for the benefit of the insomniacs.

There was, moreover, a keen attention to surroundings that would improve the patient's frame of mind. The hospitals, despite the cells for the insane, were usually spacious, monumental structures with fountains and gardens. Remarkable evidence of this aspect of the Islamic asylums is found in Evilyā Çelebi's description of the mental hospital that was founded in Edirne (Adrianople) by Bayezid II (AD 1481–1512). To the right of the Bayezid Mosque was an insane asylum, as well as a medical school; in a beautiful garden. The asylum was a massive domed structure; the winter rooms looked out on to the rose garden and inward to the fountain and pool.

Some rooms are heated in the winter according to the nature of the sick; they lay in beds provided with ample blankets and rest themselves on silk pillows, and moan and groan. In the spring, at the time of madness, those from the city who are lovesick and melancholy are put into some of the rooms. Those brought to the asylum by the police are restrained and fettered by gilded and silver chains around their necks. Each one roars and sleeps like a lion in his lair. Some fix their eyes on the pool and fountain and repeat words like a begging derwish. And some doze in the rose garden, grape orchards and fruit orchards . . . and sing with the unmelodious voices of the mad.

In his very informative report of this hospital, Çelebi mentions another type of psychic treatment: in the spring, flowers were dispersed as a type of olfactory therapy, but many of the patients ate the flowers or trampled on them. He mentions that the people of Edirne came to see the senseless, but he does not seem to imply that this visitation was some kind of Turkish Bedlam; rather, it was beneficial for the inmates. Such visits do not seem to have been unusual in Islamic hospitals, judging from the well-known visits of sultans such as Ibn Tūlūn, to their hospitals, and from stories, such as the Three Madmen's Tale in *The thousand and one nights* and the central episode in the *Maqāmāt* of al-Hamadhānī. The most surprising thing to Çelebi was the provision by the sultan in the asylum's endowment for three singers and seven musicians who were to visit the hospital three times a week. They played six different melodies, and many of the insane were reported to have been relieved. The inmates were also carefully fed, and two days a week the pharmacy was opened to all the sick of the city who received drugs and potions free. . . .

▲

The Maya's Own Words

Thomas B. Irving, ed.

The arrival and subsequent conquest of native populations by the Spanish brought about the worst epidemiological event in the history of the world. New World populations had virtually no immunity to the host of infectious diseases that came from the Old World, which resulted in a catastrophic die-off of the native populations. Smallpox in its various forms was the most virulent disease; measles was a close second, but in addition, malaria, influenza, typhus, and numerous other diseases killed thousands of people, often in tandem. No one could stop the wildfire spread of such diseases because physicians had no vaccines, no modern medications, and no accurate knowledge of how disease spread.

The Aztecs and Maya believed that sickness was caused by divine action and that the gods had abandoned them. Their political structures, economies, religion, and entire culture collapsed as a result of the unstoppable **epidemics.** *Other results included culture shock, severe depression, and disruption of the family among the survivors. The following three selections evoke the sense of despair that these peoples felt as their world collapsed and as they remembered a happier day before the foreigners came.*

▲

Reprinted by permission of Labyrinthos Press, from "Foreigners and Illness," in *The Maya's Own Words,* ed. Thomas Irving (Lancaster, CA: Labyrinthos Press, 1985), 71.

The Spanish Conquest

Foreigners and Illness

When King Lahuh-Noh, the eldest son of Cablahuh-Tihash, was reigning, some Yaquis arrived as ambassadors from King Montezuma of Mexico. . . .

| Ten years later | a plague appeared, O my sons! On the day One Ah the cycle was completed, while the plague was raging. First people fell ill of a cough, then they suffered nosebleeds and could not pass urine. The number of dead in that period was quite frightening. That is when Prince Vakaki-Ahmak died. When the plague held sway long shadows and complete night gradually enveloped our fathers and grandfathers, and ourselves as well, O my sons! . . .

▲

The Book of Chilam Balam of Chumayel

RALPH L. ROYS, ED.

▲

. . . There was then no sickness; they had then no aching bones; they had then no high fever; they had then no smallpox; they had then no burning chest; they had then no abdominal pains; they had then no consumption; they had then no headache. At that time the course of humanity was orderly. The foreigners made it otherwise when they arrived here. . . .

▲

The Broken Spears

The Aztec Account of the Conquest of Mexico

MIGUEL LEON-PORTILLA, ED.

▲

The Plague Ravages the City

While the Spaniards were in Tlaxcala, a great plague broke out here in Tenochtitlan. It began to spread during the thirteenth month and lasted for seventy days, striking everywhere in the city and killing a vast number of our people. Sores erupted on our faces, our breasts, our bellies;

we were covered with agonizing sores from head to foot.

The illness was so dreadful that no one could walk or move. The sick were so utterly helpless that they could only lie on their beds like corpses, unable to move their limbs or even their heads. They could not lie face down or roll from one side to the other. If they did move their bodies, they screamed with pain.

A great many died from this plague, and many others died of hunger. They could not get up to search for food, and everyone else was too sick to care for them, so they starved to death in their beds.

Some people came down with a milder form of the disease; they suffered less than the others and made a good recovery. But they could not escape entirely. Their looks were ravaged, for wherever a sore broke out, it gouged an ugly pockmark in the skin. And a few of the survivors were left completely blind.

The first cases were reported in Cuatlan. By the time the danger was recognized, the plague was so well established that nothing could halt it, and eventually it spread all the way to Chalco. Then its virulence diminished considerably, though there were isolated cases for many months after. The first victims were stricken during the fiesta of Teotlecco, and the faces of our warriors were not clean and free of sores until the fiesta of Panquetzaliztli. . . .

▲

Public Health in Aztec Society

HERBERT R. HARVEY, PH.D.

Whenever people are crowded into densely populated cities, public health issues become extremely important, and the Aztec capital city of Tenochtitlán was no exception. The highly centralized administration of the Aztec Empire was responsible for a number of public health services such as clean streets, safe drinking water, garbage and sewage removal, and disposal of the dead. Public health measures were administered better than in European cities of the same period, and the Spaniards marveled at the cleanliness of the city on the lake. In addition to such sanitation measures, the Aztec state promoted the availability of a wide variety of herbal remedies for the urban population, a practice unknown in Europe at the time. Overall, the population of Tenochtitlán was better served in matters of public health than were citizens of Madrid or any other sixteenth-century European capital city.

▲

The resident population of Tenochtitlan-Tlatelolco in 1519 is estimated to have been 150,000 to 200,000, and the combined city occupied an area of 15 square kilometers. Population density, therefore, was in the neighborhood of 1,000 per square kilometer. In addition to this was a large transient population, which may well have exceeded 50,000 on major market days. Such population densities can, in themselves, create problems that adversely effect the quality of life.

The physical appearance of the Aztec capital stimulated comment from 16th century observers. From their direct observations certain inferences can be made regarding management of the urban environment, in particular the sector related to the maintenance of public health. There is little

Reprinted by permission of The New York Academy of Medicine, from Herbert R. Harvey, "Public Health in Aztec Society," *Bulletin of the New York Academy of Medicine* 57, no. 2 (1981): 157–64.

question that public health was a state concern in prehispanic times and that public health measures were not only applied to immediate local jurisdictions of the major powers in the Valley of Mexico, but also were probably extended to the provinces. . . .

The first Spanish eyewitnesses of the Aztec capital and other cities of Mexico were especially impressed by their beauty and orderliness. Bernal Díaz reported of Tenochtitlan that ". . . where there were not these stones it was cemented and burnished and all very clean, so that one could not find any dust or straw in the whole place." Motolinía noted that "the streets and highways of this great city were so clean and well swept that there was nothing to stumble over, and wherever Moteczuma went, both in this city and anywhere else, the road was swept and the ground so firm and smooth that even if the sole of the foot were as delicate as the palm of the hand, it would not be hurt by going unshod."

According to Torquemada, 1,000 men were regularly employed to sweep the island city, dampen the dust of its streets, and maintain its canals. This he contrasts with the condition of Mexico City in his own day. He also noted the native practice of planting aromatic trees along the thoroughfares and the maintenance of public parks for recreation purposes. In general, it appears that the Aztecs had a disdain for unpleasant odors. Streets were illuminated at night and patrolled.

Potable water was a major concern in the island environment. According to Durán's account, Tenochtitlan acquired the rights to pipe water from Chapultepec during the reign of Chimalpopoca. Two clay conduits stretched between Chapultepec and Tenochtitlan. While one was in use the other was being cleaned. Fresh water was also transported to the city in canoes and distributed by canoe to those portions of the city not served by the aqueduct. Fresh water was directly piped into homes of the nobility, where it was stored in ponds in the gardens. This practice of water storage still survives in the rural areas, and *ajolotes* (a type of salamander) are kept in the water to keep it clean.

Unfortunately, chroniclers paid little attention to the mechanisms of disposal of garbage and sewerage. Bernal Díaz did describe, however, the practice of placing privies along all of the roads for use of the public in transit. He further noted that this kept human excrement from being lost. Human excrement was, according to Bernal Díaz carted off in canoe loads for use in salt-making and tanning. With Aztec disdain for noxious odors and their emphasis on cleanliness of public places, it seems reasonable to infer that some system of human waste disposal was operative, especially in view of the large amount of traffic required to supply the cities. While human waste had some market value in salt-making and tanning, it may also have had market value as fertilizer. In any case, the importance of Bernal Díaz' observation is that there were economic as well as sanitary reasons for providing for the disposition of human wastes.

Sahagún describes a soil, *axixtlalli:* "This is land which had been urinated upon, which is greasy . . . he makes urinated soil . . . ." This suggests a practice of restricting locations for bodily functions. He also describes *tlalauiyac,* a mellow soil, one fertilized with human excrement. Whether human excrement was used commercially as a fertilizer or incidentally, much of it was returned to the soil, and so the pathogens contained therein often survived. This could well have been a basic factor in the reported high incidence of such intestinal maladies as diarrhea and dysentery, both endemic to the area.

For late prehispanic period times, Sanders estimates a diet based 80% on the consumption of corn and **amaranth**. This diet could be expected to yield an average of 150 grams of excrement per person per day, or for a city of 200,000 people, 30,000 kilos daily. In terms of volume, 150 grams equals approximately 150 cubic centimeters. The amount of human excrement generated in Tenochtitlan-Tlatelolco, therefore, was roughly 30 cubic meters per day, enough to spread 15 hectares with a layer 2 cm. thick. What is important is that the problem of human waste disposal handled routinely is manageable even under primitive conditions.

Some of the nutrients from human waste found their way to the lakes, whether placed directly through dumping in the marshes or indirectly through run-off. The limnological descriptions of the lakes suggest eutrophic (or polluted) waters. Fish, for example, are described as small, and algae and other lower life forms were regularly harvested. Algae were a source of protein in the diet. Tenochtitlan was only one of the many cities in a densely populated valley that contributed to lake pollution. However, it does appear that the amount of pollution may have been minimized through some controlled system of waste disposal.

Disposal of the dead, always a problem for urban concentrations, was by cremation. The exceptions were those who died a violent death, those who died of incurable diseases, and those under 17 years of age. These were buried rather than cremated. To exempt from cremation those who died of incurable diseases was perhaps not the best public health measure, but the widespread practice of cremation had value.

It is apparent in its management of the urban environment that the Aztec state functioned to control or to eliminate potential sources of health hazards such as the water supply, garbage and sewerage disposal, and the maintenance of public places. Consistent with this was also its efforts in famine control.

Numerous statements by native informants recorded in the *Relaciones Geográficas* and other sources of the later 16th century speak of prehispanic dietary austerity. In fact, these informants attribute many of their maladies to overeating. Given the pressure on the food supply, it is quite likely that the average diet in prehispanic times was minimal, and famines not uncommon. Eventually, the famine threat was reduced through the introduction of state-run granaries, from which reserves regions with food shortages could be supplied. Famine control was a function of the Aztec state, and, perhaps with it or as a result of it, a certain measure of dietary control developed. There were prohibitions on the consumption of meat by commoners except on feast days, and al-

coholic beverages were restricted, even the nutritious *pulque*.

As to the general state of health in late prehispanic times, Cook observed that "The archaeological and historical record indicates a race which was remarkably free from devastating epidemics and from generalized chronic **endemic** ailments. There are few cases of serious or widespread illness in historic times and within at least two hundred years of the conquest, all of these can be classified as secondary to physical exposure and starvation." It is true that famines were remembered and that widespread prehispanic epidemics, if such occurred, were not often reported. Because of the widespread practice of cremation, there is very little archaeological evidence within the heart of the empire that allows for inferences one way or another.

The epidemiology of prehispanic Mexico is conjectural, but native remedies, in particular medicinal plants and herbs, reflect the categories of ailments and health conditions commonly treated. Diarrhea and dysentery head the list, with unidentified fevers of various types and respiratory infections crowding for second place. Even today, in modern Mexico, these head the list.

A significant activity of the Aztec state was the collection of medicinal plants and experimentation with herbal cures. For example, Cortés himself was struck by the size and extent of the botanical gardens of Huaxtepec. The efficacy of native curing practices was tested early by the Spaniards, and was much esteemed. Many remedies quickly diffused to Europe and became common in the European pharmacopoeia of the late 16th and subsequent centuries.

While documentary sources describing preconquest pharmacological practices are not abundant, it is reasonable to conclude from such direct mention as is available, together with associated practices, that the Aztecs were in the process of assembling the folk procedures and remedies from all over their realm, codifying these, and experimenting with them. The native record of this process, whether orally maintained or recorded in writing, was lost in the conquest. However, some glimpse of the magnitude of the effort can be gained from native specialists recorded by Sahagún and Juan Badiano. Both sources reveal the concerted effort that was under way to match the curative properties of plant and animal substances with specific medical conditions requiring treatment.

The Spanish Crown was significantly impressed by what it had learned of medical practices in its overseas colony to dispatch the physician Francisco Hernandez to New Spain in 1571. Hernandez was charged to make a systematic study of the medical botany of New Spain. In addition, the *Relaciones Geográficas* also included direct questions relating to the state of health within the various jurisdictions surveyed and the remedies invoked in curing. The result, from all sources, is a substantial body of description of medicinal plants with their curative properties and methods of application, suggesting that the Mexican pharmacopoeia of late prehispanic times had a strongly empirical basis.

On the other hand, most natural calamities that befell individuals were associated with the domain of one or another supernatural being. Likewise, most illnesses were linked to particular deities or classes of deities. Thus, the root cause of illness or injury was ultimately supernatural. Mexican preventive medicine involved both avoiding certain activities and practicing certain others. When an individual became ill or was injured, he might seek the help of a special practitioner, a diviner or soothsayer, to help select the proper rituals that might be required as part of the cure or for future prevention. The ritual aspects of curing are well described in the sources. However, what the sources do not reveal are the conditions which called for ritual solutions. That is, was ritual behavior required for ordinary common ailments? Also, how did it fit with empirical diagnoses and treatment? Clearly, an individual suffering from an infection was treated with specific medicines, combined perhaps with heat treatment in sweat baths, and possibly dietary prescriptions. The treatment was empirical; the cause supernatural. Because the ritual dimensions of curing have been more amply described, there has

been a tendency, from the 16th century to the present, to overlook the "scientific" knowledge of prehispanic Mexican medical practice—that which had a therapeutic effect in restoring the individual to a healthy state.

Ortiz de Montellano . . . examined the therapeutic quality of 25 selected medicinal plants which were used in prehispanic times and whose modern botanical identification can be reliably determined. He concluded, after chemical analysis, that ". . . 16 would produce most of the effects claimed in native sources, 4 may possibly be active, and 5 do not seem to possess the activity claimed by native informants." For example, *carica papaya* (Aztec *chichi hualxochitl*) may be taken internally as a digestant, because papase is a protein digestant, and externally for rash because it is an ". . . enzyme which topically will remove clotted blood, purulent exudate, and necrotic tissue from surface wounds and ulcers." Sources describe the latex of unripened fruit for external application and of the ripe fruit for internal digestion.

The significance of the native materia medica is that not only could it have been and, in many instances, probably was an effective empirical treatment, but that the state was involved in the improvement of knowledge and scientific practice related to curative medicine. This was a public health service of the prehispanic government. It also suggests that illness in prehispanic Mexico was sufficiently troublesome as to involve the state.

Herbs were widely traded. Thus, Cortés noted that "There is a street set apart for the sale of herbs, where can be found every sort of root and medical herb which grows in the country. There are houses like apothecary shops, where prepared medicines are sold, as well as liquids, ointments, and plasters . . . ." Other observers describe the market in even greater detail, and the diversity of the herb traffic commanded their attention. Many herbs were of local or otherwise rare provenience, so that the major market centers served as focal points for the distribution of products collected from even the most remote provinces. The relative economic importance of the herb trade in the overall marketing network can hardly be overestimated. With the widespread emphasis on medicinal plant cures, the economic importance of the herb trade must have been sizable. Unfortunately, specific artifacts associated with the preparation of plant cures have not been identified so that there has been little reflection of this archaeologically.

Modern descriptions of folk medicine in various localities do not reflect the imposing materia medica of prehispanic times associated with the Aztec state, nor should they. Most folk practices utilize herbal cures from locally available plants. The Hippocratic system of disease classification into hot-cold categories is not uniform from one locality or one region to the next, although the Hippocratic theory of disease causation is so widespread in Latin America that some would like to attribute its origin to convergence. The variation precisely reflects what might be expected of indigenous medicine. That is, for the same ailment different localities have devised their own cures—some of them effective. Different localities have in the past subscribed to the logic of the Hippocratic idea and idiosyncratically applied it to their own situation. The Hippocratic idea merely classified illness and its treatment into a logical framework. The Aztec materia medica at the time of the Spanish conquest was a codification of the widespread variation in folk medicine then prevailing.

The medical practitioner in ancient Mexico was held in high esteem. It was a profession learned through practice and by formal instruction. Both men and women practiced, and there appears to have been a considerable degree of specialization. The extent of state regulation of medical practitioners must be inferred. Sources hint at supervision, perhaps close supervision, since state-run hospitals, according to Las Casas, were found in all the major cities. Motolinía adds the observation that they went to the country in search of the sick. While Motolinía and Las Casas see this practice in terms of charity or social beneficence, at the same time such a system clearly reflects the state's concern with disease control. It also reflects the preventive aspect of public health

care. Unfortunately, the practice is not described in further detail—indicating, for example, the condition required for a person to be brought (perhaps forcibly) to an urban hospital; whether quarantine of persons with certain communicable diseases was an objective or whether other objectives were sought.

The rigid code of morality which prevailed in preconquest Mexico also bears mention in terms of its impact on the state of health. Striking are the severe penalties for adultery. There seems every reason to believe that these penalties were applied. This deterrent, of course, would reduce the spread of venereal infection to a minimum. Further, good personal hygiene is a dominant theme in prehispanic culture, and a regular feature of each community or neighborhood was the public bath house or *temascal*. Bath-house attendants were well paid and held in high esteem, especially with respect to their administering medicinal baths to the sick. Bathing was the prime curative measure for many ailments. The code of cleanliness is expressed in the advice of a father to his son:

> And when already thou art to eat, thou art to wash thy hands, to wash thy face, to wash thy mouth . . . . And when the eating is over . . . thou art to pick up (fallen scraps), thou art to sweep the place where there has been eating. And thou, when thou hast eaten, once again art thou to wash thy hands, to wash thy mouth, to cleanse thy teeth.

The general state of health of the native population seriously deteriorated following the Spanish conquest. In the 16th century epidemics were commonplace. Diseases hitherto unknown, such as small pox and typhus, ravaged native populations. Mortality rates soared and the population declined. However, there has been a tendency in the literature to overstress the impact of new diseases in populations lacking immunities. Unquestionably, many other variables played a direct or contributory role, factors such as malnutrition, deteriorating social conditions, poor sanitation, questionable medical procedures, and the like. The indigenous system of public health which had served well to manage large populations broke down and was not replaced. The Spaniards ignored many aspects of urban maintenance, for example, cleaning of the canals. The stench of the canals subsequently became a chronic issue at city hall. Finally, the Spaniards replaced sometimes good, but at worst ineffective, medical practice, for assuredly bad practices.

KEY TERMS

Amaranth, 149 • Atrabilious, 134 • Calculus, 135 • Cineritial, 137 • Emunctory, 138 • Endemic, 150 • Epidemics, 146 • Epistaxis, 137 • Ichorous, 137 • Igneity, 138 • Non-naturals, 144 • Oliguria, 137 • Theriacs, 145 • Vesical, 136

QUESTIONS TO CONSIDER

1. The Muslim Empire is credited with preserving a great deal of knowledge from the Greek and Roman civilizations. How might the forthcoming advances in European medicine have been altered had these classic writings been lost?

2. In the Americas, the supernatural explanation of the cause and cure of disease was universal. The American peoples also had no history of exposure to epidemic disease. Would the lack of such a stressor have had any effect on their worldviews, their religious beliefs, or their medical practices?

3. The sledgehammer effect of the epidemics of smallpox, measles, and other infectious diseases on the Native American cultures from Canada to Tierra del Fuego is difficult to imagine. If an unknown and highly infectious disease were to attack a modern nation such as the United States, how might people react? Would social norms collapse as they did among the Aztecs and Incas? How would our explanations of events differ from theirs?

4. As Ibn Sina clearly demonstrated, examination of a patient's urine could tell the physician a great deal about the ailments presented, a premise still borne out by the fact that one of the most routine tests run in modern doctors' offices is the simple urinalysis. How different is Ibn Sina's uroscopy from modern urinalysis, in terms of what the physician describes and the problems that could be diagnosed from the examination? Do any points of comparison exist?

5. Al-Zahrawi devised many of his own instruments, which he illustrated in his treatise *Al-Tasrif (On Surgery)* and which are shown in Figure 7–1. Can you see any resemblance between modern surgical instruments and these tenth-century tools, some of which are still in use in modified form? For what procedures do you think they might have been used?

RECOMMENDED READINGS

Cook, N. David. *Born to Die: Disease and New World Conquest, 1492–1650.* Cambridge: Cambridge University Press, 1998.

————. *Demographic Collapse: Indian Peru, 1520–1620.* Cambridge: Cambridge University Press, 1981.

Cook, N. David, and W. George Lovell, eds. *Secret Judgments of God: Old World Disease in Colonial Spanish America.* Norman: University of Oklahoma Press, 1992.

Cook, Sherburne F., and Woodrow Borah. *Essays on Population History.* 3 vols. Berkeley: University of California Press, 1971–1979.

Crosby, Alfred W., Jr. *The Columbian Exchange: Biological and Cultural Consequences of 1492.* Westport, CT: Greenwood Press, 1972.

Duffy, John. *Epidemics in Colonial America.* Port Washington, NY: Kennikat Press, 1972.

Maimonides, Moses. *Two Treatises on the Regimen of Health.* Philadelphia: American Philosophical Society, 1964.

McNeill, William H. *Plagues and Peoples.* Garden City, NY: Anchor/Doubleday, 1976.

Razi, Abu Bakr Muhammad ibn Zakariya (Rhazes). *A Treatise on Smallpox and Measles.* Birmingham, AL: Classics of Medicine Library, 1987.

Rosner, Fred, and Suessman Munter, trans. and ed. *The Medical Aphorisms of Moses Maimonides.* New York: Yeshiva University Press, 1970.

Sahagún, Bernardino de. *Florentine Codex: General History of the Things of New Spain.* 13 vols. Santa Fe, NM: School of American Research and University of Utah, 1950–1969.

Spink, M. S., and G. L. Lewis. *Albucasis On Surgery and Instruments.* Berkeley: University of California Press, 1973.

Ullman, Manfred. *Islamic Medicine.* Edinburgh, Scotland: Edinburgh University Press, 1978.

Waserman, M. *Pre-Columbian Medicine: Historical Sources.* Washington, DC: National Institutes of Health, 1981.

Weisman, Abner I. *Medicine before Columbus: As Told in Pre-Columbian Medical Art.* New York: Pre-Cortesian Publications, 1979.

Chapter Eight

The Renaissance and the Scientific Revolution

Technical and Theoretical Change

INTRODUCTION

Between 1400 and 1800, the study, if not always the practice, of medicine underwent revolutionary changes as its modernization began. Beginning in the Renaissance, humanist scholars sought definitive editions and translations of the works of the classical Greek, Roman, and Arabic authors. Probably the most significant advances in Western medicine during the Renaissance came in the areas of anatomy and physiology and involved a breaking away from the old Greco-Islamic traditions. With this breaking away came a new emphasis on the importance of human dissections. Art and anatomy went hand in hand in Leonardo da Vinci's sketches, and Vesalius's classic work, *De Humani Corporis Fabrica* (1543), permanently made illustration an essential part of anatomy textbooks.

In the seventeenth and eighteenth centuries, the parameters of medical research changed again as medicine was caught up in the Scientific Revolution. Men such as William Harvey, who definitively proved his theories on the circulation of blood, were committed to scientific concepts such as precise measurements and quantitative methods. Once the experimental method became a permanent part of medical research, new theories and discoveries came at avalanche speed. On the basis of clinical research, careful note taking, and repeated experiments, Edward Jenner epitomized the new framework of medical research when in 1798 he published his findings on a new and safe way to prevent smallpox.

Yet, to envision this period as a time when medicine was able to cure more patients and alleviate more suffering would be highly inaccurate. Nearly all the advances of the Renaissance and the Scientific Revolution were made by the elite of the medical establishment—university-trained physicians—often within a university setting. In this respect, Jenner, a rural English doctor, was the exception. Even though the use of the printing press meant that publication of new research and theories could reach a much larger audience than ever, this audience did not include the individuals who provided the limited health care available to the overall European population. The gap between pure science and applied science, between the theory of medicine and the practice of medicine, was never wider.

TIME LINE

1300–1650 C.E.	The Renaissance—these dates are only approximate; this period has no specific start and finish dates
1452	Gutenberg invents the printing press, which is essential to the proliferation of knowledge
1490–1495	Leonardo da Vinci (1452–1519) composes his famous *Sketchbooks*
1497	Hieronymus Brunschwig (Germany) publishes the first known work on the surgical treatment of gunshot wounds
1500	Jakob Nufer (Switzerland) performs the first recorded cesarean section on a living woman; successful procedures remain rare
1518	Royal College of Physicians is founded in London
1520	Paracelsus (1493–1541) begins using opium, which he calls *laudanum*, in a number of his formularies; opium had been used as a painkiller for centuries, but his use broadens its applications
1530	Paracelsus suggests mineral substances such as mercury and antimony as remedies, arguing that chemical compounds were far more effective than those made from plants or animals; Fracastoro (1478–1553) publishes "On Syphilis," the poem that gave the name to that disease
1543	Vesalius (1514–1564) publishes *De Humani Corporis Fabrica (On the Fabric of the Human Body)*, the first accurate work on human anatomy
1545	Paracelsus, sometimes known as "The Martin Luther of Medicine," boldly denounces Galen, even burning copies of his works; Ambroise Paré (1510–1590) publishes his work advocating the use of soothing medications instead of hot-iron cautery in treating wounds
1546	Fracastoro publishes *De Contagione (On Contagion)*, in which he states that diseases are caused by tiny seeds (seminaria) that can be passed from person to person
1553	Michael Servetus (1511–1553) publishes a work stating that blood circulates from the heart to the lungs; his theology conflicts with John Calvin's, and he is burned at the stake for unorthodox views

1614	Santorius Sanctorius's *De Statica Medicina* is the first study of metabolism
1624–1689	Thomas Sydenham lives—known as "The English Hippocrates," he urges the use of observation of the patient and disease rather than simply reading books, and states that diseases are not simply groups of symptoms but specific entities
1628	William Harvey (1578–1657) publishes *De Motu Cordis (Movement of the Heart and Blood in Animals)*, in which he proves the circulation of blood
1645	Daniel Whistler publishes the first medical description of rickets, although the deficiency was undoubtedly present for many years previously
1651	William Harvey describes human embryonic organ development
1655	Johan Schulte describes the procedure for mastectomy
1670	Thomas Willis rediscovers the connection between sugar in urine and diabetes; the Greeks and Chinese had been aware of this connection
1717	Lady Mary Montagu brings the Turkish method of inoculation for smallpox back to England; has her children inoculated
1736	Claudius Aymand (UK) performs the first successful appendectomy; success rate for this procedure remains extremely low
1738	Hermann Boerhaave (the Netherlands) dies (born 1668)—the first to recommend postmortem examination as a way to determine specific causes of death
1747	James Lind (1716–1794) discovers that consumption of citrus fruit can prevent scurvy; publishes his findings in *A Treatise on the Scurvy* in 1753
1752	William Smellie publishes the first scientific approach to obstetrics
1763	First U.S. medical society is founded, in New London, Connecticut
1765	First medical school in North America is founded as the College of Physicians of Pennsylvania
1774	Franz Mesmer (Germany) uses *mesmerism*, a healing therapy based on the idea of animal magnetism, to aid in curing disease
1775	Sir Percival Pott suggests the link between cancer and environmental chemicals
1785	William Withering publishes on the use of digitalis (foxglove) in the treatment of heart disease
1798	Edward Jenner (1749–1823) publishes his discovery of a vaccination for smallpox in *An Inquiry into the Causes and Effects of the Variolae Vaccinae . . . Known by the Name of Cow Pox*

▲

The Forging of the Renaissance Physician

Miguel A. Faria, Jr., M.D.

Beginning in the fourteenth century, the Renaissance brought with it considerable activity in science and medicine; new discoveries and the rediscovery of knowledge from classical Greece and Rome, much of it from the Muslim world. It was also a time of intense development of fine art and many inventions, as exemplified by the work of men such as Leonardo da Vinci. Some of the most famous names in the history of medicine come from this period: Fernel, Fracastoro, Paracelsus, Vesalius, and Paré, to name a few. As described in this selection, the contributions of such men not only advanced medical knowledge, but also paved the way for major developments in the nineteenth century.

▲

Part III: The Physicians and the Period of Rebirth

In The Beginning

The renaissance was a remarkable epoch in Western Civilization. It was truly an intense period of rebirth which led the way from the scholasticism of the late Middle Ages to the intellectual and scientific achievements of the Age of Enlightenment. The intellectual explosion of the Renaissance affected all areas of learning and human endeavor: sculpture, painting, poetry, writing, philosophy, astronomy, and medicine—all of which were deeply imbued by this revolution in learning. . . .

. . . The Renaissance brought new ideas and doctrines that challenged the old rules and traditional institutions which had dominated European culture and intellectual life for a millennium. Revolutionary discoveries in medicine and astronomy were at last within man's grasp. The Renaissance also witnessed the growth of the humanities and philosophic controversies. . . .

The Rulers and Patrons

This was an age when autocratic rulers wrestled and vied for power in a world surrounded by treacherous waters and centered in earthly intrigue. . . . This was the time of Martin Luther (1483–1546) and his 95 Theses nailed on the door of the Castle-Church in Wittenberg (1517). This precipitated the Protestant Reformation, and its antithesis, the Counter-Reformation. . . .

Fernel, Fracastoro, and the Contagion

During this exalted period, many great medical men dedicated their lives to translating ancient manuscripts and commenting on the newly discovered medical works. Translations of works from the Greek into Latin as well as into the vernacular languages was performed by Islamic, Jewish, and Christian physicians. Works of Galen, Hippocrates, Plato, and Dioscorides were popularized. Others attempted to reconcile the Humoural doctrines to

Reprinted by permission of the Medical Association of Georgia, from Miguel A. Faria, "The Forging of the Renaissance Physician: A Philosophic and Historic Perspective," *Journal of the Medical Association of Georgia* 81, no. 4 (1992): 165–76.

newly-discovered facts and observations. . . . The progressive idea of the specific nature of disease came into vogue. The concept of the contagion as material particles was advanced. Propagation of disease by contact from contagious sources became evident in variola, the bubonic plagues, measles, and syphilis.

Jean Fernel (1497–1588) was one of many celebrated Renaissance physicians. He trained in Paris and compiled his great treatise, *A Universal Medicine,* in which he proposed that the study of medicine be divided into three categories: physiology, pathology, and therapeutics. He summarized all of the known medical knowledge of his time. His book is credited with planting the seeds of curiosity and thirst for knowledge in his contemporaries which led to an avalanche of medical theories.

Fernel, along with Paré and Paracelsus, advanced the idea of the contagious nature of diseases by different causes. In 1494, after Spanish troops returned from the New World, there was an outbreak of an epidemic of a new disease in Naples. This disease was subsequently called the French Disease after it became widespread in Europe disseminated by the victorious French troops who had battled the Spaniards in Naples. Mercurials were first used as ointment and found to be effective against this malady, which was later called syphilis. Paracelsus has been given the credit for this therapy, which has been described by a contemporary as: "spend one hour with Venus and the rest of your life with Mercury . . ." in reference to its method of transmission and the required long-term treatment.

Girolamo Fracastoro (1478–1553) was another great Renaissance physician who along with Jean Fernel suggested that syphilis was a venereal disease and recommended mercurials for treatment. In 1547, Fracastoro wrote on contagious diseases and separated the bubonic plague from typhus and meningitis while providing excellent clinical descriptions as well as prognosis of these diseases. He believed in transmission by human contact, or by contaminated objects and air. He was a Renaissance physician in both the modern and historic sense. He even wrote a poem about a shepherd afflicted with syphilis for which he is still remembered. His treatise on infectious diseases was ahead of its time, and perhaps if it had been pursued further it could have propelled bacteriology into a true science three centuries earlier. . . . Fracastoro was also a proponent of the heliocentric theory proposed by fellow physician Copernicus.

Quarantining those afflicted was found to be an effective way to treat contagious diseases which up through this time had been decimating the populations of Europe and Asia in both sporadic outbreaks as well as in endemic transmission. Hygiene, diet, clean water, disinfection with sulfur vapors, and burial of contaminated bodies outside the city became commonplace during epidemic diseases of the Renaissance. . . .

The theory of specificity of disease promoted by Paracelsus essentially substituted the theory of the "doctrine of signature" which had established that a medicament of nature by its external appearance was endowed by nature with the proper qualities for the treatment of diseases. For example, digitalis was discovered and used for heart ailments because of the shape and form of the leaves of the plant from which it was extracted. Botany and chemistry flourished in man's search for remedies. Many treatises on therapeutics were published encompassing a compilation of all of the known Greek pharmacopeia, and some even included the new Islamic additions. The old "science" of alchemy which had been essentially forgotten in Europe during the Middle Ages was rediscovered and popularized during this time.

The Nonconformist: Paracelsus

The main figure associated with the vivification of Alchemy was the controversial Paracelsus (Theophrastus Bombastus von Hohenheim, 1493–1541) of Basel. He blended not only magic with mysticism but also alchemy with medicine.

And controversial he was. . . . [H]e was said to have been censored for teaching in the vernacular, and worse, "he often could be found lecturing roaring drunk in lecture halls . . ." and forever battering the walls of the establishment.

He opposed the medieval reliance on the work of Galen and Avicenna, and instead, he emphasized observation, experimentation, and empiricism. He has been called the Father of **Iatrochemistry** for his application and use of chemistry in the practice of medicine. He challenged the traditional theories of the imbalance of the Humours and the axiom of *Contraria-Contrariis-Curantur.* He vehemently espoused the active intervention of the physician during the crisis of disease. He believed in simple Christianity and the virtues of herbs and drugs as a product of God's creation and affirmed that physicians do God's work. Paracelsus was a proponent of the modern examination of the urine as opposed to the old misleading science of uroscopy. Perhaps his major achievement is that of his regard for surgery and medicine on an equal footing. In fact, he performed his own surgery and thus he described himself as a doctor in medicine and surgery, helping to raise the status of his surgical colleagues as well as those who practiced both. . . .

The Genius: Andreas Vesalius

If Paracelsus was the most controversial and impetuous proponent of the new learning of the Renaissance, Andreas Vesalius (1514–1564) was the greatest anatomist of the era. . . . In his *De Humani Corporis Fabrica* (*On The Fabric of the Human Body,* 1543), Vesalius gave the world one of Western Civilization's greatest masterpieces. As professor of anatomy . . . , he had ample opportunity for human dissection and anatomical studies that led to this monumental work. In *Fabrica,* he laid the foundation for modern scientific anatomic investigation. The treatise also for the first time publicly contradicted and corrected previous anatomic concepts established and accepted as dogma since Galen's time. Though Vesalius revered Galen, he recorded what he saw in his anatomic dissections instead of accepting the inaccuracies and errors contained in the copied and recopied ancient manuscripts. With the publication of *Fabrica,* Vesalius . . . literally revolutionized the field of anatomy. By actual dissection, Vesalius revealed simple truths that contradicted not only anatomic misconceptions but also philosophic notions. He challenged Aristotle's doctrine that stated that thought and personality were in the heart; Vesalius believed them to be a function of the brain.

Some of the truths that Vesalius revealed by his anatomic works were arrived at by simple observations. For example, he nullified the belief that men have one rib less than women which was assumed by the biblical account of the creation of Eve. Vesalius simply counted the ribs of male and female cadavers in the dissection room and reached the incontrovertible truth. He also debunked the erroneous idea that men have more teeth than women.

The illustrations in the *Fabrica* were not only precise and accurate but also genuine artistic masterpieces. Moreover, the illustrations were closely integrated with the text, making the book highly effective. Each body system was described with their organs and their interrelation and function. The chambers of the heart were described, and previous errors corrected. . . .

Nevertheless, the publication of this book led to a violent academic quarrel between the medical establishment headed by one of the Renaissance's great anatomists, Jacob Sylvius (1478–1555), and the young Vesalius. Sylvius followed Galen's teachings, whose anatomy he accepted without reservation, and he could therefore not accept Vesalius's revolutionary findings. Vesalius's revelations were too much for the medical world even for this period. The fuming controversy was fortunately ameliorated by his temporary good fortune of being installed as personal physician to the Emperor Charles V, and when the Emperor retired, Vesalius became the physician to his son, Phillip II, King of Spain.

. . . [H]uman corpses for cadaveric dissection were difficult to obtain, and body snatching became a necessity even for conscientious anatomists.

Consequently, the quest for human corpses for anatomic dissection was such that anatomists were "forced to violate the sanctity of the grave and the threat of excommunication." Vesalius himself recalled one night when he remained hidden outside the city walls and then cut from the gallows the corpse of an executed prisoner to be used for anatomic dissection. It was said that Cosimo de Medici, Grand Duke of Tuscany, offered Dr. Fallopio two condemned criminals for anatomic work. Allegedly, he told the professor, "kill them in any manner you wish and then dissect them." . . .

Vesalius's unhappiness was not to end with his medical controversy but was to culminate with an even greater calamity. The story goes that he was to dissect the corpse of a Spanish nobleman who had died in his care. Allegedly, when he opened the chest, he found that the heart was still beating. Some authorities deny this occurrence as an abominable calumny perpetrated by his many unforgiving enemies. Nevertheless, following this unfortunate event, his life was endangered by the Inquisition. He was saved again by royal favor, and his penitence was to make a pilgrimage to Jerusalem where he lived for many years. He finally decided to return to Padua where he had been offered a professorship, but he never made it back. He was only 50 years old when he died on his return trip on the Greek island of Zakymthos in 1564. He is now considered the Father of Anatomy and is warmly remembered for his anatomic masterpieces and scientific legacy. . . .

Part IV: Physicians for All Seasons

Ambroise Paré—Barber Surgeon

Considered the greatest surgeon of the Renaissance, Ambroise Paré (1510–1590) was born in Laval in Northern France. From his humble beginnings, Paré, the barber surgeon, elevated himself to a distinguished medical/surgical career during the zenith of the Renaissance. He came to be revered by the nobility and peasants alike. He served as personal physician to five successive French kings.

In 1533, at the age 23, Paré went to Paris and trained as house surgeon at Hotel Dieu, the first municipal hospital said to have been founded by St. Landry in 660 A.D. He learned to do cadaveric dissections and was taught by Jacob Sylvius, who had also taught Vesalius at Padua. After completing his training, Paré was certified for the private practice of surgery. His plans to practice were suddenly interrupted, however, when he was recruited by Colonel de Montejan, commander of the French infantry. . . . It was subsequently in the battlefields of the various wars between the Emperor and the King of France that Paré was to gain most of his surgical experience and expertise for which he became famous.

It was in the Battle of Chateau de Villane, where the French sustained heavy losses during the siege and storming of the town of Turin, that one of Paré's most celebrated discoveries took place. It was said that he ran out of the boiling oil that was used to neutralize wounds contaminated with gunpowder (which was thought to be poisonous. He improvised by applying a salve of egg white, rose oil, and turpentine. The next morning, he found that those soldiers who had been treated with the salve spent the night well and experienced less pain and inflammation, whereas those treated with the boiling oil experienced fever, aches, and swelling about their wounds. From then on, Paré felt that it was "cruel to burn poor people who had suffered shot wounds."

Paré abandoned the surgical instructions then in vogue by the authoritative Giovanni de Vigo, a papal surgeon who taught the traditional idea that gunshot was poisonous and thus recommended cauterization of gunshot wounds. During this time, he not only tended wounds but also drained abscesses and reduced fractures.

After serving 2 years with distinction as military surgeon, Paré was allowed to return to Paris. . . .

In 1541, Paré joined the College of Barber Surgeons after passing its entrance examination. He wrote a dissertation on gunshot wounds that was used for the treatment of wounds in subsequent wars. He created an uproar, however, by insisting that gunpowder was not poisonous and that cautery by boiling oil in the treatment of wounds was harmful. In 1549, he wrote another book based on the anatomic dissections of Vesalius whom he greatly admired. In 1561, *Universal Surgery* followed, describing further refinements in surgical principles and techniques.

Paré's surgical successes led to fame and fortune but not to peace and tranquility. After King Francis I died in 1547, . . . Paré was soon summoned for further service to his country. At the siege of Metz, he practiced trephination for head wounds and perfected his technique of amputations. Despite the rigors of war and the muddy and bloody circumstances of the battlefield, he remained committed to the care of his soldiers. He was obsessed with cleanliness and sanitation and even prescribed dietary regimes [*sic*] of hyperalimentation for the wounded. . . .

Within months after Metz, Paré was in another besieged town, Hesdin, where the situation was so hopeless for the French army that Paré, as an officer, voted with the majority to surrender. He was imprisoned and obliged to treat the leg ulcers of his captor, Lord Vaudeville (1553). After an arduous but successful ordeal, Paré was released by the Knight and rewarded for his treatment with a trumpet-blowing escort to the camp of Henry II. Paré was subsequently appointed "Surgeon In-Ordinary" to the King, but he resented that he was no more than a Master Barber Surgeon in professional circles. This situation was corrected in 1554, when he passed a rigorous examination and was granted a license as a member of the confraternity of St. Côme. . . .

Paré like Vesalius waged war against obsolete methods of treatment even when he had to go against the medical establishment. Paré's magnum opus was his *Les Oeuvres* (*Collected Works*: first edition, 1575) which was published at age 65. In his *Works,* he described techniques for bladder operations, artificial eyes and limbs, the suturing of wounds, and other innovative surgical procedures which were described and illustrated in considerable detail. His *Works* went through several editions. In one of the later editions, he got into trouble for not asking permission to include information from the Parisian medical society. He also offended the Establishment for vehemently condemning the use of "unicorn's" horn and tissue from Egyptian mummies as pharmaceuticals. He went on to describe prostatism as a cause of painful urination, and the effects of syphilis on arterial walls including the development of aneurysrns. He showed midwives how to stop **puerperal** hemorrhaging. He advocated prompt caesarean section as soon as the mother died to save the baby, and conversely, urged abortion to remove a dead fetus from a living woman. He popularized the use of [the] truss in the management of hernias. . . .

Perhaps his greatest single contribution was to introduce the use of ligatures for controlling hemorrhaging during surgery, which was one of the worst surgical problems of his day. Until then, the sole means to stop bleeding was the cautery iron which had been used extensively by Arabian physicians. Responding to the inquisitorial interrogation of the Parisian medical society, Paré said, "You say that tying up the blood vessels after an amputation is a new method, and should therefore not be used. That is a bad argument for a doctor."

Because of his advances in the discipline of surgery during the Renaissance, as well as his indomitable moral courage and great technical skills, he has been deservedly called "the Father of Modern Surgery." Near death, Paré bequeathed to his family, "his wealth, property and honor" and to his profession "a burning against mystification and the Ivory Tower." Some aphorisms ascribed to Paré include: "I bandaged him but God cured him," "It is better to prescribe a dubious drug than to leave the patient without help," and "Always give the patient hope even when death is near." . . .

Epilogue

The explosion of ideas during the Renaissance created tidal waves of expanding knowledge that poured over the world for the next 300 years. These waves of knowledge flowed naturally into the Age of Reason and the Enlightenment. In the 19th Century, two of the greatest accomplishments in medical history occurred: the germ theory of disease and the discovery of general anesthesia. These advances were essential steps for the forthcoming and even greater achievements of scientific medicine in the 20th Century.

As we have seen, the Renaissance was a giant step forward in the acquisition of medical knowledge, but within the context of medical history, it represented the placement of just one of the blocks (albeit a giant one) in building the pyramid of medical knowledge. From the intuitive medicine of primitive society to the scientific medicine of today, the Renaissance represented a spectacular moment. . . .

▲

Comparative Drawings

LEONARDO DA VINCI AND ANDREAS VESALIUS

Some of the most important advances in medical knowledge during the Renaissance were in anatomy, a field in which little had changed throughout the Middle Ages. In part because human dissections were uncommon in medieval medical schools, not much had been done to develop knowledge beyond Galen's teachings. One of the first individuals to portray the human body more accurately was not a man of medicine, but rather a true Renaissance scholar and artist: Leonardo da Vinci. His Sketchbooks, *which predate any changes in medical textbooks, reveal considerable detail of skeletal and muscular structures. Da Vinci's famous masterpieces were based on his dissections of both animals and human cadavers, the work of a man of science as well as of the arts. Although his drawings of internal organs contain inaccuracies, many of his sketches are extremely accurate and detailed.*

The Sketchbooks *were not published until long after da Vinci's death; nevertheless, they point the way toward increasingly accurate anatomical knowledge in the service of fine art. Less than thirty years after his death, a professor of surgery at the University at Padua, Andreas Vesalius, published one of the most important anatomical texts in medical history:* De Humani Corporis Fabrica (On the Fabric of the Human Body; *1543). The extremely detailed and accurate drawings in the seven books composing the* Fabrica *are works of art as much as scientific illustrations. Many are based on preliminary sketches by Vesalius, although the identity of the actual artists responsible for these drawings is still controversial. The text is Vesalius's and was produced on the recently invented printing press, while the corresponding illustrations were done as woodcuts. The* Fabrica *and its accompanying volume, the* Epitome, *rapidly became the definitive anatomical textbooks used by university-educated physicians.*

Rather than a reproduction of text from the Sketchbooks *and the* Fabrica, *this selection is a study in contrasts: Plates from da Vinci and Vesalius demonstrate the different ways of portraying human anatomy. The reader is encouraged to compare the works of these two authors in terms of both accuracy and artistry, and to consider the role of art in the portrayal of the human body.*

▲

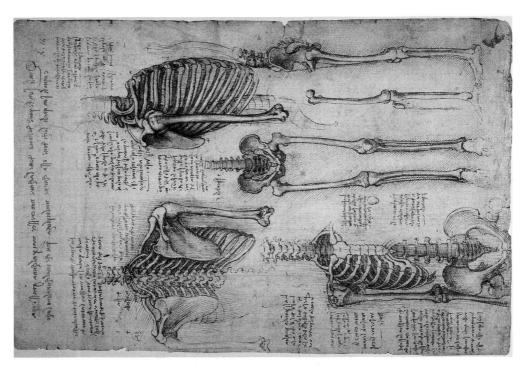

FIGURE 8–2 The Skeletal System, by da Vinci

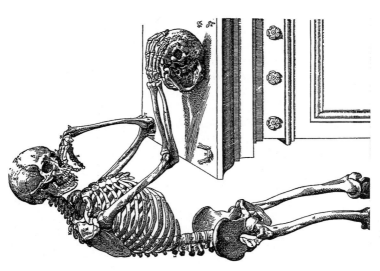

FIGURE 8–1 The Skeletal System, by Vesalius

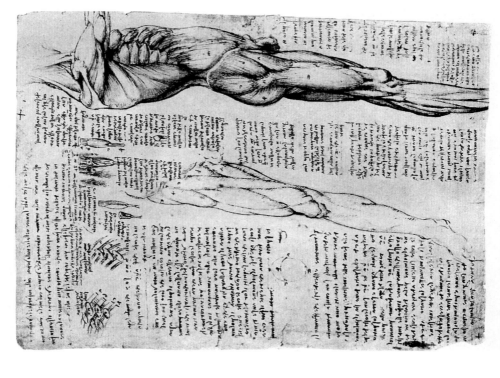

FIGURE 8–4   The Muscular System, by da Vinci

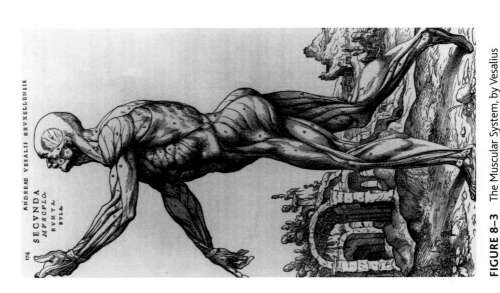

FIGURE 8–3   The Muscular System, by Vesalius

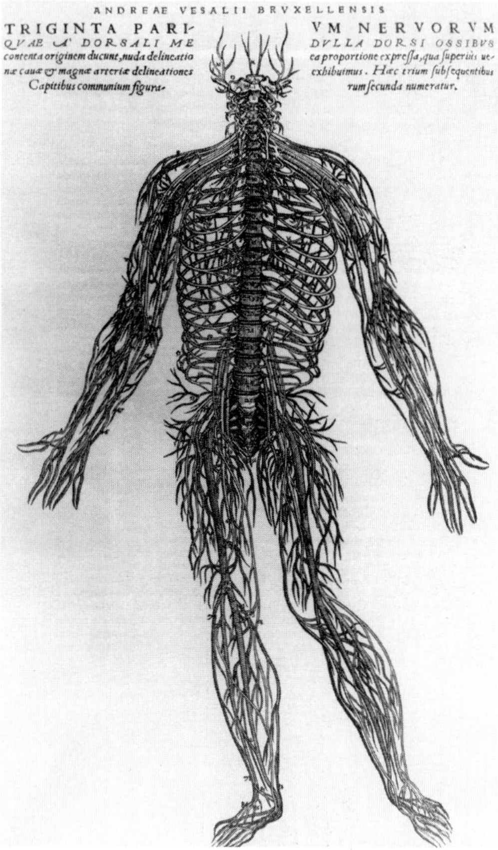

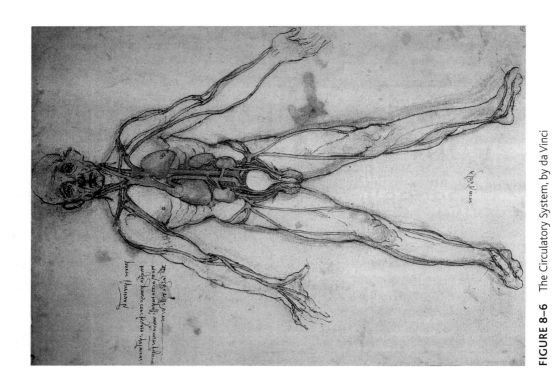

FIGURE 8–6   The Circulatory System, by da Vinci

FIGURE 8–5   The Circulatory System, by Vesalius

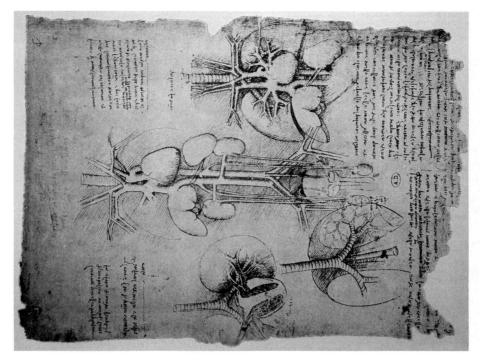

FIGURE 8–8 The Internal Organs, by da Vinci. [The heart and the circulation, facsimile of the Windsor book (pen and ink on paper), Vinci, Leonardo da (1452–1519)(after)/Bibliotheque des Arts Decoratifs, Paris, France, Archives Charmet/Bridgeman Art Library.]

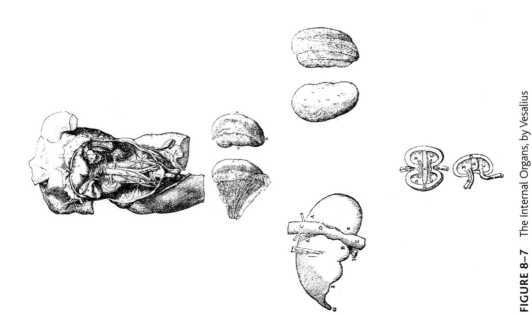

FIGURE 8–7 The Internal Organs, by Vesalius

▲

On the Motion of the Heart and Blood in Animals

WILLIAM HARVEY

Another discovery that modernized anatomy and physiology and contradicted Galen's established teachings was William Harvey's revelations about the circulation of blood, published in his De Motu Cordis *in 1628. Revolutionary as his findings were, Harvey's statement that blood is conserved and circulates throughout the entire body was based on solid scientific observation. Although challenges to Galen's model of the movement of blood had been posed earlier, none was accepted until Harvey provided a comprehensive model for circulation that was measurable and repeatable across species lines. Nevertheless, his work was not immediately accepted; in fact, it was violently attacked by the medical establishment for decades after its publication. Eventually, it was recognized as accurate, and William Harvey remains one of the most important figures in the history of physiology.*

▲

CHAPTER VIII

Of the Quantity of Blood Passing Through the Heart from the Veins to the Arteries; and of the Circular Motion of the Blood

Thus far I have spoken of the passage of the blood from the veins into the arteries, and of the manner in which it is transmitted and distributed by the action of the heart; points to which some, moved either by the authority of Galen or Columbus, or the reasonings of others, will give in their adhesion. But what remains to be said upon the quantity and source of the blood which thus passes is of a character so novel and unheard-of that I not only fear injury to myself from the envy of a few, but I tremble lest I have mankind at large for my enemies, so much doth wont and custom become a second nature. Doctrine once sown strikes deep its root, and respect for antiquity influences all men. Still the die is cast, and my trust is in my love of truth and the candour of cultivated minds. And sooth to say, when I surveyed my mass of evidence, whether derived from vivisections, and my various reflections on them, or from the study of the ventricles of the heart and the vessels that enter into and issue from them, the symmetry and size of these conduits,—for nature doing nothing in vain, would never have given them so large a relative size without a purpose,—or from observing the arrangement and intimate structure of the valves in particular, and of the other parts of the heart in general, with many things besides, I frequently and seriously bethought me, and long revolved in my mind, what might be the quantity of blood which was transmitted, in how short a time its passage might be effected, and the like. But not finding it possible that this could be supplied by the juices of the ingested aliment without the veins on the one hand becoming drained, and the arteries on the other getting ruptured through the excessive charge of blood, unless the blood should somehow find its way from the arteries into the veins, and so return to the right side of the heart, I began to think whether there might not be a MOTION, AS IT WERE, IN A CIRCLE. Now, this I afterwards found to be true; and I finally saw that the blood, forced by the action

From *On the Motion of the Heart and Blood in Animals* by William Harvey, trans. by Robert Willis (Arnherst, NY: Prometheus Books). Published 1993.

of the left ventricle into the arteries, was distributed to the body at large, and its several parts, in the same manner as it is sent through the lungs, impelled by the right ventricle into the pulmonary artery, and that it then passed through the veins and along the vena cava, and so round to the left ventricle in the manner already indicated. This motion we may be allowed to call circular, in the same way as Aristotle says that the air and the rain emulate the circular motion of the superior bodies; for the moist earth, warmed by the sun, evaporates; the vapours drawn upwards are condensed, and descending in the form of rain, moisten the earth again. By this arrangement are generations of living things produced; and in like manner are tempests and meteors engendered by the circular motion, and by the approach and recession of the sun.

And similarly does it come to pass in the body, through the motion of the blood, that the various parts are nourished, cherished, quickened by the warmer, more perfect, vaporous, spirituous, and, as I may say, alimentive blood; which, on the other hand, owing to its contact with these parts, becomes cooled, coagulated, and so to speak effete. It then returns to its sovereign, the heart, as if to its source, or to the inmost home of the body, there to recover its state of excellence or perfection. Here it renews its fluidity, natural heat, and becomes powerful, fervid, a kind of treasury of life, and impregnated with spirits, it might be said with balsam. Thence it is again dispersed. All this depends on the motion and action of the heart.

The heart, consequently, is the beginning of life; the sun of the microcosm, even as the sun in his turn might well be designated the heart of the world; for it is the heart by whose virtue and pulse the blood is moved, perfected, and made nutrient, and is preserved from corruption and coagulation; it is the household divinity which, discharging its function, nourishes, cherishes, quickens the whole body, and is indeed the foundation of life, the source of all action. But of these things we shall speak more opportunely when we come to speculate upon the final cause of this motion of the heart.

As the blood-vessels, therefore, are the canals and agents that transport the blood, they are of two kinds, the cava and the aorta; and this not by reason of there being two sides of the body, as Aristotle has it, but because of the difference of office, not, as is commonly said, in consequence of any diversity of structure, for in many animals, as I have said, the vein does not differ from the artery in the thickness of its walls, but solely in virtue of their distinct functions and uses. A vein and an artery, both styled veins by the ancients, and that not without reason, as Galen has remarked, for the artery is the vessel which carries the blood from the heart to the body at large, the vein of the present day bringing it back from the general system to the heart; the former is the conduit from, the latter the channel to, the heart; the latter contains the cruder, effete blood, rendered unfit for nutrition; the former transmits the digested, perfect, peculiarly nutritive fluid. . . .

▲

The Apologie and Treatise

AMBROISE PARÉ

Gunpowder was a relatively new invention for Europeans when Ambroise Paré served as a military surgeon. Although his assumptions about the origin of gunpowder were incorrect, Paré well understood the dangers of the wounds that it caused. He did not believe the accepted theory, however, that it was a poisonous substance that had to be burned out of the wound

Reprinted from Geoffrey Keynes, ed., *The Apologie and Treatise of Ambroise Paré* (New York: Dover, 1968), 137–38.

by application of either boiling oil or a red-hot iron. One day when the fighting was so severe that his supplies were limited, Paré tried an alternative method of wound treatment that proved far gentler to the patient. Although his method met stiff resistance from other surgeons, Paré became famous for its use. He has been called "The Father of Modern Surgery" for a number of new ideas and procedures—from the use of prostheses to new methods of wound surgery—always implemented in his effort to modernize and improve on obsolete methods.

▲

Part II: Surgical Writings

Of Wounds Made by Gunshot, Other Fierie Engines, and All Sorts of Weapons

The First Discourse Wherein Wounds Made by Gunshot Are Freed from Being Burnt or Cauterized According to Vigoes Methode

In the yeare of our Lord 1536. *Francis* the French King, for his acts in warre and peace stiled the Great, sent a puissant Army beyond the Alpes, under the governement and leading of *Annas* of Mommorancie high Constable of France, both that he might releeve *Turin* with victualls, souldiers, and all things needefull, as also to recover the Citties of that Province taken by the Marquis of *Guast* Generall of the Emperours forces. I was in the Kings Army the Chirurgion of Monsieur of *Montejan* Generall of the foote. The Imperialists had taken the straits of *Suze,* the Castle of *Villane,* and all the other passages; so that the Kings army was not able to drive them from their fortifications but by fight. In this conflict there were many wounded on both sides with all sorts of weapons, but cheefely with bullets. I will tell the truth, I was not very expert at that time in matters of Chirurgery; neither was I used to dresse wounds made by Gunshot. Now I had read in *John de Vigo* that wounds made by Gunshot were venenate or

poisoned, and that by reason of the Gunpouder; Wherefore for their cure, it was expedient to burne or cauterize them with oyle of Elders scalding hot, with a little Treacle mixed therewith. But for that I gave no great credite neither to the author, nor remedy, because I knew that causticks could not be powred into wounds, without excessive paine; I, before I would runne a hazard, determined to see whether the Chirurgions, who went with me in the army, used any other manner of dressing to these wounds. I observed and saw that all of them used that Method of dressing which *Vigo* prescribes; and that they filled as full as they could, the wounds made by Gunshot with Tents and **pledgets** dipped in this scalding Oyle, at the first dressings; which encouraged me to doe the like to those, who came to be dressed of me. It chanced on a time, that by reason of the multitude that were hurt, I wanted this Oyle. Now because there were some few left to be dressed, I was forced, that I might seeme to want nothing, and that I might not leave them undrest, to apply a digestive made of the yolke of an egge, oyle of Roses, and Turpentine. I could not sleepe all that night, for I was troubled in minde, and the dressing of the precedent day, (which I judged unfit) troubled my thoughts; and I feared that the next day I should finde them dead, or at the point of death by the poyson of the wound, whom I had not dressed with the scalding oyle. Therefore I rose early in the morning, I visited my patients, and beyound expectation, I found such as I had dressed with a digestive onely, free from vehemencie of paine to have had good rest, and that their wounds were not inflamed, nor turnifyed; but on the contrary the others that were burnt with the scalding oyle were feaverish, tormented with much paine, and the parts about their wounds were swolne. When I had many times tryed this in divers others, I thought thus much, that neither I nor any other should ever cauterize any wounded with Gun-shot. . . .

▲

An Inquiry into the Causes and Effects of the Variolae Vaccinae . . . Known by the Name of Cow Pox

EDWARD JENNER

One of the few pathogens that attack only humans, with no other hosts or vectors, smallpox is highly contagious and carries a high mortality rate. It was apparently a fairly mild disease in Europe until a virulent form made it far more serious in the early seventeenth century. Before then, it was the disease most responsible for the decimation of the Native American peoples and others when they first came into contact with Europeans, because they had no acquired immunity to the disease. Although officially eradicated in the 1970s, smallpox remains a deadly potential weapon in the new era of biowarfare.

Edward Jenner, a rural English doctor, observed in 1796 that people who had been infected with a less severe disease called cowpox *did not become infected with smallpox when they were exposed to it. He kept careful case notes of a number of such individuals and deduced that giving a person a case of cowpox, what we now call a* vaccination, *immunized them against smallpox. Although he was wrong about the origin of cowpox, believing that it came from an equine disease, his conclusions were undoubtedly correct. Within a few years of the publication of his* Inquiry into the Causes and Effects of the Variolae Vaccinae *in 1798, vaccination replaced the far riskier procedure of inoculation, which involved the use of live smallpox matter, and rapidly became widespread. Edward Jenner is one of a small handful of individuals who may be said to have prevented the deaths of millions of future individuals from a killer disease.*

▲

. . . There is a disease to which the Horse, from his state of domestication, is frequently subject. The Farriers have termed it *the Grease*. It is an inflammation and swelling in the heel, from which issues matter possessing properties of a very peculiar kind, which seems capable of generating a disease in the Human Body (after it has undergone the modification which I shall presently speak of), which bears so strong a resemblance to the Small Pox, that I think it highly probable it may be the source of that disease.

In this Dairy Country a great number of Cows are kept, and the office of milking is performed indiscriminately by Men and Maid

Reprinted with permission from Edward Jenner, *An Inquiry into the Causes and Effects of the Variolae Vaccinae* (*1798*). The Classics of Medicine Library. New York: Gryphon Editions, 1976.

Servants. One of the former having been appointed to apply dressings to the heels of a Horse affected with *the Grease,* and not paying due attention to cleanliness, incautiously bears his part in milking the Cows, with some particles of the infectious matter adhering to his fingers. When this is the case, it commonly happens that a disease is communicated to the Cows, and from the Cows to the Dairy-maids, which spreads through the farm until most of the cattle and domestics feel its unpleasant consequences. This disease has obtained the name of the Cow Pox. It appears on the nipples of the Cows in the form of irregular pustules. At their first appearance they are commonly of a palish blue, or rather of a colour somewhat approaching to livid, and are surrounded by an **erysipelatous** inflammation. These pustules, unless a timely remedy be applied, frequently degenerate into **phagedenic** ulcers, which prove extremely troublesome. The animals become indisposed, and the secretion of milk is much lessened. Inflamed spots now begin to appear on different parts of the hands of the domestics employed in milking, and sometimes on the wrists, which quickly run on to suppuration, first assuming the *appearance* of the small vesications produced by a burn. Most commonly they appear about the joints of the fingers, and at their extremities; but whatever parts are affected, if the situation will admit, these superficial suppurations put on a circular form, with their edges more elevated than their centre, and of a colour distantly approaching to blue. Absorption takes place, and tumours appear in each **axilla.** The system becomes affected—the pulse is quickened; and shiverings, with general lassitude and pains about the loins and limbs, with vomiting, come on. The head is painful, and the patient is now and then even affected with delirium. These symptoms, varying in their degrees of violence, generally continue from one day to three or four, leaving ulcerated sores about the hands, which, from the sensibility of the parts, are very troublesome, and commonly heal slowly, frequently becom-

ing phagedenic, like those from whence they sprung. The lips, nostrils, eyelids, and other parts of the body, are sometimes affected with sores; but these evidently arise from their being needlessly rubbed or scratched with the patient's infected fingers. No eruptions on the skin have followed the decline of the feverish symptoms in any instance that has come under my inspection, one only excepted, and in this case a very few appeared on the arms: they were very minute, of a vivid red colour, and soon died away without advancing to maturation; so that I cannot determine whether they had any connection with the preceding symptoms.

Thus the disease makes its progress from the Horse to the nipple of the Cow, and from the Cow to the Human Subject.

Morbid matter of various kinds, when absorbed into the system, may produce effects in some degree similar; but what renders the Cow-pox virus so extremely singular, is, that the person who has been thus affected is for ever after secure from the infection of the Small Pox; neither exposure to the variolous effluvia, nor the insertion of the matter into the skin, producing this distemper. . . .

CASE II

Sarah Portlock, of this place, was infected with the Cow Pox, when a Servant at a Farmer's in the neighbourhood, twenty-seven years ago.

In the year 1792, conceiving herself, from this circumstance, secure from the infection of the Small Pox, she nursed one of her own children who had accidentally caught the disease, but no indisposition ensued. —During the time she remained in the infected room, variolous matter was inserted into both her arms, but without any further effect than [an **efflorescence** only, taking on an erysipelatous look about the centre, appearing on the skin near the punctured parts]. . . .

CASE VI

It is a fact so well known among our Dairy Farmers, that those who have had the Small Pox either escape the Cow Pox or are disposed to have it slightly; that as soon as the complaint shews itself among the cattle, assistants are procured, if possible, who are thus rendered less susceptible of it, otherwise the business of the farm could scarcely go forward.

In the month of May, 1796, the Cow Pox broke out at Mr. Baker's, a Farmer who lives near this place. The disease was communicated by means of a cow which was purchased in an infected state at a neighbouring fair, and not one of the Farmer's cows (consisting of thirty) which were at that time milked escaped the contagion. The family consisted of a man servant, two dairymaids, and a servant boy, who, with the Farmer himself, were twice a day employed in milking the cattle. The whole of this family, except Sarah Wynne, one of the dairymaids, had gone through the Small Pox. The consequence was, that the Farmer and the servant boy escaped the infection of the Cow Pox entirely, and the servant man and one of the maid servants had each of them nothing more than a sore on one of their fingers, which produced no disorder in the system. But the other dairymaid, Sarah Wynne, who never had the Small Pox, did not escape in so easy a manner. She caught the complaint from the cows, and was affected with the symptoms described [previously] in so violent a degree, that she was confined to her bed, and rendered incapable for several days of pursuing her ordinary vocations in the farm.

March 28th, 1797, I inoculated this girl, and carefully rubbed the variolous matter into two slight incisions made upon the left arm. A little inflammation appeared in the usual manner around the parts where the matter was inserted, but so early as the fifth day it vanished entirely without producing any effect on the system. . . .

CASE XVII

The more accurately to observe the progress of the infection, I selected a healthy boy, about eight years old, for the purpose of inoculation for the Cow Pox. The matter was taken from a sore on the hand of a dairymaid, who was infected by her master's cows, and it was inserted, on the 14th of May, 1796, into the arm of the boy by means of two superficial incisions, barely penetrating the cutis, each about half an inch long.

On the seventh day he complained of uneasiness in the axilla, and on the ninth he became a little chilly, lost his appetite, and had a slight head-ach. During the whole of this day he was perceptibly indisposed, and spent the night with some degree of restlessness, but on the day following he was perfectly well.

The appearance of the incisions in their progress to a state of maturation were much the same as when produced in a similar manner by variolous matter. The only difference which I perceived was, in the state of the limpid fluid arising from the action of the virus, which assumed rather a darker hue, and in that of the efflorescence spreading round the incisions, which had more of an erysipelatous look than we commonly perceive when variolous matter has been made use of in the same manner; but the whole died away (leaving on the inoculated parts scabs and subsequent eschars) without giving me or my patient the least trouble.

In order to ascertain whether the boy, after feeling so slight an affection of the system from the Cow-pox virus, was secure from the contagion of the Small-pox, he was inoculated the 1st of July following with variolous matter, immediately taken from a pustule. Several slight punctures and incisions were made on both his arms, and the matter was carefully inserted, but no disease followed. The same appearances were observable on the arms as we commonly see when a patient has had variolous matter applied, after having either the Cow-pox or the Small-pox. Several months afterwards, he was again inoculated with variolous matter, but no sensible effect was produced on the constitution. . . .

⋏

Why Can't a Woman Be More Like a Man? A Renaissance Perspective on the Biological Basis for Female Inferiority

Michael T. Walton, PhD, Robert M. Fineman, MD, PhD, and Phyllis J. Walton, JD

Aristotle's declaration that woman is a defective and inferior form of man was widely believed throughout Europe until the eighteenth century. Galen in turn had adopted the same statement, giving medical support to the cultural belief of the inferiority of women. Even during the Renaissance, when old ideas were routinely disproved and displaced by modern theories, these old Aristotelian-Galenic statements were not challenged. In the sixteenth century, however, the theory was refined somewhat, so that the belief was that some females could go beyond their gender identity and become men. The era of the "rebirth" of knowledge clearly did not include challenging the theory of the naturally superior male and the inferior female.

⋏

In Greek legend, Teiresias, a male, was turned into a female and then back into a male. As a born again male, he testified that women have more joy in sex. His testimony on the joy of being a woman notwithstanding, the written record from the ancient world through the Renaissance assumed that women were inferior to men. Plato . . . in his *Timaeus* taught that cowardly or immoral men were reborn as women. St. Paul who died circa 66 CE, set the tone for Christianity by stating, "Let your women keep silence in the churches . . . they are commanded to be under obedience . . . and if they will learn anything, let them ask their husbands at home. . . ." Western Europeans justified the assumption of female inferiority with biomedical doctrines that passed from the Greeks through the Middle Ages to the Renaissance. As in so many things, Renaissance thinkers built, with some originality, on received biological notions concerning women.

I

A point of departure for biological ideas of female inferiority is Aristotle's . . . *Generation of Animals.* For Aristotle, generation was analogous to baking in an oven. The amount of heat and moisture involved determined the quality of the finished product. In a discussion of human generation, Aristotle posited that the "female takes longer to develop" in the womb because the female is colder by nature. After parturition, the female develops more quickly due to her colder nature; that is, she has less to develop because her organs remain internalized. The female deficiency of heat is what prevents her from becoming the perfect form intended by nature: a male. The failure of the female to fully realize her "telos" or true end, meant that "we should look upon the female state as being, as it were, a deformity, though one which occurs in the ordinary course of nature." Of course, this is quite opposite to our contemporary understanding of sex differentiation, which is based on active biochemical steps needed for male differentiation. In our modern view, men are deviations from the female.

Aristotle presented his biological ideas of female inferiority within the context of the doctrine of vital heat that was almost universally accepted by Graeco-Roman physicians and persisted until it was discarded in the eighteenth century. Ancient Greek schools of medicine, whether Hippocratic or Methodist, relied on qualitative explanations of physiological function. Each individual had a temperament based on a combination of qualities. Apparently no ancient medical school rejected Aristotle's characterization of the human female as "colder" than the male. Indeed, Galen . . . , the prince of ancient physicians, elaborated ideas of female inferiority within his highly developed system of physiology that was based on extensive anatomical research.

Galen taught that the female, because of her smaller size and internal, less perfect, testes generated "a scantier, colder, and wetter" semen. "The Creator, in his wisdom" made the female less perfect than the male because her interior organs ensured that generation could take place. Given that Galen disagreed with Aristotle on many points (e.g., he disproved Aristotle's notion that intellect resides in the heart by demonstrating that the brain controls the nervous system), Galen's agreement with *the* Philosopher on the nature of the female, however, ensured the acceptance of the idea that the female is a defective male.

II

Throughout the Middle Ages, theologians placed women below men. As clerics were influenced by the philosophy of Aristotle, his explanation of the defective physical nature of females was integrated into a religious understanding of the inferior nature of women. In his *Summa Theologiae,* Thomas Aquinas . . . stated that the active reproductive force—the male—seeks to create its perfect likeness. Only a weakness in the male force, or the

material upon which it works, prevents the perfect realization and creates a female.

If Aquinas, in a religious work, used physiological terms to explain the inferiority of women, physicians attached no comparable theological language to their descriptions of the female and her nature. Medieval medicine was thoroughly Aristotelian-Galenic in its language and doctrines, despite the fact that most of Galen's anatomical works were unavailable until the fourteenth century and later. The cold nature of the female was a given, and was important primarily in explaining reproduction and female diseases. Organ function and the role of bodily fluids were described in terms of qualities and attractive or expulsive virtues. Thus, testes are described as hot and moist in the thirteenth century *Anatomie Nicolai,* while the uterus is cold and dry. Because the left side of the body is colder than the right side, males generated by the left testis or in the left side of the uterus will be weak or effeminate.

Soon after its rediscovery in the later Middle Ages, Galen's *On the Usefulness of Parts* became readily available in Latin. The anatomical portions of Guy de Chauliac's . . . surgical treatise, the *Inventarium,* provided a detailed condensation of Galen's teachings which made physicians and surgeons more sophisticated anatomically. However, the qualities and functions of the heart, liver, brain, testes, uterus, etc., while more detailed, in no way contradicted the received wisdom of the past. Surgeons and physicians were taught to understand that repair of the body and healing came through restoration of qualitative humoral balance. Therefore, the high medieval medical tradition was a passing on of ancient ideas and their consolidation with ancillary information from earlier and contemporary authors. This did nothing to change the intellectual perception of the status of women.

III

The Aristotelian-Galenic notion of female inferiority passed into the Renaissance from the Middle Ages and also directly from rediscovered ancient texts. The popular collection of medieval medical tracts printed as the *Fasciculus Medicinae* in Venice in 1491 stated unequivocally that "nature always intends to make a male and never a female, for the female is an accidentally defective male and a monster of nature as is clear in the book [Aristotle's] *On Animals*. . . . " The *Fasciculus* sits squarely in the medieval tradition, but its use of Aristotle does not differ essentially from that of the sixteenth century Aristotelian humanist Andreas Cesalpino. . . .

Like other orthodox physicians, Cesalpino, most noted for his pre-Harvean doctrine of diurnal circulation of the blood, viewed the female sexual organs as internalized male organs. In his *Artis medica* . . . , he wrote, "the husband's testicles and generative organ extend from without, while the woman's are situated within . . . the testes and the seminal vessels are like the horns of the uterus." Furthermore he notes that "the woman's temperament is cold and humid, which if lessened and the spirit depressed, creates an ambiguous girl or an effeminate male called an Hermaphrodite." . . .

Indeed, the perceived difference in male and female temperament which resulted in the production of external (perfect) or internal (imperfect) genitalia was so common that it is found in virtually every discussion of sex difference. This is due in no small measure to Galen's and Aristotle's agreement on the qualitative aspects of the male and female natures. That agreement was not only seen in the works of *the* Philosopher and *the* Physician, but also in digests of their works by Renaissance scholars. Nicholas Regia's epitome of Galen's *On the Usefulness of Parts,* which was prepared for medical students, points to female inferiority in a marginal note and in the text. "The female, however, is less perfect, primarily because she is colder . . . the female's testes are lesser and imperfect, and the seed in them is sparse, being cold and moist."

IV

In the sixteenth century, a fascinating change occurred in medical discussions regarding the development of males and females. Observations buttressed assertions. Before, it had been sufficient to assert that females were males who were not quite "finished" due to their lack of vital heat. Now we see reports of "cases" of women going beyond their femaleness and becoming males.

Ambrose Paré . . . , in his treatise on monsters, reports four cases of women who developed into men. Three cases were contemporary, one observed by Paré himself, and one was found in Pliny the Elder. . . . The first case drawn from Amatus Lusitanus . . . was of Maria Pateca who, *at the appointed age for her courses to flow, had instead of them a man's yard {penis}, laying before {that} time hid and covered, so that of a woman she became a man; and therefore laying aside her woman's habite, was cloathed in man's, and changeing her name, was called Emanuel . . . and married a wife; but Lusitanus saith he did not certainly know whether he had anie children.*

The second case was reported by a royal official Anthonie Loqueneux who said that in 1560 he saw a man in Reimes *who was taken for a woman until the fourteenth year of his age; for then it happened as he played somewhat wantonly with a maid which laie in the same bed with him, his members (hitherto lying hid) started forth and unfolded themselves: which when his parents knew (by the help of Ecclesiastick power) they changed his name from Joan to John, and put him in men's apparel.*

Paré recalled that while he served the court of Charles IX, he met a man named Germane Garnierus "but by some [in jest or in ridicule?] Germane Maria (because in times when he was a woman he was called Marie)" *who was taken for a girl until the fifteenth year of his age, whilest he . . . pursued hogs . . . he leaped violently over a ditch, whereby it came to pass that the states and foldings beeing broken, his hidden members suddenly broke forth, but not without pain; going home, he weeping complained to his mother that his guts came forth . . . the whole business being brought before the Cardinal Bishop of Lenucure, an assemblie being called, he received the name and habite of a man.*

Paré found in Pliny the Elder an account of the child of a man named Cassinus who was born a girl and became a boy, but that the soothsayers had him removed to a "desert island because they thought such monsters did alwaies shew or portend some monstrous thing."

V

From a modern medical perspective, we believe that Paré's cases are examples of a well-documented condition called female **peripubertal virilization** secondary to **hyperandrogenism**. This belief is, of course, tentative because of the terse nature of Paré's reports. In hyperandrogenism, the increased production of male hormone in affected females may be caused by more than a half dozen different conditions. Most cases involve increased androgen production in the ovaries, adrenal glands, or in both glands. Some of the more common underlying causes are simple virilizing adrenal **hyperplasia,** sex chromosome abnormalities associated with abnormal gonadal development and function, polycystic ovaries, and adrenocortical and ovarian tumors.

As normal sex differentiation in humans is followed by growth and development after birth, individuals who would normally continue as females take on male characteristics as androgen levels increase. Their anatomy, biochemistry, and physiology become "out of sync." This is due to the fact that females develop in the absence of testicular hormones, but retain the potential in the presence of such hormones to respond and develop the male characteristics Paré and Pliny the Elder described. We presume that these cases represent females with peripubertal virilization and not hermaphrodites because: (a) they occurred at puberty, and (b) Renaissance medicine was well aware of hermaphrodites. Paré and his contemporaries described many hermaphrodites, and in a society that knew of alchemical hermaphroditic images such a defect was almost always noted at birth. As Paré does not report any question of genital abnormalities until puberty, we are comfortable with our assumption. However, we cannot be totally sure in lieu of more precise data which will never be available.

Given our assumption of the diagnosis of peripubertal virilization and without going into a lengthy discussion on hyperandrogenism found in modern texts, one further observation can be made. None of Paré's case reports state that the girls who turned into men became fully functioning, fertile males. This is consistent with modern scientific doctrines. While these girls may have suffered from acute and/or chronic testosterone overproduction, at least they did not pass it on to their children because they most likely functioned as infertile males.

VI

Returning to Paré and his time, it appears that Paré did not need to await modern medical theory to explain his cases. He found them quite intelligible in the context of Renaissance medicine. He wrote, *Certainly women have so manie and like parts lying in their womb, as men have hanging forth; . . . onely a strong and livilie heat seem's to be wanting, which may drive forth that which lie's hid within: therefore in {the} process of time, the heat being increased and flourishing, and the humiditie (which is predominant in childhood) overcome, it is not impossible that the virile members . . . may be put forth; especially if to that strength of the growing heat som vehement concussion or jactation of the bodie be joined.*

Traditional ideas of qualities, vital heat, and anatomical analogues were combined by Paré to explain in natural, biomedical terms how women became men. The upshot of the cases, however, was a proof of Aristotle's contention that women are but defective males. Paré ends his discussion, *Therefore, I think it manifest by these experiments and reasons; that it is not fabulous that some women have been changed into men: but you shall finde, in no historie men, that have degenerated into women; for nature alwaies intends and goes from the imperfect to the more perfect, but not basely from the more perfect to the imperfect.*

Conclusion

The traditional biological doctrine of female inferiority found strong proof in Paré's study of females who turned into males. Without access to modern genetic-endocrinological knowledge, Paré's cases seem to have no other solution. Indeed, before recent Swedish surgical innovations, there was no instance of men "degenerating" into women. For the Renaissance and beyond, women were destined to be viewed as defective men and, therefore, inferior because the doctrines and observations of science, religion, and philosophy offered no other "reasonable" explanation.

Key Terms

Axilla, 172 • Efflorescence, 172 • Erysipelatous, 172 • Hyperandrogenism, 177 • Hyperplasia, 177 • Iatrochemistry, 160 • Peripubertal virilization, 177 • Phagedenic, 172 • Pledgets, 170 • Puerperal, 162

Questions to Consider

1. Examine the drawings of da Vinci and Vesalius closely. What differences do you see, both in technique and in the portrayal of the anatomy? Can you spot any errors? What would explain the differences between the two artists?(*Remember:* Vesalius was not the artist who drew these plates.)

2. A clear prejudice against women existed in Renaissance medicine. Given the advances in anatomical knowledge at the time, how can we explain the continued adherence to the ideas of Aristotle and others in an era of pursuit of new knowledge?

3. Making a list of accomplishments and discoveries that occurred in science and medicine during this period is easy. However, in medicine, the "bottom line" is patients and their care. How much difference in the actual treatment of trauma and illness do you think these developments made at the time? Which of these men whose writings we have studied would have had an impact on medical care? Why did all these advances not have a greater impact at the time?

4. "I dressed him and God healed him," said Paré about his astounding results of less-drastic wound care. Were Renaissance and early modern science and medicine still inextricably linked to a magicoreligious belief system? Or, was Paré just being extremely humble? Do modern researchers announcing a major breakthrough react as he did?

5. Unquestionably, Edward Jenner's discovery of the vaccination against smallpox was one of the most outstanding advances of the eighteenth century. His *Inquiry* describes a careful set of clinical trials of his method on human patients, many of them children. How would his methodology be critized today? Would it have even been possible in modern research? Why or why not?

Recommended Readings

Leonardo da Vinci

Belt, Elmer. *Leonardo the Anatomist.* New York: Greenwood Press, 1969.
Crispino, Enrica, ed. *Leonardo: Art and Science.* Firenze, Italy: Giunti, 2000.
Mathe, Jean. *Leonardo da Vinci: Anatomical Drawings.* Geneva, Switzerland: Liber, 1984.
O'Malley, Charles D. *Leonardo da Vinci on the Human Body: The Anatomical, Physiological and Embryological Drawings of Leonardo da Vinci.* New York: Gramercy Books, 2003.

William Harvey

Bylebyl, Jerome J. *William Harvey and His Age: The Professional and Social Context of the Discovery of the Circulation.* Baltimore: Johns Hopkins University Press, 1979.

Gregory, Andrew. *Harvey's Heart: The Discovery of Blood Circulation.* Cambridge, UK: Icon Books, 2001.

Keynes, Geoffrey. *A Bibliography of the Writings of Dr. William Harvey, 1578–1657.* 3rd ed. Winchester, UK: Norman, 1989.

Edward Jenner

Adler, Robert E. *Medical Firsts: From Hippocrates to the Human Genome.* Hoboken, NJ: Wiley, 2004.

Barzin, H. *The Eradication of Smallpox: Edward Jenner and the First and Only Eradication of a Human Infectious Disease.* San Diego: Academic Press, 2000.

Saunders, Paul. *Edward Jenner: The Cheltenham Years, 1795–1823: Being a Chronicle of the Vaccination Campaign.* Hanover, NH: University Press of New England, 1982.

James Lind

Lind, James. *A Treatise on the Scurvy.* 3rd ed. Birmingham, AL: Gryphon Editions, 1980.

Paracelsus (Philippus Aureolus Theophrastus Bombastus von Hohenheim)

Debus, Allen G. *The French Paracelsians: The Chemical Challenge to Medical and Scientific Tradition in Early Modern France.* Cambridge: Cambridge University Press, 1991.

Grell, Ole Peter. *Paracelsus: The Man and His Reputation, His Ideas and Their Transformation.* Leiden, the Netherlands: Brill, 1998.

Pagel, Walter. *Paracelsus: An Introduction to Philosophical Medicine in the Era of the Renaissance.* 2nd ed. Basel, Switzerland: Karger, 1982.

Scholz, William Gerhild. *Parcelsian Moments: Science, Medicine, and Astrology in Early Modern Europe.* Kirksville, MO: Truman State University Press, 2002.

Temkin, C. Lilian. *Four Treatises of Theophrastus von Hohenheim, Called Paracelsus,* Baltimore: Johns Hopkins University Press, 1941.

Ambroise Paré

Hamby, Wallace B. *Ambroise Paré: Surgeon of the Renaissance.* St. Louis, MO: Green, 1967.

Packard, Francis R. *Life and Times of Ambroise Paré, with a New Translation of His Apology and an Account of His Journeys in Divers Places.* New York: Blom, 1971.

Paré, Ambroise. *Ten Books of Surgery, with the Magazine of Instruments Necessary for It.* Athens: University of Georgia Press, 1969.

———. *The Collected Works of Ambroise Paré.* Pound Ridge, NY: Milford House, 1968.

Andreas Vesalius

Lind, L. R. *The Epitome of Andreas Vesalius.* Cambridge, MA: MIT Press, 1969.

O'Malley, Charles D. *Andreas Vesalius of Brussels, 1514–1564.* Berkeley: University of California Press, 1964.

Saunders, J. B. *The Illustrations from the Works of Andreas Vesalius of Brussels.* New York: Dover, 1973.

Chapter Nine

Europe, 1500–1800

Health, Disease, Trauma, and Society

INTRODUCTION

The seventeenth and eighteenth centuries in Europe saw both considerable change and intransient lack of improvement in medicine. On the positive side of the equation was the development of a new interest in some aspects of public health, which resulted in attention to some of the more pressing social ills of European society. On the negative side were such matters as an extremely high infant mortality rate, reduced life expectancy, near-constant warfare on the continent, and continued waves of epidemics.

Somewhere in the middle of the tally sheet were the developments in academic medicine. A number of continued advances were made in the scientific quest for knowledge about the human body and the impact of disease and trauma on it. However, new inventions that have become nearly synonymous with medical practice—the stethoscope and the microscope—were not put into common use until the nineteenth century. The discovery of novel plants and animals in the New World brought a variety of new remedies, perhaps the most important of which was quinine for the treatment of malaria.

This rosy picture is mitigated, however, by a number of negative points about the theory and practice of medicine. The university-trained physicians became so embroiled over different theories, methodologies, and systems of medicine that they lost sight of the relationship between scientific medicine and improved medical care for people. Instead, they spent long hours vehemently arguing the pros and cons of iatrochemistry versus iatrophysics. Regardless of the ideological system, the treatment of disease became ever more drastic—such as bleeding a patient until he or she fainted from blood loss and prescribing toxic dosages of medications, to name only a few. Physicians focused on the theory of medicine to explain the value of such drastic treatments, completely overlooking the patient's health and comfort. Perhaps the only ray of hope was the teachings of Thomas Sydenham, "The English Hippocrates," who emphasized the importance of clinical medicine and patient care.

So what did these physicians' attitudes mean for the patient? The care was poorer than in the past, when supportive care, rest, and diet were the norm. Most people in Europe lived in the countryside, whereas most physicians were urban professionals. Thus, the average person was far more apt to look for help from the local midwife-herbalist, or perhaps a barber-surgeon. Even access to an apothecary was uncommon.

For the individuals unfortunate enough to be confined to a public institution such as a prison, a poorhouse, or an asylum, the situation was even more grim. Conditions were terrible, and medical care was unavailable. The eighteenth century did see improvements in this area as public health became a state concern. Conditions improved slowly in the mental hospitals, even in the prisons, but reform came slowly.

Public health issues were closely linked to the Enlightenment thinkers and to the political model of absolutism. Part of the Enlightenment focused on a search for rational explanations of disease and practical ways to prevent it. Rulers came to understand that the state's greatest asset was its people and that a healthier population was more productive, which would lead to a more powerful nation. Within this philosophical context, new attention was paid to such matters as the maternal mortality rate, the need for more hospitals and dispensaries, care for the indigent, improved urban water supply and sanitation, and even— as in Prussia—the creation of a national health system.

In the long run, such measures had a greater impact on the overall health of the European population than did the trained physicians' activities. Such changes were neither quick nor easy, but as the political elite saw a reason to support them, conditions did improve.

TIME LINE

1485 C.E.	English Sweating Sickness breaks out; reappears in 1506, 1517, and 1551; actual disease remains unknown
1489–1490	Major typhus epidemic in Europe, introduced by Spaniards returning from Cyprus
1493–1494	First European outbreak of syphilis, known as the *Great Pox*, the *Neapolitan Disease, French Disease,* and so forth; it is endemic by the seventeenth century
1510	Influenza epidemic in Europe; reappears 1557–1558, 1580
1534–1536	Jacques Cartier's exploration of the St. Lawrence River—he loses a large number of his crew to scurvy
1545	Typhus epidemic in South America kills about five hundred thousand people
1618–1648	Thirty Years' War; plague, scurvy, dysentery, and typhus kill far more people than fighting does
1625	Plague breaks out in London; more than forty thousand people die
1630	Plague in Venice kills about five hundred thousand people

1647	First recorded cases of yellow fever in the Americas; introduced with African slaves
1656	Hospital General in Paris is opened as a hospital, poorhouse, and factory
1665	The Great Plague in London—more than seventy thousand people die; the epidemic was recorded in Daniel Defoe's semifactual *Journal of the Plague Year;* ended with the Great Fire in 1666
1717	Lady Mary Montagu introduces the Turkish method of inoculation for smallpox when she returns to London
1720	Last outbreak of plague in western Europe; the last outbreak anywhere in Europe is in Moscow in 1771–1772
1721	First large-scale inoculation, or variolation, campaign in the colonies; the evidence from Boston clearly proves its success
1722	At his coronation, King Louis XV of France touched about two thousand sufferers of scrofula, believing that the primary tuberculosis of the lymph nodes could be cured by the "Royal Touch"
1724	Reverend Cotton Mather publishes *The Angel of Bethesda,* an early treatise on medicine, supporting smallpox variolation
1735	First description of pellagra, by Spanish physician Gaspar Casal
1739	First obstetrics ward in England is opened
1740	Horace Walpole, while traveling in Italy, describes in a letter "a horrid thing called mal'aria. . .," giving this name to the disease
1747	World's first clinic for sexually transmitted diseases opens, in London
1752	First general hospital in North America is opened
1753	James Lind publishes his *Treatise on the Scurvy;* lime juice is made mandatory on British naval ships in 1795
1754	University of Halle graduates the first woman with the degree of medical doctor
1770	First U.S. public mental health institution opens in Williamsburg, Virginia; the public is restricted from everyday viewing of the insane at Bedlam in London, a popular pastime
1775	General George Washington orders all his troops variolated because most of his soldiers have never been exposed to smallpox
1780	Dr. Benjamin Rush describes an outbreak of "bilious **remittent fever**" in Philadelphia, now diagnosed as dengue fever
1785–1786	First diagnosed epidemic of ergot poisoning occurs in Russia (it had probably been appearing since the fifteenth century)
1791	Phillippe Pinel's *Traité médico-philosophique sur l'aliénation mentale* advocates more humane treatment of the insane
1793	Yellow fever epidemic in Philadelphia; kills 10 percent of the population

▲

A Midwife's Tale

Martha Ballard

Since the earliest recorded times, women have performed as midwives. In addition, however, they have commonly been the village herbalists, with a great deal of knowledge about the various local herbs and other natural remedies. In fact, throughout history, the midwife was frequently the closest thing to a health-care provider that ordinary people had access to. In addition to aiding women in labor, they nursed the sick, prescribed and prepared whatever remedies they had available, sat with the dying, and attended the funerals of the dead. The midwives were also wives and mothers and had to raise their families and do all the usual domestic tasks of cooking, weaving and spinning, sewing, and washing. In short, a midwife's life was one of constant hard work. Martha Ballard, a midwife in late eighteenth-century and early nineteenth-century Maine, kept a diary in which her daily entries clearly reveal the length and breadth of her daily labors.

▲

3 6* Clear & very hot. I have been pulling flax. Mr Ballard Been to Savages about some hay.

4 7 Clear morn. I pulld flax till noon. A very severe shower of hail with thunder and Litning began at half after one continud near 1 hour. I hear it broke 130 pains of glass in fort western. Colonel Howard made me a present of 1 gallon white Rhum & 2 lb sugar on account of my atendance of his family in sickness. Peter Kenny has wounded his Legg & Bled Excesivily.

5 g Clear morn. Mr Hamlin Breakfastd here. Had some pills. I was calld at 7 O Clok to Mrs Howards to see James he being very sick with the canker Rash. Tarried all night.

6 2 I am at Mrs Howards watching with her son. Went out about day, discovered our saw mill in flames. The men at the fort went over. Found it consumd together with some plank & Bords. I tarried till Evinng. Left James Exceeding Dangerously ill. My daughter Hannah is 18 years old this day. Mrs Williams here when I came home. Hannah Cool gott Mrs Norths web out at the Loome. Mr Ballard complains of a soar throat this night. He has been to take Mr gardners hors home.

7 3 Clear. I was Calld to Mrs Howards this morning for to see her son. Find him very low. Went from Mrs Howards to see Mrs Williams. Find her very unwell. Hannah Cool is there. From thence to Joseph Fosters to see her sick Children. Find Saray & Daniel very ill. Came home went to the field & got some Cold water root. Then Calld to Mr Kenydays to see Polly. Very ill with the Canker. Gave her some of the root. I gargled her throat which gave her great Ease. Returned home after dark. Mr Ballard been to Cabesy. His throat is very soar. He gargled it with my tincture. Find relief & went to bed comfortably.

8 4 Clear. I have been to see Mary Kenida. Find her much as shee was yesterday. Was at Mr McMasters. Their Children two of them very ill.

---

*The first number indicates the day of the month, the second number the day of the week. Letters indicate Sundays.

The other 2 recovering. At Mr Williams also. Shee is some better. Hear James Howard is mending. Hannah Cool came home.

9   5   Clear. I workd about house forenoon. Was Calld to Mrs Howards to see James. Found him seemingly Expireing. Mrs Pollard there. We sett up. He revivd.

10   6   At Mrs Howards. Her son very sick. Capt Sewall & Lady sett up till half after 4. Then I rose. The Child seems revivd.

11   7   Calld from Mrs Howard to Mr McMasters to see their son William who is very low. Tarried there this night.

12   g   Loury. At Mr McMasters. Their son very sick. I sett up all night. Mrs Patin with me. The Child very ill indeed.

13   2   William McMaster Expird at 3 O Clock this morn. Mrs Patin & I laid out the Child. Poor mother, how Distressing her Case, near the hour of Labour and three Children more very sick. I sett out for home. Calld at Mrs Howards. I find her son very Low. At Mr Williams. Shee very ill indeed. Now at home. It is nine O Clok morn. I feel as if I must take some rest. I find Mr Ballard is going to Pittston on Business. Dolly is beginning to weave thee hankerchiefs. Ephraim & I went to see Mrs Williams at Evining. I find her some Better.
*death of Wm McMaster**

14   3   Clear & hott. I pikt the safron. Mrs Patten here. Mr Ballard & I & all the girls attended funeral of William McMaster. Their other Children are mending. James Howard very low. I drank Tea at Mr Pollards. Calld at Mr Porters.

15   4   Clear morn. I pulld flax the **fornon**. Rain afternoon. I am very much fatagud. Lay on the bed & rested. The two Hannahs washing. Dolly weaving. I was called to Mrs Claton in **travil** at 11 O Clok Evening.

16   5   At Mr Cowens. Put Mrs Claton to Bed with a son at 3 pm. Came to Mr Kenadays to see his wife who has a sweling under her arm. Polly is mending. I returnd as far as Mr Pollards by water. Calld from there to Winthrop to Jeremy Richards wife in Travil. Arivd about 9 o Clok Evin.
Birth Mrs Clatons son

17   6   At Mr Richards. His wife Delivered of a Daughter at 10 O Clok morn. Returned as far as Mr Pollards at 12. Walked from there. Mrs Coy buryd a dafter yesterday. Mr Stanley has a dafter Dangirous. William Wicher 2 Children also.
Birth Jeremy Richard dafter

18   7   I spun some shoe thread & went to see Mrs Williams. Shee has news her Mother is very sick. Geny Huston had a Child Born the night before last. I was Calld to James Hinkly to see his wife at 11 & 30 Evening. Went as far as Mr Weston by land, from thence by water. Find Mrs Hinkly very unwell.

19   g   At Mr Hinkleys. Shee remaind poorly till afternoon then by remedys & other means shee got Easyer. I tarried all night.

20   2   Clear. Mr Hinkly brot me to Mr Westons. I heard there that Mrs Clatons Child departed this life yesterday & that she was thot Expireing. I went back with Mr Hinkly as far as there. Shee departed this Life about 1 pm. I asisted to Lay her out. Her infant Laid in her arms. The first such instance I ever saw & the first woman that died in Child bed which I delivered. I Came home at dusk. Find my family all Comfortable. We hear that three Children Expird in Winthrop last Saterday night. Daniel Stayd at Mr Cowens.

21 3 A rainy day. I have been at home knitting.

22 4 I atended funeral of Mrs Claton & her infant. Am Enformd that Mrs Shaw has Doctor Coney with her. I calld to see James Howard find him low. Mrs North also is sick. A thunder Shower this Evinng.

23 5 I sett out to visit Joseph Fosters Children. Met Ephraim Cowen by Brooks' Barn. Calld me to see his Dafters Polly & Nabby who are sick with the rash. Find them very ill. Gave directions. Was then Calld to Mrs Shaw who has been ill some time. Put her safe to Bed with a daughter at 10 O Clok this Evinng. Shee is finely.
Birth Mr Shaws Dafter

24 6 Calld from Shaws to James Hinklys wife in travil. Put her safe to Bed with a son at 7 O Clok this morn. Left her as well as is usual for her. Came to Mr Shaws receivd 6/8. Receivd 6/8 of Mr Hinkly also. Came to Mr Cowens. Find his dafters & Jedy ill. Claton & David came inn from Sandy river. People well there. Arivd at home at 5 afternoon. Doctor Coneys wife delivrd of a dafter Last Evening at 10 O Clok.
Birth James Hinkleys son

▲

Love's the Best Doctor

L' Amour Médecin

Jean-Baptiste Molière

Despite all the dramatic advances in medical research and knowledge in Renaissance and early modern Europe, patient care seemed to deteriorate during this period. Only a tiny percentage of the population had access to a doctor—a fact that in reality might have extended these people's life span. The male, urban, university-trained physician of early modern Europe received his education in the context of what we might call "heroic" medicine, setting aside Hippocrates' famous admonition to "first, do no harm" in favor of more-drastic methods. Bleeding was standard practice for nearly every ailment, and the sicker the patient, the greater the volume of blood removed. Added to this destructive practice were the emetics, enemas, and purges used in an effort to ameliorate the patient's sufferings. Understandably, many people would not call a doctor until an astrologer had pronounced that the patient would live regardless.

French dramatist and satirist Jean-Baptiste Molière apparently had personal experience with the practice of heroic medicine, and he chose to make it the subject of his play Love's the Best Doctor *(1665). His scathing dialogue shows the doctors to be insufferable pedants who were more concerned with the size of their fees and with impressing each other than with the patient's welfare.*

▲

Reprinted by permission of Penguin Books Ltd., from Jean-Baptiste Molière, *The Miser and Other Plays,* trans. John Wood (London: Penguin Books, 1953), 181–87. Copyright © John Wood, 1953.

Scene Two
Sganarelle, Lisette

LISETTE   What do you want with four doctors, master? Isn't one enough to kill the girl off?

SGANARELLE   Be quiet, Four opinions are better than one.

LISETTE   Can't your daughter be allowed to die without the help of all those fellows?

SGANARELLE   You don't mean to suggest that doctors do people in?

LISETTE   Of course they do. I knew a man who used to maintain that you should never say such and such a person perished of a fever or pleurisy but that he died of four doctors and two apothecaries.

SGANARELLE   Be quiet! We mustn't offend these gentlemen.

LISETTE   Upon my word, master, our cat fell from the housetop into the street a while back and yet he got better. He ate nothing for three days and never moved a muscle. It was lucky for him that there aren't any cat doctors or they would soon have finished him off. They would have purged him and bled him and—

SGANARELLE   Oh, be quiet, I tell you! I never heard such nonsense. Here they come.

LISETTE   Now you will be well edified. They will tell you in Latin that there is something wrong with the girl.

Enter DOCTORS TOMÉS, DES-FONANDRÈS, MACROTIN, BAHYS.

SGANARELLE   Well, gentlemen?

DR. TOMÉS   We have examined the patient with every care, and there is no doubt that she is chock full of impurities.

SGANARELLE   My daughter impure!

DR. TOMÉS   Hem! I ought to have said that there are many impurities in her system, many corrupted humours.

SGANARELLE   Ah, I understand.

DR. TOMÉS   We propose to hold a consultation.

SGANARELLE   Quick, chairs for the gentlemen.

LISETTE   [*to* DR. TOMÉS]   Ah doctor, so you are one of them, are you?

SGANARELLE   How do you come to know the doctor?

LISETTE   I saw him the other day at your niece's friend's house.

DR. TOMÉS   How is her coachman getting on?

LISETTE   Well enough, but he's dead.

DR. TOMÉS   Dead?

LISETTE   Yes.

DR. TOMÉS   It's impossible!

LISETTE   I don't know whether it's impossible or not, I only know that it's true.

DR. TOMÉS   I tell you he can't be dead.

LISETTE   Well, I tell you he is dead—and buried.

DR. TOMÉS   You are mistaken.

LISETTE   I saw it myself.

DR. TOMÉS   It is quite out of the question. Hippocrates says that such maladies last either fourteen or twenty-one days and it is only six days since he fell ill.

LISETTE   Hippocrates can say what he likes, but the fellow is dead.

SGANARELLE   [*to* LISETTE]   Be quiet, you chatterbox, and come out of here. Gentlemen, I implore you to give every attention to your consultation. Although it is not usual to pay in advance—just in case I forget—and to get the thing over—here is—*He gives money and each one receives it with his own particular gesture. Exit with* LISETTE.

The doctors sit down and each in turn gives a little cough.

DR. DES-FONANDRÉS
Paris is becoming an awfully big place! Getting about becomes a serious matter as one's practice grows.

DR. TOMÉS
Well, you know, I use a mule—a splendid animal for the job. You would hardly believe the distance she covers in a day.

DR. DES-FONANDRÉS
I have a wonderful horse. He's simply tireless, is my horse!

DR. TOMÉS
Do you know what distance my mule did to-day? I started down by the Arsenal. From the Arsenal I went to the far end of the Faubourg Saint-Germain, from there to the far end of the Marais, from the far end of the Marais to the Porte Saint-Honoré, from the Porte Saint-Honoré to Faubourg Saint-Jacques, from Faubourg Saint-Jacques to the Porte de Richelieu, from the Porte de Richelieu along here, and from here I have to go back to the Place Royale.

DR. DES-FONANDRÉS
My horse has done as much as that today, and in addition I have been out to see a patient at Ruel.

DR. TOMÉS
Well, while we are talking, what is your opinion of the controversy between Dr. Théophraste and Dr. Artimius? It seems to be dividing the whole faculty into opposite camps.

DR. DES-FONANDRÉS
I'm on Artimius's side.

DR. TOMÉS
Yes, so am I. Of course his treatment, we know, killed the patient, and Théophraste's ideas might have saved him, but Théophraste was in the wrong all the same. He shouldn't have disputed the diagnosis of a senior colleague. Don't you think so?

DR. DES-FONANDRÉS
No doubt about it! Stick to professional etiquette whatever happens.

DR. TOMÉS
Yes, I'm all for the rules—except between friends. Only the other day three of us were called in for consultation with a man outside the faculty. I held up the whole business. I wouldn't allow anyone to give an opinion at all unless things were done professionally. Of course the people of the house had to do what they could in the meantime, and the patient went from bad to worse, but I wouldn't give way. The patient died bravely in the course of the argument.

DR. DES-FONANDRÉS
It's a very good thing to teach people how to behave and make them aware of their ignorance.

DR. TOMÉS
When a man's dead he's dead and that's all it amounts to, but a point of etiquette neglected may seriously prejudice the welfare of the entire medical profession.

Enter SGANARELLE.

SGANARELLE
Gentlemen, my daughter is getting worse. Do tell me quickly what decision you have come to.

DR. TOMÉS
[*to* DES-FONANDRÉS].
Come, sir.

DR. DES-FONANDRÉS
You speak first, if you please.

DR. TOMÉS	No, no, you are too kind.
DR. DES-FONANDRÉS	I couldn't give my opinion before yours.
DR. TOMÉS	Sir—please—
DR. DES-FONANDRÉS	Please, sir—
SGANARELLE	Oh, for goodness' sake, gentlemen, cut out the ceremony. Remember the matter is urgent. *They all four speak at once.*
DR. TOMÉS	Your daughter's complaint—
DR. DES-FONANDRÉS	In the opinion of these gentlemen—
DR. MACROTIN	After much care-ful con-sult-a-tion—
DR. BAHYS	To consider—
SGANARELLE	One at a time, if you please.
DR. TOMÉS	Sir, we have been discussing your daughter's illness, and my own view is that it arises from overheating of the blood. My advice is therefore—bleeding as early as possible.
DR. DES-FONANDRÉS	In my opinion the trouble is a putrefaction of humours caused by a surfeit of er—er—something or other. My view is that she should be given an emetic.
DR. TOMÉS	In my opinion an emetic would kill her.
DR. DES-FONANDRÉS	On the contrary, I maintain that to bleed her now would be fatal.
DR. TOMÉS	You *would* try to be clever!
DR. DES-FONANDRÉS	I know what I'm talking about. I can give you points on any professional question.
DR. TOMÉS	Don't forget how you cooked that fellow's goose the other day.
DR. DES-FONANDRÉS	What about the woman *you* sent to glory only three days ago?
DR. TOMÉS [*to* SGANARELLE].	You have my opinion.
DR. DES-FONANDRÉS [*to* SGANARELLE].	You know what I think.
DR. TOMÉS	If you don't have your daughter bled without delay, you can take it she's done for. [*Exit.*]
DR. DES-FONANDRÉS	If you *do* have her bled, she won't last a quarter of an hour. [*Exit.*]
SGANARELLE	Which am I to believe? What's to be done when you get two such different opinions? Gentlemen, I implore you, set my mind at rest, give me an unprejudiced opinion as to which treatment will save my daughter.
DR. MACROTIN [*drawling*].	Sir! On these oc-cas-ions one must pro-ceed with cir-cum-spec-tion and do nothing, as one might say, in pre-cip-it-a-tion, for mis-takes thus com-mit-ted may well, as our Master Hippocrates ob-serves—have dan-ger-ous cons-equences!
DR. BAHYS [*in a quick stammering voice*].	Yes, one n.n.needs to be c.c.careful. Th.th.there's no ch.ch.child's play about such c.c.c.cases as th.th.this. And it it's no.no.not an easy m.matter to p.put th.things right if.if.if you m.m.make a m.m.m.mistake. Experimen-tum p.p.p.p.periculo-sum, y.you n.need to l.l.look before you l.l.l.leap and weigh th.things w.w.warily, consider the c.c.constitution of the p.p.patient, c.c.cause

of the m.m.malady, and the nature of the c.c.c.cure.

SGANARELLE [*aside*]. One's as slow as a funeral, t'other c.c.can't s.s.spit it out fast enough!

DR. MACROTIN [*as before*]. But, sir, to come to the point, my diagnosis is that your daughter's illness is chronic and that it may well prove dangerous if nothing is done for her, more especially as the symptoms indicate that a **fuliginous and mordicant** vapour is inflaming the cerebral membrane. This vapour, which in Greek is called Atmos, is produced by putrescent and persistent **conglutinations** concentrated in the lower abdomen.

DR. BAHYS [*as before*]. These humours are of such long standing and have been inflamed to such malignity that the vapours rise up to the very cerebral region itself.

DR. MACROTIN [*as before*]. So much so, that a tremendous purging is essential to loosen, expel, and evacuate the humours. But—as a preliminary I think it wise, if there is no objection, to administer an anodyne, that is to say, some little emollient, emulsive, detergent injection with refreshing juleps and syrups which she can mix in her drinks.

DR. BAHYS [*as before*]. Later we can come to purgings and bleedings—repeated as necessary.

DR. MACROTIN [*as before*]. All this treatment notwithstanding—it is still possible that your daughter may die, but you will at least have the satisfaction of having done something, and the consolation of knowing that she died according to the rules of the profession.

DR. BAHYS [*as before*]. H'm, yes, far better die according to rules than live on in spite of them.

DR. MACROTIN We are giving you our opinion quite unreservedly.

DR. BAHYS As one man to another.

SGANARELLE [*imitating* MACROTIN]. I am most hum-bly grateful to you. [*Imitating* BAHYS.] Th.th.thanks very m.m.much f.f.for the t.t.trouble you have taken.

Exeunt doctors.

SGANARELLE Now I'm no wiser than I was at the start—but here's an idea! I'll go buy some Orvietan. It's a remedy that has done lots of folk good.

Enter VENDOR *of quack remedies.*

SGANARELLE Sir, please give me a box of your Orvietan and I will pay you in a moment.

QUACK VENDOR [*singing*]. The wealth of every clime
    around the ocean
Could it ever pay the value
    of the remedy I'm selling?
I guarantee a cure, every
    other one excelling,
A cure for every ill, use it as
    you will,
As a medicine or lotion.

The itch,
The stitch,
The palsy,
And the gout:
Whatever be
Your troubles,
This cure
Will find 'em out!

I guarantee
A cure to every woman, every
   man
Who will try but one box of my
   Orvietan!

The cure for every ill that man
   is heir to,
And it's nothing but the truth
   that I'm a-telling.
I guarantee a cure, every other
   one excelling;
A cure for every ill, use it as you
   will,

As a medicine or a lotion.

The itch,
The stitch, etc.

SGANARELLE   Sir, I fully believe that all the gold in the world isn't really enough to buy your Orvietan, but here is my shilling. You can take it or not, as you like.

The VENDOR *sings again. Clowns and attendants on the* VENDOR *show their satisfaction in a dance which forms the Second Interlude.* . . .

▲

Scurvy's Conquest and Sailors' Health

FRANCIS E. CUPPAGE

Scurvy, a deficiency disease caused by lack of vitamin C in the diet, was one of the most serious problems facing Europeans determined to explore and conquer the rest of the world. However, it was not peculiar to the Age of Discovery but manifested anywhere the human diet was deficient, including in the lives of many children, who when weaned did not receive an adequate diet. This disease can even appear in modern-day individuals who sacrifice proper nutrition for the sake of fad weight-loss diets.

Scurvy routinely attacked sailors on long transoceanic voyages. It was thus a serious obstacle to continued exploration until the 1750s, when James Lind and other individuals proved that the use of lemons and limes could prevent the disease. The existence of vitamins per se was as yet unknown, but the fact that citrus fruit and fresh green vegetables could prevent scurvy was clear. The problem did not disappear quickly, however, because a combination of changing medical theory and a cost-conscious bureaucracy greatly delayed official adoption of the citrus remedy in the British navy for more than forty years. Even after the remedy was finally embraced, scurvy broke out numerous times—in Arctic and whaling expeditions, during World War I, and any time a human population has had insufficient vitamin C in its diet.

▲

The quincentenary of Columbus' arrival in the New World rekindled interest in the problems seamen faced during the voyages of discovery. Historical studies of early Phoenician travels throughout the Mediterranean have been followed by those of Viking and Irish transatlantic

Reprinted by permission of Blackwell Publishing, from Francis E. Cuppage, "Scurvy's Conquest and Sailors' Health," *The Historian* 57, no. 4 (1995): 695–702.

voyages to North America and of Columbus to the Caribbean. As ships increased in size and navigational skills improved, circumnavigations, beginning with the Portuguese navigator Magellan in 1519, continued with the explorers Drake, Dampier, Anson, Byron, and Wallis.

Early circumnavigational explorations were limited by the poor health of the ships' crews. Later expeditions were more successful due in part to the control of such sea diseases as scurvy. The control of scurvy, allowing for more prolonged maritime explorations, was related to the preventive health measures of Captain James Cook during his three circumnavigations from 1768 to 1780. This essay is based on Cook's written accounts that document his addition to the sailors' diets of the local fresh greens, which provided the **antiscorbutic** vitamin, ascorbic acid. . . .

Despite the benefits of opening new vistas, the sailing conditions of pre–eighteenth century voyages were abominable. A sailor's diet consisted of salted fish and meat, dried vegetables, weeviled biscuits and rancid oils, cheese, and butter. Such distilled beverages as beer, wine, and rum were abundant. While the alcohol temporarily eased the sailors' burdens, the resulting dehydration and addiction resulted in numerous accidents and poor health. The caloric content—estimated at 2,500–3,000 calories—was adequate, but the diet was sorely deficient in vitamins. In the absence of vitamin C, rampant scurvy became responsible for thousands of sailors' deaths and disabilities. On long voyages, nearly three-quarters of a ship's crew was likely to be unable to sail because of this deficiency.

A young Scottish surgeon, James Lind, determined that scurvy could be cured and prevented by the administration of orange and lemon juices. In 1742, in what has been called the first controlled clinical trial, Lind cured two sailors of scurvy with oranges and lemons, while other reputed antiscorbutics failed to cure his other patients. However, for another fifty years the Royal Navy gave no serious consideration to the use of fresh citrus for combating scurvy.

Science in the eighteenth century had only reached the humoral epoch, where most diseases were believed to be caused by an imbalance of body humors and the presence of foul air. The germ theory of contagion was yet to be formulated, and there was no appreciation of the role of essential dietary nutrients including vitamins. Ships' surgeons contributed little to the health of the men. Usually poorly trained and often disinterested in their work, surgeons practiced medicine in cramped quarters. They either prescribed herbals or surgically removed diseased parts. With infections rampant, burials at sea were commonplace.

George Anson began a circumnavigation in 1740. Intent on challenging the Spanish in the Pacific and on discovering new lands for the emerging British Empire, Anson captured the Manila treasure galleon and collected a large amount of gold and silver for the Crown. By the time he returned to England in 1742, he had lost eighty percent of his men. Most of these losses were attributed to scurvy. While Anson was a capable commander, he only vaguely conceived of preventive medicine and received little help from his ships' surgeons. Something had to be done if the British were to conquer the seas, develop trade routes to the Orient, and expand their colonial empire.

James Cook, a commoner by birth, received his education on a farm in northern England. At the age of eighteen, he went to sea in 1746. He learned seamanship and navigation while sailing on **colliers,** transporting coal from Newcastle to London in the stormy North Sea. This experience served him well. Cook joined the Royal Navy at the age of twenty-seven, when Britain was at war with France. He spent nearly a decade on ships stationed along the east coast of North America, where he accurately charted the St. Lawrence River. During this time he also learned the best traits of leadership and became known to his superiors, especially Sir Hugh Palliser, who became a prominent member of the Admiralty and one of Cook's most steadfast supporters.

The Royal Society convinced the Admiralty, in 1768, to send a scientific expedition to the Pacific Ocean in order to observe the transit of Venus across the surface of the sun. Cook was recommended to be the commander by his mentor, Palliser. Cook's extended voyage was to be the first circumnavigation expressly for scientific purposes, with observations of the planet to be made from the newly discovered island of Tahiti.

Lieutenant Cook commanded a Whitby collier that had been renamed the *Endeavour.* The astronomer, Charles Green, and the botanist/naturalist, Joseph Banks, sailed with Cook and 138 men. The *Endeavour* was supplied with standard naval provisions for eighteen months at sea. If the ship were to be at sea longer, the crew would have to obtain additional provisions from wherever they anchored. In addition to the standard rations of salted meats and dried vegetables, the Admiralty supplied Cook with a small amount of traditional antiscorbutics to try at sea. These included malt for fermenting into wort, sauerkraut, carrot marmalade, saloup, dried soup, and some concentrated lemon and orange juices. Most of these substances were later found to be deficient in vitamin C and incapable of preventing scurvy.

The *Endeavour,* leaving Britain in July 1768, reached Rio de Janeiro in early December. The Portuguese viceroy neither allowed any men ashore nor sold them any provisions because he doubted the expressed scientific nature of the voyage. After leaving Rio, the ship headed for the tip of South America at Cape Horn. At Tierra del Fuego the crew harvested the local greens that botanist Banks thought were antiscorbutic. The ship then sailed on to Tahiti. After observing the transit of Venus, the *Endeavour* sailed south to New Zealand in search of Terra Australis Incognita (the great southern continent). Cook reached the islands of New Zealand and then returned to the British Isles by the westerly route to the Cape of Good Hope at the southern tip of Africa. En route the *Endeavour* slowly explored the east coast of New Holland (later called Australia). Whenever the ship dropped anchor, Banks and the crew collected indigenous greens and added them to the crew's salads.

After running aground on the Great Barrier Reef near Tribulation Bay, Cook took possession of Australia and sailed for the Dutch East Indian harbor of Jakarta. Here many of Cook's crew developed dysentery and malaria, with more than thirty men subsequently dying. The *Endeavour* gained the Cape of Good Hope in mid March and reached Britain in June 1771, after 2 years, 9 months, and 17 days at sea. Of the initial complement of 138 men, only 41 had died during the long voyage. None of them had succumbed to scurvy.

Cook had been at home only four months when the Admiralty ordered a second circumnavigational voyage. Its primary mission would be a definitive search for Terra Australis Incognita. The strong belief in a continent at the South Pole stemmed from the assumption that it was needed to balance the northern hemisphere's landmass in order for the earth to spin properly on its axis. Since Cook did not wish to repeat such a long voyage with only one ship, two Whitby colliers were selected. Each ship was provisioned for thirty months at sea and provided with antiscorbutics similar to those on the first voyage. Better navigational instruments were added, including the Kendall chronometer, which could be used to determine longitude accurately.

The *Resolution* and the *Adventure* left Britain in July 1772, rounded the Cape of Good Hope, and made several southerly passes in search of the southern continent. When the ships were separated by fog in the Antarctic Ocean and again off the coast of New Zealand, the *Adventure* returned to England. The *Resolution,* with Cook in command, crossed the Antarctic Circle three times, and wintered at Ship's Cove in New Zealand and among the South Pacific islands during the southern winters. Cook sailed as far south as 71 degrees latitude without finding the continent since each time he was stopped by pack ice. On several occasions he obtained fresh water from icebergs. Finally, the *Resolution* returned to the British Isles in July 1775, after 3 years and 18 days at sea. Although Cook did not find Antarctica, he postulated that there was land at the South Pole. The many large "ice islands" they had sailed among, he believed, originated from a large landmass that was uninhabitable because of its ice and freezing temperatures.

Cook's long sea voyage was the first without significant scurvy. While there had been several cases of the disease, serious scurvy had been prevented by the consumption of local fresh greens collected at numerous sites of anchorage.

The Admiralty convinced Cook that his next expedition should aim at locating a passage to the East Indies and Orient via the North American continent. Parliament had a standing offer of £20,000 for any British subject travelling on a British ship who found the Northwest Passage. Cook, now forty-eight, was given two ships: the *Resolution* and a second collier, the *Discovery*. Because of the scientific nature of the voyage, French and American colonists agreed to grant protection to Cook and his ships.

The two ships, leaving in July 1776, were reprovisioned at the Cape of Good Hope and then sailed on to Australia and New Zealand. At Queen Charlotte Sound, they obtained more antiscorbutic greens, some of which they harvested from their previously planted gardens, made repairs, and then left for the Northern Pacific. The *Resolution* and the *Discovery* visited the Friendly, Society, and Tonga Islands and rediscovered the Hawaiian Islands, naming them the Sandwich Islands. The ships' crews wintered and reprovisioned in Hawaii before sailing for the west coast of North America. In early March 1778, they took possession of the Oregon coast for George III, and began their search up the west coast. Crossing the Bering Strait without finding a passage to the Atlantic, they were halted in August by pack ice in the Arctic Ocean. They headed south to winter in the Sandwich Islands before venturing north again.

Cook reprovisioned at Hawaii's Kealakekua Bay, having been received as a god by the natives. Leaving Hawaii in February 1799, the *Resolution* sprung its foremast in a gale, and Cook returned to Hawaii for repairs. The natives, fearing a further depletion of their supplies, stole one of the *Discovery's* cutters and killed Cook. Now under Charles Clerke's command, the two ships sailed northward but were again blocked by pack ice in the Arctic. After turning south, they made their way back via the Siberian coast, China, and the Cape of Good Hope, and arrived in Britain in October 1780, after a voyage of 4 years, 2 months, and 22 days. The crews of both ships were in good health. While the Northwest Passage had not been located, the voyage was seen as successful in that no cases of scurvy had appeared on either ship during the entire voyage.

The three circumnavigational voyages from 1768 to 1780 were historically significant for several reasons. They led to the opening of new lands for colonization and trade, provided descriptions of native cultures, developed theories of Polynesian migration, and delineated new flora and fauna. Moreover, the preservation of the sailors' health by controlling scurvy would enable future expeditionary voyages to make more important discoveries.

While it is customary to assume that lemons, oranges, and limes were the antiscorbutics that had maintained the health of Cook's sailors, none of these were generally available. Cook deemphasized citrus juices in favor of malt wort, which was ineffective, and sauerkraut, which may have had some antiscorbutic effect. It is likely that the prevention of scurvy on the voyages was more related to the harvesting and consuming of local greens, as suggested by botanist Banks on the first voyage, since nearly all growing plants contain quantities of vitamin C.

Cook stopped at local anchorages as often as possible for water, greens, fish, fowl, and meat, and for the brewing of tea and spruce beer, so it is likely that the greens provided the source of the vitamins. Other antiscorbutics provided by the Admiralty were of little value since prolonged boiling and long storage depleted their vitamins. Cook began his voyages with young, healthy sailors and helped to maintain the men's health by using the three-watch system, by reducing overcrowding, by ventilating the ships' lower decks, and by providing clean, warm clothing for his sailors.

Lind, the Scottish doctor, originally used citrus juices to prevent and treat scurvy, while Cook used indigenous greens to contain the disease. Although sporadic scurvy occurred in later whaling voyages and during arctic explorations, scurvy was prevented whenever fresh citrus fruits and greens containing antiscorbutic amounts of vitamin C were used. The prevention of this devastating deficiency disease allowed for overseas exploration, colonization, and trade, all of which altered global history.

The English Sweating Sickness, 1485 to 1551

Guy Thwaites, Mark Taviner, and Vanya Gant

The fifteenth- and sixteenth-century disease known as The Sweat, *or* English Sweating Sickness, *remains one of the mysteries of medical history. Only five epidemic episodes were recorded, its symptoms match no known modern disease, and it vanished after 1551. The symptomology was generally nonspecific: fever, pains, coma, and death. It apparently had a high mortality rate. Its only unusual symptom was a foul-smelling perspiration, which gave the disease its name. It attacked primarily adult males; a much lower incidence occurred among women, children, and persons who were elderly.*

Modern medical historians have postulated a number of culprits, but no modern disease fits the epidemiological profile of The Sweat exactly. Whether it was a unique illness that flared up for a time in England and then disappeared or a disease that mutated into something completely different remains a matter of conjecture. In the meantime, it joins such epidemics as the Athenian Plague, afflictions unknown to modern people.

In the summer of 1485, a rapidly fatal infectious fever struck England: "A newe Kynde of sickness came through the whole region, which was so sore, so peynfull, and sharp, that the lyke was never harde of to any mannes rememberance before that tyme."

Sudor Anglicus, later known as the English sweating sickness, was characterized by sudden headaches, myalgia, fever, profuse sweating, and dyspnea. Four additional epidemics were reported in the summers of 1508, 1517, 1528, and 1551, after which the disease abruptly disappeared. Contemporary observers distinguished the condition from plague, malaria, and typhus. Later suggestions included influenza, food poisoning, an **arbovirus,** and an **enterovirus** as possible causes. We here review the clinical and epidemiologic features of the English sweating sickness and draw some tentative conclusions about a viral cause.

Clinical Features

The only physicians to provide us with eyewitness accounts of the clinical features of the English outbreaks of the sweating sickness are Thomas Forestier and John Caius. This scarcity of clinical descriptions reflects a medical culture that was far from 20th-century conventions of diagnosis. Also, published dialogue among physicians in England was limited by a relatively undeveloped printing industry. Forestier recorded his observations of the 1485 epidemic in two treatises. His shorter account, in English, summarized contemporary observations on the rapidity and violence of the new disease. His other account, written in Latin for fellow physicians, includes the following description:

> The exterior is calm in this fever, the interior excited . . . the heat in the pestilent fever many times does not appear excessive to the doctor, nor the heat of the sweat itself particularly high. . . . But it is on account of the ill-natured, fetid, corrupt, putrid, and loathsome vapors close to the region of the heart and of the lungs whereby the panting of the breath magnifies and increases and restricts of itself.

John Caius of Gonville Hall, Cambridge, who was president of the Royal College of Physicians, devoted an entire book to the 1551 epidemic. This was the first monograph in English to deal exclusively with one disease. It includes the following vivid description:

> First by peine in the backe, or shoulder, peine in the extreme parts, as arme, or legge, with a flusshing, or wind as it semeth to certaine of the patientes, fleing the same. Secondly by the grief in the liver and nigh stomach. Thirdly, by peine in the head, and madness of the same. Fourthly by a passion of the hart . . . it lasteth but one natural day.

Caius was describing a typical viral **prodrome** of myalgia and headache, progressing to abdominal pain, vomiting, increasing headache, and delirium. There followed cardiac palpitation, **tachycardia,** and worsening **tachypnea** with chest pain, prostration, possible paralysis with **agonal** breathlessness, and death—sometimes within 12 to 24 hours of the onset of symptoms. Forestier's emphasis on "the panting of the breath" and the "difficulty of breathing" suggests an important pulmonary component to the sweating sickness. Caius concurs: "the patientes breathed rapidly and heavily of necessity . . . with a whining, sighing voice."

Other historical commentators have also highlighted the importance of pulmonary involvement. The 19th-century German historian Hirsch noted: "Among other serious symptoms mentioned were colliquative sweating and extreme breathlessness. Death would then occur with the symptoms of dyspnoea and generalised paralysis." Similarly, Hecker described the disease as "the result of a commotion excited on the part of the lungs, which was critical with respect to the disease itself."

Epidemiology of the Sweating Sickness

Meaningful epidemiologic analysis requires a statistical basis; however, until the institution of the parish registers in 1538 there was only testamentary evidence. Gottfried's study of the mortality patterns in East Anglia and Hertfordshire uses testamentary evidence for the 1485 outbreak. He characterizes the epidemic as widely scattered and patchy in its geographic distribution, with a rapid appearance, a short and violent course, and an equally rapid disappearance in any one locality. For the 1551 epidemic, more extensive records are available from surviving parish registers. They document a transient rise in mortality only in July and August of that year, with no significant increase in annual mortality. The overall effect of the sweating sickness was limited despite the often hyperbolic narratives. Lack of data makes it difficult to estimate the case fatality rate, and any variation in case fatality and virulence is impossible to assess without data on nonfatal cases. All reports nevertheless attest to the sweating sickness's consistently high mortality: "It killed some within three hours . . . for in some one toune halfe the people died, and in some other toune the thirde parte, the Sweate was so fervent and infeccious."

All accounts agree as to the summer preponderance of the sweating sickness. All five epidemics occurred in July, August, and early September and disappeared with the onset of winter. Providing any further evidence that annual fluctuations in climate were related to epidemic years is problematic. For the years before the advent of data on temperature and rainfall, annual variations in climate cannot be assessed accurately.

Narrative accounts recorded in Holinshed's *Chronicles of England, Scotland and Ireland* and in correspondence reported a distinct age and sex predisposition: "It is to be noted, that this mortalitie fell chieflie or rather upon men, and those of the best age as between thirtie and fortie years. Few women, nor children, nor old men died thereof."

These narrative accounts emphasized the susceptibility of upper-class men. Such epidemiologic characteristics, however, rely heavily on observer interpretation. The preponderance of wealthy male victims in narrative accounts probably reflects the high profile of these men within society rather than an actual susceptibility to the sweating sickness. The most meaningful figures for any epidemiologic analysis are those for the 1551 epidemic from parish registers. These too, unfortunately, have their limitations. We have no information on age distribution, since the age at death was not recorded. Of the surviving registers dating back to 1551, many are later 16th-century transcripts that do not always include the cause of death. The best analysis of the epidemiology of the 1551 outbreak of the sweating sickness uses only Devon registers; a systematic search through all other surviving registers for the summer of 1551 might shed further light on the affected population.

The Sweating Sickness as an Infectious Disease

From our research of the available evidence relating to both the clinical features and the epidemiology of the sweating sickness, we conclude that it was a rapid and usually fatal infectious illness with a marked pulmonary component. The summer preponderance and scattered rural nature of the sweating sickness led Wylie and Collier to suggest that the infectious agent was likely to have its reservoir in a mammalian or avian host. They concluded that "an arbovirus [with a rodent reservoir and an arthropod vector] is the most probable agent of the English sweating sickness." Rodent populations are

largest in late summer or early autumn, coinciding with the peak incidence of the disease. Indeed, as early as 1906, Chantemesse et al. blamed field mice for carrying the disease. Most arboviruses, however, run clinical courses distinct from that of the sweating sickness and are often associated with exanthematous or hemorrhagic signs. Such cutaneous signs are notably absent from all accounts of the disease. "It was a pestilent fever, but not seated in the veins or humors, for that there followed no carbuncle, no purple or livid spots, or the like." A viral hemorrhagic fever therefore seems most unlikely.

We agree that it is likely that the sweating sickness was caused by a virus with a rodent vector. If it was indeed a viral pulmonary disease, then its clinical and epidemiologic features seem most closely to resemble those of the hantavirus pulmonary syndrome, which was first recognized in the southwestern United States in May 1993. The syndrome consists of a brief and nonspecific prodrome of fever, myalgia, and headache and rapidly progressive noncardiogenic pulmonary edema, requiring mechanical ventilation in 88 percent of patients within 24 hours of admission. Furthermore, those who died despite ventilation did so within approximately 72 hours. Infection is acquired by inhalation of rodent excreta, and rodents act as the reservoir for hantaviruses. The hantavirus pulmonary syndrome outbreak of 1993 occurred after an unusually warm and wet spring, when the rodent population density was much greater than usual because of the plentiful food supply. To date, the modern outbreaks of hantavirus pulmonary syndrome have been rural; the prevalence of seropositivity relates to exposure to rodents, which is associated with living or working in rodent-infested homes.

Conclusions

Without molecular confirmation from the tissues of victims, our etiologic hypothesis about the English sweating sickness remains speculative. Tissues from some victims may someday be available. Caius confirms that Henry Brandon, the Duke of Suffolk, and his brother Charles died of the sweating sickness during the epidemic of 1551. Thomas Wilson, their tutor, described their death and their burial in the parish church cemetery of St. Mary's, in what is now Buckden village, in Huntingdonshire. Although information relating to DNA sequences has been successfully obtained by polymerase-chain-reaction techniques from 7000-year-old human tissue, we doubt that hantaviral RNA might similarly be identified. This does not preclude the possibility that other DNA-based candidate pathogens for the sweating sickness will be identified, however.

Poisons of the Past

Mary K. Matossian

A significant number of women in early modern Europe were imprisoned, tortured, and even executed during the witch hunts. The New World colonies were not immune to this phenomenon, as the Salem witchcraft trials witness. A number of reasons for this violence have been evinced, primarily from social psychology and cultural anthropology perspectives. However, as the author of this selection suggests, the origins of the accusations that powered the persecutions may have been medical—the result of ingestion of toxic mold on rye, which produces nearly every symptom mentioned in the records of the proceedings. Ultimately, however, we may never be able to isolate a single cause of the witch hunts but must look for a constellation of factors. In the meantime, the case for ergot poisoning appears to be an excellent step in the right direction.

CHAPTER V

Witch Persecution in Early Modern Europe

It is difficult to think clearly about bizarre behavior, for it tends to arouse anxiety. Anyone who has ridden on a city bus with one or more harmless but obviously disoriented or disturbed persons will realize that others on board feel uncomfortable. Naturally people get even more uncomfortable when confronted with a whole crowd of psychotics. Even when one contemplates *past* insanity it is difficult to maintain objectivity. The urge to ride a hobbyhorse of some kind—moral, religious, intellectual, or political—is strong. To avoid this inclination one must define clearly what it is one is trying to understand. When witchcraft is the topic of investigation, the kinds of behavior that incriminated the accused must be identified and examined.

Anyone who has consulted the records of witchcraft persecution realizes that actual harm was done, and the harm fit a pattern. "Outbreaks" of witchcraft were often accompanied by outbreaks of central nervous system symptoms; tremors, anesthesias, paresthesias (sensations of pricking, biting, ants crawling on the skin), distortions of the face and eyes gone awry, paralysis, spasms, convulsive seizures, permanent contraction of a muscle, hallucinations, manias, panics, depressions. There were also a significant number of gangrene cases and complaints of reproductive dysfunction, especially agalactia (inability of a nursing mother to produce enough milk). Animals behaved wildly and made strange noises; cows too had agalactia. Not every victim of "bewitchment" had all the symptoms, but most had abnormal experiences and behaved in abnormal ways.

The victim of persecution was a person accused of causing these symptoms in another. These symptoms were real. Certainly it was possible to "frame" someone for witchcraft, but that does not mean that all episodes of bewitchment can be ascribed to invention. Many of those affected were young children who could not be accused of feigning possession or having malicious plans to "get even" with a neighbor, and many died of their symptoms. The cause of harm was not known, but harm there was.

This pattern of symptoms, furthermore, was distributed in a nonrandom way in space and time. The characteristics of the nonrandom distribution will be described below. Only by linking the pattern of symptoms with a distinct epidemiology can we hope to find a reliable explanation.

The investigators who have looked into witchcraft persecution have proposed no adequate explanation for its epidemiology. They have not attempted to explain why witches were persecuted in one place and not another, at one time and not another. It simply will not suffice to discuss widespread beliefs about witches, tensions between factions in a witch-persecuting community, ruling-class repression, or legal and judicial arrangements for dealing with witchcraft. These were continuous cultural and social realities that did not vary in space and time as the distribution of "bewitchment" varied. One cannot explain a variable with a constant.

Of course, beliefs about witches, laws, court procedures, and social structures have been studied and should be studied to understand the social response to cases of "bewitchment." How the symptoms were perceived and interpreted was *culturally mandated*. They were seen through a screen of preconceptions.

Moreover, the persons accused of witchcraft were not chosen at random; nor were their persecutors from a random selection of community members. The existing body of witchcraft persecution theory tries to explain these nonrandom distributions of witches and persecutors of witches, but it does not explain the nonrandom distribution of witch-hunts. To blame witch accusers and courts for witchcraft persecution is to mistake an effect for a cause. Witches were persecuted because harm had befallen a community, not just because there were people vulnerable to indictment and other people prone to indict them.

Spatial Distribution of Witch Persecution

The location of witch trials in Early Modern Europe . . . reveals that a large proportion of trials were concentrated in alpine areas of France and central Europe and in the Rhine Valley. In all these areas rye was the staple cereal. Temperatures in the coldest month (usually January) were below freezing, and at higher altitudes they might be colder. Witch trials were also more common in wet areas. The area of highest concentration of trials was both cold and wet. The . . . middle Rhône Valley (southeastern France) and the two circles in southwestern France encompass areas in which summer temperature tends to be ideal for production of ergot alkaloids (17.4°–18.9° C).

Some other examples of the significance of spatial distribution may be found in the British Isles. In Scotland, witch persecution was concentrated in the northeast, along the coast—the country's main rye-growing area.

The absence of persecution is also significant. There were few witch trials in Ireland, for example. One was held in Kilkenny in 1578, but the record is lost. In 1661 in the Puritan (English) colony of Youghal, there were victims of the bewitchment syndrome and a trial followed; likewise on Island Magee off County Antrim there was a trial in 1711. It may be relevant that the Irish at this time consumed mainly dairy products and oats, which may explain why they were not very susceptible to "bewitchment."

In Spain, witch trials occurred only in Galicia, a damp region in the northwest corner, and in the Pyrenees. Trials were rare in Italy and Scandinavia as well—countries that were warm and dry or that were in the cold northern tier.

Temporal Distribution of Witch Persecution

It is generally agreed that between the end of the fifteenth century and 1560 the incidence of witch trials was low. There were some trials in the Pyrenees and Barcelona in 1507, 1517, and the 1520s. Epidemics of central nervous system disorders, not involving charges of witchcraft, were also rare. This was a period of warm weather.

In the 1560s the climate of Europe grew cooler and wetter. In Essex, France, Galicia, Switzerland, and southwestern Germany the incidence of trials increased.

The best place for statistical testing of the relationship between witch persecution and ergotism is Swabia, in southwestern Germany. Erik Midelfort, using primary sources, compiled an annual index of the number of trials from 1550 to 1689. There is also an index of rye prices in Augsburg, which indicates the amount of pressure on the poor to eat grain of questionable quality. Moreover, other researchers have compiled an index of tree-ring widths in a nearby part of Switzerland that gives an indication of spring and summer temperatures during the period of persecution.

I discovered that the higher the rye prices in Augsburg, the more the witch persecution in Swabia. . . . The colder the spring and summer temperatures in Switzerland, the more the persecution . . . *63.3 percent of the variance in witch persecution could be predicted by temperature and price combined.*

The timing of witch persecution in eastern Europe was quite different. In Russia, the highest incidence of trials occurred in the period 1650–1700, and there were no trials before 1623. The mean winter temperature index for Russia in 1640–1749 (at longitude 35° E) was −11.1, compared to the 1100–1969 mean of −4.0, which indicates that cold winters predicted witch trials.

In Poland, 81 percent of all witch trials occurred between 1700 and 1750. Simultaneously, Germany, Sweden, the Baltic countries, and Russia, which, like Poland, were rye-dependent, were reporting epidemics of ergotism. These epidemics were distributed as follows: in 1650–1699 there were four; in 1700–1750, thirteen; and in 1751–1800, eight. The peak in symptoms of "bewitchment" in Poland and the peak in symptoms of ergotism reported by the neighbors of the Poles coincide. I suggest this is so because they had a common etiology.

Witch Persecution in Essex County, England

Many scholars have investigated witch persecution in England. G. L. Kittredge surveyed all published sources; K. V. Thomas studied the context of folk belief; and C. L. Ewen made an overall survey of the English court records. Alan MacFarlane did an exhaustive study of the court records in Essex and evaluated various theories of witch persecution. Essex was the only county in England with quarter-session records that went back as early as 1556; the next earliest series went back only to 1589, after the peak in witch persecution had passed; only four other counties had any records for the sixteenth century; and there were none surviving for sixteenth-century London.

MacFarlane showed that there was no evidence of a pagan cult in Essex, with fluctuating levels of activity, that might explain the incidence of witch persecution there. He found that Puritans were no more likely to persecute witches than were non-Puritans. Neither alleged witches nor their intended victims had any characteristic religious beliefs.

His examination of possible economic influences on the incidence of witch persecution yielded ambiguous results. On the one hand, he thought alleged witches tended to be poorer than their victims, although he gave no exact figures. In many cases an accusation of witchcraft was made after the "witch" had asked the "victim" for an economic favor; the victim having refused, the witch wished him ill. Moreover, in the period 1560–1650 the traditional means of helping the poor were "strained," according to MacFarlane. But he could find no correlation in Essex between the incidence of witch persecution on the one hand and, on the other, changes in population density, wheat prices, or the fortunes of the cloth industry. The central region of Essex, which was least troubled by poverty, had a high incidence of witch persecution.

MacFarlane rejected the notion that the incidence of witch persecution could be explained by an increasing incidence of illness, physical or mental. In three sample villages he found no correlation between mortality and witch accusations. Unfortunately, he had no morbidity statistics to consult. In his mind there were no connections between witch accusations and any particular disease. But Mac-Farlane, like most English scholars, did not consider that ergotism might have been present in Essex. He did not question the assertions of earlier authors, notably Charles Creighton, J. C. Drummond, and A. Wilbraham, that ergotism was insignificant in England and that little rye was consumed.

One reason Essex may have been the site of particular excitement over witches was the fact that it was a rye-growing center in a time of expanding markets, both within the county and in London. In order to expand production the farmers of Essex reclaimed marshland. According to Eric Kerridge, reclamation took on greater impetus after 1560. This was particularly true of the Vale of London, in southwestern Essex, and along the Essex coast. One of the crops sown on recently drained marshland was rye, which flourished in the sour soil as other cereals could not. Moreover, this is the part of England with the highest mean July temperature (17° C in the twentieth century), the most favorable for ergot alkaloid production.

Are there traces of the symptoms of ergot poisoning in the Essex court records? Yes, and some symptoms were specific to severe ergotism:

1. *Permanent constrictures:* [A] boy whose feet became "crooked and useless"; a child's hand "turned where the backes shoulde bee, and the backe in place of the palmes"; a man with "mouth drawne awrye, well neere uppe to the upper parte of his cheeke"; and a case in which "the right arme tirynge clene contrarie, and the legg contrarie to that, and rysinge double to the hed of the childe."

2. *"Fits":* [I]n three reports victims suffered violent "fits," which in common usage of the time usually meant symptoms of the central nervous system.

3. *Gangrene:* [O]ne person's right thigh reportedly "did rot off."

These reports represented only a small proportion of all injuries attributed to witchcraft. Most of the other reported symptoms could have been symptoms of ergotism, but they neither proved nor disproved the case in themselves: they merely contributed to the larger picture. These symptoms included lameness; loss of sight, hearing, and speech; nausea; fainting; making animal noises; hallucinations ("a dazzling" in the eyes); suicide; and sudden death.

Similar symptoms were noted in scattered court records and narratives in various parts of England where witches were persecuted. C. L. Ewen said that the greatest stir in witchcraft cases was caused by "the convulsive, hysterical, and epileptic seizures popularly termed 'fits.'" Michael MacDonald . . . noted that Richard Napier (1597–1634) regarded as bewitched patients who had plucking sensations, convulsions, "fits," and lingering symptoms generally.

We have details of three case studies of bewitchment in England, none of which, unfortunately, occurred in Essex. They do serve, however, to make clear what English people in the sixteenth and seventeenth centuries meant when they spoke of bewitchment. The first was the case of Warboys village in Huntingdonshire. Here, in 1589, Robert Throckmorton's five daughters, seven maidservants, and others in the village suffered from fits, hallucinations, and temporary blindness, deafness, and numbness. In addition, many cattle in the area died. The second was the case of Joan Harvey of Hockham, Norfolk, in the year 1600. Her symptoms included fits, spasms, the sensation of being "nipped," bloody spots on her skin, temporary blindness, deafness, and numbness, lameness, manic behavior, lying senseless, and hallucinations. Norfolk, like Essex, was an important rye-growing center. The third case was an epidemic in Fewstone, Norfolk, which started in October 1621. The common symptoms included fits, hallucinations, and trances. One victim of alleged bewitchment had gangrene, and another threatened to commit murder and suicide. The symptoms noted in case histories are typical of dystonic ergotism.

Generally, the victims of bewitchment were a generation younger than the accused witches. As noted before, ergotism affects children and teenagers most often and most severely. In a rapidly growing population such as that of Essex in the late sixteenth century there are more young people; as a result, the at-risk population for ergotism is greater than in a slow-growing, stable, or declining population. In 1584 Reginald Scot, speaking of England generally, said that witchcraft accusations were linked with the occurrence of "apoplexies, epilepsies, convulsions, hot fevers, worms, etc." in children. According to MacFarlane,

> While suspected witches were characteristically middle-aged or old, their victims appear to have been younger adults. The Assize indictments often stated, in the case of children, the age of the victim; in a number of instances the victim was said to be the "son of" or "daughter of" another person. It seems likely that this was only recorded when the victim was a child. . . . As well as these cases, there were sixty in which the victim was described as the "son" or "daughter" of another. Comparing these ninety-two victims with a total of 341 victims altogether, it would seem that over two-thirds of those believed to be bewitched were adults. . . . Unfortunately it has been impossible to collect information on the exact age of the accusers; only indirect evidence, such as the presence of young children in the family of the bewitched, remains. This gives the impression that they were quite often a generation younger than the accused.

That the victims of both bewitchment and ergotism were among the youngest members of the community supports the hypothesis that ergotism was a cause of the kind of behavior that was blamed on witchcraft.

Another piece of epidemiological evidence for this conclusion is the time of year of accusation. Indictments for witchcraft in Essex were about evenly distributed throughout the year, but were somewhat more frequent between February and June. This pattern differed from the classic pattern of an ergotism epidemic identified on continental Europe, in which the disease peaked in August and September, immediately after a rye harvest. This is because the continental epidemics occurred in communities heavily dependent on rye alone; the inhabitants began to eat the new crop as soon as it was harvested. The English people, however, had a more varied diet; in time of scarcity they could turn to barley, oats, and legumes. Moreover, judging from the practices of English settlers in New England, rye might stay in the barns until February or later before it was threshed and consumed. Ergot can remain chemically stable for up to eighteen months.

Also, witch persecution was less common in certain sections of Essex than in others, and these areas were at less risk for ergotism. Relatively little rye was grown in the northwest corner, a region of chalky hills, and in this area persecution was rare. Another part of Essex with relatively little persecution was around Colchester: little rye was grown there. The southeastern coastal area of Essex, bordering on the Thames estuary, was almost free of witch persecution: wheat was the most important crop in this area. But there was a high incidence of witch persecution in the southwestern section (Vale of London) and northeastern section of Essex—lowland areas with wet, sandy soils, where ergot was more likely to form on rye and where rye was cultivated intensely.

The incidence of witchcraft accusations was related, in addition, to long-term trends. Witch trials in Essex fell mainly between 1560 and 1619, with a concentration in the 1580s and 1590s. During this period the best predictor of trials was wet growing seasons . . . , but changes in diet in the later years may have had an even greater effect. With the growth of the London market in the late sixteenth century, some farmers prospered (and were thus able to afford white wheat bread) and some lagged behind. The poor ate oats, barley, and other cereals, but could not afford either wheat or rye. According to William Harrison, writing in 1587 after cereal prices had risen, "If the world lasts awhile after this rate, wheat and rye will be no grain for poor men to feed on, and some caterpillars [pillagers] there are can say so much already." According to Kerridge, around 1620 the people of southeastern England had largely lost the habit of eating rye. In Scotland, however, where rye consumption continued during the seventeenth century, ergot symptoms and witchcraft accusations continued.

The Social Response

The distribution of witch accusers and persecutors depended on the social structure of the region involved, and no European-wide generalizations can be made. The distribution of the *accused,* on the other hand, was nonrandom and tended to be the same in all rural areas.

Witches had wortcunning, knowledge of the medicinal properties of herbs. The role of the healer was a perilous one, for people were afraid of his or her seemingly magic power over a living body. They might think that someone who could cure disease by magic could also cause it by magic. Restoring health was "white" magic, taking it away was "black" magic. Like any physician today, a witch could be blamed when things went wrong, and in some ways witchcraft accusations may have been analogous to malpractice suits against physicians.

Among the symptoms healers of the Early Modern Era could sometimes relieve were the very symptoms associated with both ergotism and bewitchment. Motherwort and mistletoe, for example, were effective against some kinds of convulsions and spasms. It is not unlikely that, where ergotism was mistaken for bewitchment, the targets of witch-hunts were often among those herbalists who had had some success in quieting nervous disorders. On the other hand, witches could not be accused of causing bubonic plague and were not so accused, for they had no means to cure it. The same was true of other diseases for which they had no cure. Witches were usually accused of causing diseases which, in some cases, they knew how to cure or relieve.

Accused witches might admit to curing disease while denying that they caused it or that they used magic to cure it. One accused Essex witch, Ursula Kemp, declared that though she could "un-witch," she could not "witch." In Scotland in 1620, Alexander Drummond was accused of using magic to cure "frenzies, the falling evil [epilepsy], persons mad, distracted or possest with fearful apparitions, and St. Antonie's fire [gangrenous ergotism]." He admitted curing people, but said he used no magic.

In summary, in Early Modern Europe witchcraft persecution occurred at a time of widespread impairment of the health of people and animals. The distribution of illness, often interpreted as a sign of bewitchment, mimics the pattern of the incidence of ergotism: it was most common in alpine areas and those with summers in the $17.4°–18.9°$ C temperature range; a majority of the victims were children and teenagers; and rye was a dietary staple in the areas affected.

Why did witchcraft persecution peak in the period 1560–1660? Perhaps the weather was to blame. This was a cold century. The Thames River froze over in 1565, 1595, 1608, 1621, 1635, 1649, and 1655; it has not done so since. Cold winters traumatize rye and increase the risk of ergot alkaloid formation. Such alkaloids may have caused the symptoms of "bewitchment." When the incidence of these symptoms increased, so did the incidence of witchcraft persecution. We today should avoid the mistake made by the witch-burners of long ago by not overlooking a physical cause for events that mystify us.

KEY TERMS

Agonal, 195 • Antiscorbutic, 191 • Arbovirus, 194 • Colliers, 191 • Conglutinations, 189 • Enterovirus, 194 • Fornon, 184 • Fuliginous and mordant, 189 • Prodrome, 195 • Remittent fever, 182 • Tachycardia, 195 • Tachypnea, 195 • Travil, 184

QUESTIONS TO CONSIDER

1. The expression "old wives' tale" is often heard in response to reports of the efficacy of a natural-based remedy that has been known for a long time. Yet, consider how often such remedies have worked, even when no one necessarily knew why. The use of foxglove (digitalis) for heart problems, and consumption of fresh vegetables and fruits, especially citrus (vitamin C), to prevent scurvy are two well-known examples. What other old wives' tales have been proven useful by science?

2. Historical epidemics such as The Sweat and the Athenian Plague have never been scientifically and reliably identified. Considerable evidence now reveals that even the Black Death was in fact *not* bubonic plague, at least as we now know it. However, aside from providing a publication subject for revisionist historians, why does this fact matter? Of what value is identifying these ancient epidemics? What lessons can be learned by the modern epidemiologist?

3. What are the linkages today between new findings in the laboratory and the treatment of patients? Why do you think doctors of the past were so reluctant to try new methods and ideas? Is the field of medicine simply one in which new ideas must be derided, even ridiculed for a time, before they become part of patient care? If so, why?

4. What is the greater lesson to be learned from the possible link between ergot poisoning and the witch persecutions? What does Matossian want the reader to take away from that particularly dark chapter of history?

RECOMMENDED READINGS

Alexander, John T. *Bubonic Plague in Early Modern Russia: Public Health and Urban Disaster.* Oxford: Oxford University Press, 2002.

Bourgeois, Louise. *Midwifery and Medicine in Early Modern France.* Exeter: University of Exeter Press, 1996.

Brown, Stephen R. *Scurvy: How a Surgeon and a Gentleman Solved the Greatest Medical Mystery of the Age of Sail.* New York: Thomas Dunne Books, 2004.

Carmichael, Ann. *Plague and Poor in Renaissance Florence.* Cambridge: Cambridge University Press, 1986.

Cohn, Samuel K., Jr. *The Black Death Transformed: Disease and Culture in Early Renaissance Europe.* London: Arnold, 2003.

Defoe, Daniel. *A Journal of the Plague Year.* New York: Norton, 1992.

Healy, Margaret. *Fictions of Disease in Early Modern England: Bodies, Plagues, and Politics.* New York: Palgrave, 2002.

Hunter, Lynette, and Sarah Hutton, eds. *Women, Science, and Medicine, 1500–1700.* Phoenix Hill, Gloucestershire, UK: Sutton, 1997.

Lindemann, Mary. *Medicine and Society in Early Modern Europe.* Cambridge: Cambridge University Press, 1999.

Park, Katherine. *Doctors and Medicine in Early Renaissance Florence.* Princeton, NJ: Princeton University Press, 1985.

Chapter Ten

The Nineteenth Century

The Development and Spread of Western Medicine

INTRODUCTION

In the nineteenth century, Western medicine became modernized in the context of an entirely new paradigm—the germ theory of disease—which would affect every branch of the field. However, this modernization was not the only change that occurred; innovations and discoveries were reported in surgery; in medical education; in gastroenterology, dentistry, obstetrics, epidemiology, and pathological anatomy; and in many other specialties. New equipment was developed, new hospitals were built, new professional organizations were formed, and new textbooks were written. Not a year passed without reports of improvements in the theory and practice of medicine. The Bacteriological Revolution, beginning with Louis Pasteur's and Robert Koch's discoveries, set Western medicine on a path of dynamic change. Bacteriology, virology, parasitology, immunology, and microbiology all grew out of the Bacteriological Revolution, and by the end of the century, a significant number of pathogens and vectors had been labeled in the etiology of many infectious diseases.

Two of the most important discoveries in nineteenth-century medicine were the developments in antisepsis and anesthesia, both of which revolutionized the practice of surgery. Semmelweis's 1847 mandate of hand washing in Vienna's obstetric wards and the resultant drastic decrease in the mortality and morbidity rates of **puerperal fever** demonstrated a simple way to reduce infection. Twenty years later, Englishman Joseph Lister published his findings on the efficacy of wound disinfection with carbolic acid, proving that killing infective agents present on a wound and preventing their new growth resulted in a much higher surgical survival rate. In 1844 and 1846, U.S. dentists Horace Wells and Thomas Morton demonstrated the anesthetic quality of nitrous oxide, which was soon replaced by chloroform and ether. These two momentous breakthroughs made new surgical techniques possible by deadening pain and preventing infection, the two greatest obstacles facing surgeons. The era of modern surgery began at this point.

Some of the improvements in medical knowledge and patient care were linked to the many wars that erupted in the nineteenth century. The Napoleonic Wars, Crimean War, U.S. Civil War, Franco-Prussian War, Spanish-American War, and others were closely connected with epidemics including malaria, yellow fever, typhoid fever and dysentery, and typhus. Many advances in the laboratory did not make their way to the battlefield quickly. In particular, anesthesia and antisepsis methods were often unknown or unavailable. Improvements that *were* seen included the use of ambulances to remove wounded individuals from the battlefield and better hospital care because of the efforts of nursing staffs led by women such as Florence Nightingale, Dorothea Dix, and Clara Barton. Perhaps two of the best results from the warfare experience were the Geneva Convention, which established international rules for the treatment of wounded soldiers, and the creation of the International Red Cross.

The latter part of the nineteenth century was also the Age of Imperialism, as capitalism in the Atlantic world drove the industrial countries in an insatiable competition for overseas colonies. Because so many of the colonial possessions of England, France, Belgium, Germany, Italy, and the United States were located in the tropics, both soldiers and civilians who became the colonial elite had to deal with new diseases. The nascent field of tropical medicine emerged as a full-fledged specialty because of the need to control diseases with which the Europeans had little experience. Such diseases included **schistosomiasis; African sleeping sickness,** or trypanosomiasis; **leishmaniasis;** and **elephantiasis,** as well as old enemies such as yellow fever and malaria.

The new science-based medicine was touted as a great benefit for the colonial peoples, as Europeans attempted to justify, at least in their own minds, their takeover of huge portions of the world. The argument seemed logical: Peoples who had suffered for countless generations from these tropical diseases could benefit from modern medical care, vaccines, and better sanitation. However, the medical component of imperialism did not improve the standard of living in Asia and Africa. In fact, conversely, infectious diseases could travel faster and farther because of modern transportation. People like the Hawaiians and Fiji Islanders nearly vanished because of their exposure to temperate-zone diseases to which they had no immunity. The number of epidemics increased, and the colonial peoples were submerged in a level of poverty unlike any they had ever seen.

Thus, the medical history of the nineteenth century shows a decidedly bifaceted picture. On one hand, Western medicine became permanently linked to science, with all the discoveries and innovations that came with this link. On the other hand, not everyone benefited from these advances, and poverty, war, and pestilence continued to stalk most of the world.

TIME LINE

(note: The following time line is by no means complete, but is rather a sampling of the hundreds of advances in this period.)

1812 C.E.	Benjamin Rush writes the first U.S. textbook on psychiatry— *Medical Inquiries and Observations Upon the Diseases of the Mind;* Bellevue Hospital is founded in New York City

1816	René Théophile Laënnec (France) invents the stethoscope; publishes his findings in 1819
1817	James Parkinson (UK) publishes *An Essay on the Shaking Palsy*—the first clinical description of parkinsonism
1822	William Beaumont begins experiments on digestion by testing digestive activity in gunshot victim Alexis St. Martin's stomach; publishes findings in 1833
1825	Pierre Bretonneau (France) performs the first successful tracheotomy to treat diphtheria; in 1826, he publishes a description of the disease and names it
1831	Samuel Guthrie discovers chloroform, which will become an important anesthetic in the next two decades
1832	British Medical Association is formed
1835	Charles Pravaz (France) invents the hypodermic syringe
1839	Baltimore College of Dental Surgery is founded—first dental school in the world
1843	Oliver Wendell Holmes recommends that doctors wash hands and wear clean clothes to cut down on the incidence of puerperal fever
1844	Horace Wells is the first person to use nitrous oxide (laughing gas) as a dental anesthetic
1845	Rudolph Virchow (Germany) first describes leukemia
1846	William Morton uses ether as an anesthetic in general surgery for the first time
1847	American Medical Association (AMA) is founded; James Simpson (Scotland) initiates the use of chloroform in childbirth, which becomes a common practice; Ignaz Semmelweiss (Hungary) proves puerperal fever is contagious—orders doctors to wash their hands before going into hospital wards
1849	Elizabeth Blackwell receives her doctor of medicine (MD) degree in New York—first woman in the United States to do so
1850	Women's Medical College of Philadelphia is founded
1852	American Pharmaceutical Association is founded
1854	John Snow proves cholera is waterborne by disabling London's Broadstreet pump and mapping the incidence of the disease in the city
1858	*Gray's Anatomy* is first published; becomes a standard text
1860	Florence Nightingale (UK) founds the Nightingale School for Nurses, thus establishing nursing as a woman's profession

1861	Louis Pasteur (France) proves that disease is caused by germs in his *On the Extension of the Germ Theory to the Etiology of Certain Common Diseases;* germ theory revolutionizes medicine
1863	Pasteur proves that bacteria are destroyed by heat, which makes the safe use of commercially produced milk through pasteurization possible
1865	Joseph Lister (UK) uses carbolic acid as a surgical disinfectant; reduces surgical death rate from 45 percent to 15 percent
1869	Gerhand Hansen (Norway) discovers the leprosy bacillus
1872	Jean Charcot (France) uses hypnosis in therapy; teaches the method to Freud in 1885
1874	London School of Medicine for Women is founded
1876	Robert Koch (Germany) discovers the anthrax bacillus, which gives credence to the new germ theory of disease; six years later, he also discovers the tuberculosis bacillus
1879	Albert Neisser (Germany) discovers the gonorrhea bacillus
1881	Carlos Finlay (Cuba) suggests *Aedes aegypti* mosquitoes carry yellow fever, but he is ignored until 1900; Edwin Klebs discovers the typhoid bacillus—also works on tuberculosis, malaria, anthrax, and syphilis
1883	Koch discovers the cholera vibrio; proves it is spread by water and food
1884	Carl Koller (Austria) first uses cocaine as a local anesthetic
1885	Pasteur develops and successfully uses the rabies vaccination
1886	Ernst von Bergmann (Germany) introduces steam sterilization in surgery
1887	Almoth Wright (UK) develops the typhoid vaccine
1888	Eugen Fick (Switzerland) and Edouard Kalt (France) almost simultaneously invent the contact lens; Pasteur Institute is founded
1890	Emil von Behring (Germany) and Shibasaburo Kitasato (Japan) codevelop the tetanus and diphtheria vaccinatons; William Halstead introduces the use of sterile rubber gloves in surgery; William James publishes *Principles of Psychology,* which becomes a standard text; Koch discovers tuberculin and despite huge popular acclaim of the substance as a cure for human tuberculosis, it is found to be useless —public reaction shows the level of popular fear of the disease
1893	William Osler (Canada) publishes *The Principles and Practice of Medicine,* which becomes a standard text in the United States; Johns Hopkins Hospital is established for teaching and research; Daniel Williams performs the first open-heart surgery, in the United States
1894	Alexandre Yersin (France) and Shibasaburo Kitasato independently discover the plague bacillus, which is named after Yersin

1895	William Roentgen (Germany) discovers x-rays
1897	Ronald Ross (UK) finds the malaria parasite in the *Anopheles* mosquito; shows transmission is by mosquito bite
1898	*Tropical Diseases—A Manual of the New Diseases of the Warm Climates,* by Patrick Manson (UK), is published; becomes a basic manual on tropical diseases and parasitology
1900	Sigmund Freud (Germany; 1856–1939) publishes *Interpretation of Dreams;* Walter Reed proves the yellow fever pathogen is carried by *Aedes aegypti* mosquitoes—a major step in controlling the disease; Karl Landsteiner (Austria) shows that ABO blood types are not compatible

Notes on Nursing

What It Is, and What It Is Not

Florence Nightingale

Florence Nightingale is without doubt one of the most famous women in the history of medicine. Born to a wealthy British family, she devoted her life to the nursing profession, despite her family's disapproval, because the occupation was regarded as disreputable. When the English became embroiled in the Crimean War in 1853, she was asked to go to the hospital at Scutari in the Crimea to take charge of nursing the enormous number of wounded soldiers. Amid chaos, confusion, and outright resistance by military leaders, she and her nurses cleaned up the hospital, reduced the mortality rate, and provided compassionate care to scores of intensely grateful patients.

After her return to England, Nightingale took a much more behind-the-scenes approach to nursing reform, and the profession was changed forever. In her letters and other writings, Nightingale made clear what nursing involved, how it must be done, and why women were admirably suited to the profession. As a result, nursing became an acceptable occupation outside the home for middle-class women. In 1859 she opened the Nightingale School of Nursing and shortly thereafter started a visiting nurse program that provided desperately needed care for the urban poor. Although she faced considerable opposition and resistance, her reclusive nature presented relatively little threat to the male medical establishment and politicians, so that she was able to accomplish such reforms. Her monumental achievements came at a time when women were not considered capable of such efforts.

Reprinted from Florence Nightingale, *Notes on Nursing: What It Is, and What It Is Not* (Cutchogue, NY: Buccaneer Books, 1976), 7–12.

Shall we begin by taking it as a general principle —that all disease, at some period or other of its course, is more or less a reparative process, not necessarily accompanied with suffering: an effort of nature to remedy a process of poisoning or of decay, which has taken place weeks, months, sometimes years beforehand, unnoticed, the termination of the disease being then, while the antecedent process was going on, determined?

If we accept this as a general principle, we shall be immediately met with anecdotes and instances to prove the contrary. Just so if we were to take, as a principle—all the climates of the earth are meant to be made habitable for man, by the efforts of man—the objection would be immediately raised,—Will the top of Mount Blanc ever be made habitable? Our answer would be, it will be many thousands of years before we have reached the bottom of Mount Blanc in making the earth healthy. Wait till we have reached the bottom before we discuss the top.

In watching diseases, both in private houses and in public hospitals, the thing which strikes the experienced observer most forcibly is this, that the symptoms or the sufferings generally considered to be inevitable and incident to the disease are very often not symptoms of the disease at all, but of something quite different—of the want of fresh air, or of light, or of warmth, or of quiet, or of cleanliness, or of punctuality and care in the administration of diet, of each or of all of these. And this quite as much in private as in hospital nursing.

The reparative process which Nature has instituted and which we call disease, has been hindered by some want of knowledge or attention, in one or in all of these things, and pain, suffering, or interruption of the whole process sets in.

If a patient is cold, if a patient is feverish, if a patient is faint, if he is sick after taking food, if he has a bed-sore, it is generally the fault not of the disease, but of the nursing.

I use the word nursing for want of a better. It has been limited to signify little more than the administration of medicines and the application of poultices. It ought to signify the proper use of fresh air, light, warmth, cleanliness, quiet, and the proper selection and administration of diet—all at the least expense of vital power to the patient.

It has been said and written scores of times, that every woman makes a good nurse. I believe, on the contrary, that the very elements of nursing are all but unknown.

By this I do not mean that the nurse is always to blame. Bad sanitary, bad architectural, and bad administrative arrangements often make it impossible to nurse. But the art of nursing ought to include such arrangements as alone make what I understand by nursing, possible.

The art of nursing, as now practised, seems to be expressly constituted to unmake what God had made disease to be, viz., a reparative process.

To recur to the first objection. If we are asked, Is such or such a disease a reparative process? Can such an illness be unaccompanied with suffering? Will any care prevent such a patient from suffering this or that?—I humbly say, I do not know. But when you have done away with all that pain and suffering, which in patients are the symptoms not of their disease, but of the absence of one or all of the above-mentioned essentials to the success of Nature's reparative processes, we shall then know what are the symptoms of and the sufferings inseparable from the disease.

Another and the commonest exclamation which will be instantly made is—Would you do nothing, then, in cholera, fever, &c.?—so deep-rooted and universal is the conviction that to give medicine is to be doing something, or rather everything; to give air, warmth, cleanliness, &c., is to do nothing. The reply is, that in these and many other similar diseases the exact value of particular remedies and modes of treatment is by no means ascertained, while there is universal experience as to the extreme importance of careful nursing in determining the issue of the disease.

The very elements of what constitutes good nursing are as little understood for the well as for the sick. The same laws of health or of nursing, for they are in reality the same, obtain among the well as among the sick. The breaking of them produces only a less violent consequence among the

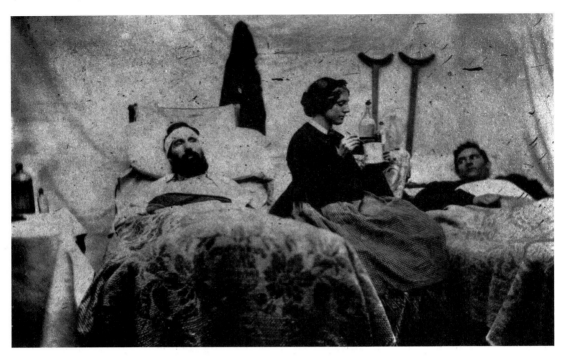

FIGURE 10–1   Civil War Nursing
Pioneering work in the field of professional nursing by women such as Florence Nightingale, Clara Barton, and Dorothea Dix found direct application during the U.S. Civil War. Civilian women worked in Union and Confederate hospitals, caring for the wounded within strict guidelines about what they could do and how they had to appear. In this photo, nurse Anne Belle, dressed properly, prepares to feed a patient, one of her many duties.

former than among the latter,—and this sometimes, not always.

It is constantly objected,—"But how can I obtain this medical knowledge? I am not a doctor. I must leave this to doctors."

Oh, mothers of families! You who say this, do you know that one in every seven infants in this civilized land of England perishes before it is one year old? That, in London, two in every five die before they are five years old? And, in the other great cities of England, nearly one out of two? "The life duration of tender babies" (as some Saturn, turned analytical chemist, says) "is the most delicate test" of sanitary conditions. Is all this premature suffering and death necessary? Or did Nature intend mothers to be always accompanied by doctors? Or is it better to learn the piano-forte than to learn the laws which subserve the preservation of offspring?

Macaulay somewhere says, that it is extraordinary that, whereas the laws of the motions of the heavenly bodies, far removed as they are from us, are perfectly well understood, the laws of the human mind, which are under our observation all day and every day, are no better understood than they were two thousand years ago.

But how much more extraordinary is it that, whereas what we might call the coxcombries of education—*e. g.*, the elements of astronomy—are now taught to every school-girl, neither mothers of families of any class, nor school-mistresses of any class, nor nurses of children, nor nurses of hospitals, are taught anything about those laws which God has assigned to the relations of our bodies with the world in which He has put them. In other words, the laws which make these bodies, into which He has put our minds, healthy or unhealthy organs of those minds, are all but unlearnt. Not but that these laws—the laws of life—are in a certain measure understood, but not even mothers think it worth their while to study them—to study how to give their children healthy existences. They call it medical or physiological knowledge, fit only for doctors.

Another objection.

We are constantly told,—"But the circumstances which govern our children's healths are beyond our control. What can we do with winds? There is the east wind. Most people can tell before they get up in the morning whether the wind is in the east."

To this one can answer with more certainty than to the former objections. Who is it who knows when the wind is in the east? Not the Highland drover, certainly, exposed to the east wind, but the young lady who is worn out with the want of exposure to fresh air, to sunlight, &c. Put the latter under as good sanitary circumstances as the former, and she too will not know when the wind is in the east. . . .

▲

Pasteur and Rabies

An Interview of 1882

JOHN ILLO, TRANS. AND ED.

The greatest achievement of nineteenth-century medical history was Louis Pasteur's development of the germ theory of medicine. Few events in medical history provoked such a drastic rethinking of the theory and practice of the healing arts as did the acceptance of germ theory. Pasteur became a national and international hero for his work, and also became embroiled in a heated competition with the other great figure of the Bacteriological Revolution—Robert Koch.

Yet, despite all the publicity and honors heaped on him, Pasteur remained a quiet individual, more comfortable working in his laboratory than in the limelight. His genius apparently showed in his gaze, however, because the reporter who recorded this interview described it as "impaling." The interview was conducted after Pasteur had achieved some of his most famous accomplishments: his work in the wine and silkworm industries, his new process of pasteurization, and his research refuting the ancient theory of spontaneous generation. At the time, Pasteur was heavily involved in the research that eventually made him a household name—his discovery of the vaccine for rabies, a universally fatal disease for which no cure existed.

The work of Pasteur and Koch introduced an entirely new paradigm in medical research and paved the way for literally thousands of new discoveries in following years. Their work was based on science, the experimental method, and quantification. As a result, medicine became permanently tied to the laboratory and the calculator.

▲

The following interview was conducted in 1882, when Pasteur was sixty. In his long career, besides his discoveries in chemistry and crystallography, he had been successful in preventing the spoiling of wine and beer, in treating the diseases of silkworms, and in vaccination for fatal diseases among livestock, achievements of great importance to the economy of France. He had been received into the Académie Française on 27 April 1882. He was at work on what would be the crowning achievement of his life, a cure for rabies. He attained it within three years. . . .

The interview was conducted by Clément Bertie-Marriott, a French journalist who used the pseudonym d'Alberty. . . . D'Alberty was not an Aristotle, but he was not a fool. And yet in the present interview he seems more impressed by Pasteur's reputation and the *bizarrerie* of his laboratory than by the significance of his work, though d'Alberty may have been writing for the tastes of his readers. . . .

Every year at the same season a terror strikes Paris. The sun burns ever and ever hotter. Rabies draws near, and gains force. Every dog becomes an object of suspicion—the poor dog, good as he is.

I thought it might be interesting and useful to visit M. Pasteur, one of the greatest scientists of our time, and to ask him the results of his remarkable research. . . .

The Academician was seated at a table littered with vials, instruments, and cages of small animals.

His grey eyes, somewhat vague, produced a strange fascination—I think that a mouse might feel the same way when he is impaled by a cat. . . .

"I've just come from Aubenas," said M. Pasteur, "and I'm most happy to see you. . . . [T]he most touching moment of my life was the welcome—cordial, enthusiastic—of all those fine people who, with all their hearts, thanked me for my discoveries—because for six years I lived among them, spending my days and nights seeking the means of helping them in their condition. I left my health behind me there. . . . **A hemiplegia** paralyzed half my body, but I restored the life and activity of that great silk industry, which is one of the glories of our country and one of the sources of its commercial wealth.

"Fifteen years ago, when it was learned that I had the imagination to make observations on liquids extracted from butterflies, and in this way to distinguish the good eggs of silkworms from the bad, everyone shrugged their shoulders. To place microscopes and delicate scientific instruments in the hands of peasants on a farm—what a daydream! That was impractical! Experience has replied victoriously. The microscope has become a commonplace instrument in silkworm nurseries, especially in the hands of women, who are particularly adept in this sensitive work.

"And so, as I said in the preface of my book on silkworms, 'the role of the infinitely small appeared to me to be infinitely great, whether because of various contagious diseases, or because it contributes to the decomposition and return to the atmosphere of all that has lived.'

"It is by this method that I found the causes of diseases in wine and beer, a true theory of the formation of vinegar, and, consequently, I made intelligible the sure method of preserving organic materials and transporting them without risk of their decomposing.

"Before me, the production of these infinitely small things called microbes, bacteria, etc. . . . was left to chance. The role they played was unknown, and was assigned to *spontaneous generation.* . . .

"Nevertheless, this propagation is the cause, if not of all, certainly of a great number of contagious diseases, and particularly of those that decimate barnyards, stables, sheepfolds. These beings, invisible to the naked eye, constitute viruses of extreme danger, which often cause death, as is proved by anthrax. . . .

"I discovered that, by the process of culture, it was possible to render these microscopic beings harmless. I found that viruses attenuated by cultures became preservatives, true vaccines that resist the development of viruses that are lethal in nature, if inoculations were given in advance.

In that way I invented anthrax vaccination in large animals.

"I hope in the same way to arrive at the discovery of a vaccine against plague, yellow fever, rabies, etc.

"But of course," M. Pasteur added, "I'd forgotten that M. Chamberland has told me that you wish to see my experiments with rabies. If you please, we'll go down to the section containing animals inoculated with rabies, and you will soon understand my procedures."

We come into a large cellar that receives air and light by wide ventilators. All along the walls are ranged great round iron cases of modern construction.

In each of the cases is a dog. There are bulldogs, poodles, terriers, griffons, etc. Above each container is a label indicating the date on which rabies was inoculated into the animal.

"Up to this point," M. Pasteur told me, "this is what I was able to discover—not much—but it was the first step to be taken. Before me, it was believed that rabies could not be transmitted except by saliva, and people were astonished to see dogs bitten by rabid dogs remaining healthy for long periods, and sometimes all their lives, without showing symptoms of the disease. I discovered the virus of rabies in the brain of the dog, in the spinal marrow, and generally throughout the nervous system. A drop of this virus, protected from contact with microbes of the outside air, and introduced into the brain of a healthy dog, will communicate rabies, and he will die of it within 15 days.

"Look—here is one in which the virus was inoculated 10 days ago. Put your foot near his cage. You see, he licks your shoe. In two days he will be dead. He is in the period of affectionateness which usually precedes by two or three days the period of violence, in which he bites everything around him. Here's another—kick his cage. See—he leaps at you. Hear that hoarse doleful barking—he has hallucinations and recognizes no one. It's been 14 days since he was inoculated. He will die tomorrow.

"Humans have the same symptoms, with the exception that the time of incubation is usually between 30 and 40 days, and that they have a horror of water, a phenomenon that is never produced among dogs.

"We have seen men who didn't die after being bitten by rabid dogs. That's because the saliva underwent the influence of the air, and a kind of struggle ensued between the microbes of the virus and the microbes of the surrounding air. This last sometimes neutralizes or modifies the effect of the virus. But with the virus in the pure state in which I extract it from the brain of one of my dogs, after a specific time of delay, death is certain, and up to now no palliation has been found for this pitiless disease.

"I still have hope, and if my life is spared, I believe that by analogy and experiment, I will attain to the discovery of a remedy.

"But before reaching the goal, I must obtain precise recognition of the organic constitution of the microbes of this virus. For these invisible beings differ among themselves as much as a man differs from a horse, and a horse from an elephant. They undergo influences just as diverse, and what diminishes the strength of one augments the strength of others. It's just in that way that I proceeded with anthrax, which killed thousands of sheep in a few days before the discovery of my vaccine, which is nothing other than the attenuated virus itself. By exposing the virus to a temperature of 40° for a certain time, the microbes grew weak, so that when they were in the body of the animal, they transmitted only a very slight anthrax, and forever protected the animal from epidemic.

"The vaccine that I obtain against anthrax offers another guarantee from that of Dr. Jenner against small-pox. The latter vaccine is taken from a heifer. It is a disease of an animal that is inoculated in a human. When the disease in cows will have disappeared—how can we preserve humans from small-pox? Thus, my dispute with Dr. Jules Guérin, who, right in the midst of a meeting of l'Académie, challenged me to a duel because I had told him that he did not understand a word of what he was asserting.

"Here are cocks, hens, guinea pigs, rabbits, mice, monkeys. I transmit to them all the serious diseases that may become epidemic, in order to study the disease in all their phases and to find a counter-poison, or at least a derivative.

"Let's move on to this small room. Look at these—a thousand little vials. They all contain the germs or viruses of dreadful diseases. There is enough here to kill all of Paris, and to give birth to the most murderous epidemics. Here I must maintain the temperature of an oven in order to keep all these germs in good condition."

Having made the tour of the room while holding a handkerchief to my nose, so strong was the odour, I was not unhappy to reach the door and find myself once again in the blossoming garden that adjoins the laboratory.

I had just had before my eyes the essence of all the diseases that decimate humanity. In spite of myself, I imagined that I might well have encountered some microbe escaped from its prison. . . .

The Medical Challenge of Military Operations in the Mississippi Valley During the American Civil War

Frank R. Freemon, MD

The U.S. Civil War was a devastating event, perhaps the first modern war and the last major war before the general acceptance of the germ theory of medicine. Casualties on both sides were extremely heavy; some 620,000 men, about one in four of the fighting force, died in the four-year conflict. Yet, battlefield injuries, horrendous as they were with the use of new weaponry, were not the principal cause of the deaths. Infectious disease, the "Third Army," killed far more men than minie balls, bayonet wounds, and other trauma combined.

Conditions in the camps were terrible. Lack of sanitation and clean water; the prevalence of mosquito-infested swamps nearby; lack of pest control of fleas, lice, and ticks; and chronic malnutrition all contributed to the overall mortality rate. Common diseases such as measles, whooping cough, and mumps spread through the troops easily because so many men came from isolated rural areas where they had never been exposed to such infections. Typhoid fever and dysentery were endemic. Pneumonia was probably the single greatest killer. Malaria attacked nearly every soldier, incapacitating even when it did not kill.

In fact, as demonstrated in this selection, the two endemic problems of malaria and dysentery played an important role in determining the outcome of the war. Because of a shortage of quinine, the relative effectiveness of both Union and Confederate forces was compromised in the Mississippi Valley campaign. Had more soldiers been available on one side or the other, the outcome of that campaign, and the war, might have been different.

Reprinted by permission of *Military Medicine:* International Journal of AMSUS, from Frank R. Freemon, "The Medical Challenge of Military Operations in the Mississippi Valley During the American Civil War," *Military Medicine* 157, no. 9 (1992): 494–97. Copyright © 1992 *Military Medicine:* International Journal of AMSUS. All rights reserved.

Introduction

At the end of the Civil War, John William Draper set to work to write, in three huge volumes, the history of that struggle. . . . According to Draper, the Northern public in 1861 was gripped by two major obsessions. These obsessions became the great war-ideas that emanated from the people and drove military strategy. The war-idea of the East called for the military occupation of the Confederate capital. . . . The great war-idea of the West demanded the free flow of the Mississippi River from the American heartland to the sea.

The barrier to the accomplishment of the war-idea of the East was the Confederate Army. While the military leaders of the North listed the destruction of the Confederate military force as the primary objective, military strategy revolved around the popular idea of seizing the Confederate capital, home of arch-rebel Jefferson Davis. For 4 years, the powerful Union Army of the Potomac and the great Confederate Army of Northern Virginia pounded each other back and forth from Washington to Richmond.

The barrier to the opening of the Mississippi, however, was primarily medical rather than military. It was well known in the middle of the 19th century that the Mississippi Valley was an area afflicted by a high rate of disease. The terminology of the period described the region as suffering from a "sickly climate," especially during the "sickly season" of late summer and fall. . . . The major illness that afflicted the population of this region was malaria, spread by the hoards of mosquitoes bred in the brackish waters of the Mississippi from New Orleans to Wisconsin. . . . In addition to malaria, the lower Mississippi Valley experienced outbreaks of the terrifying and deadly disease of yellow fever.

After the capture of New Orleans by U.S. Navy vessels steaming up from the Gulf of Mexico and of Memphis by vessels following the Mississippi southward from Cairo, Illinois, these two cities were turned into supply bases and hospital centers. The Memphis hospital system of 5,000 beds occupied virtually every downtown building. In New Orleans, several federal hospitals were opened; in addition, Union soldiers were treated by Southern civilian physicians at Charity Hospital, with the U.S. Army paying the hospital daily charges.

New Orleans harbored a potential medical disaster: yellow fever. Like malaria, this disorder was spread from the afflicted to the healthy by the bite of mosquitoes. However, malaria was an indolent disease that caused much sickness but few deaths, while yellow fever was often fatal. . . .

The Vicksburg Campaign

With Memphis and New Orleans in Union hands, the stage was set for the greatest struggle in the Mississippi Valley, the campaign for the Confederate stronghold of Vicksburg. . . .

The mission of taking Vicksburg was assigned to the Army of the Tennessee. . . . This army, numbering about 155,000 men, was under the command of Ulysses S. Grant. The opposing Confederate force, named the Army of Mississippi and East Louisiana, was commanded by John C. Pemberton until May, when he was superseded by Joseph E. Johnston. . . . The Vicksburg defenders under Pemberton engaged Grant at the Battle of Champion's Hill, but were defeated and streamed back into Vicksburg where they were surrounded. The city surrendered on July 4, 1863.

Throughout the campaign, about one in four Union soldiers of the Army of the Tennessee was on the sick and disabled list. These soldiers were in convalescent camps, were with their units but not fit for duty, or were evacuated to general hospitals. No soldiers from the Vicksburg siege were evacuated farther than the medical base of operations in Memphis by special order of General Grant. Of the 30,000 to 40,000 soldiers on the list of sick and wounded at any time, only a handful were wounded. The Union wounded numbered a few hundred every month of the campaign except May, when the heavy operations at Champion's Hill and Vicksburg produced 6,000 wounded soldiers. Despite this sudden jump in the number of wounded, the total number of sick and wounded was less in May than in April, because of a decreasing number of those sick.

The opposing Confederate forces numbered about 45,000 at the beginning of 1863. Combing the surrounding countryside for recruits and bringing in local garrisons raised the total troop concentration to nearly 65,000 by summer. . . . At the beginning of the campaign about one-third of the Confederate force was sick; this proportion rose to almost one-half by July 1863. A large number of sick were evacuated from the Department of Mississippi and East Louisiana to general hospitals in Alabama. . . . As with the Northern forces, only a handful of the disabled were wounded.

The two major illnesses afflicting the forces of both sides were symptomatic, non-specific diarrhea and malaria. These disorders were subdivided according to the **nosologic** system devised by the English physician William Farr, used by both Northern and Southern medical authorities. Diarrhea was subdivided into acute diarrhea, chronic diarrhea, acute dysentery, and chronic dysentery. . . . Malaria was subdivided into five types of **intermittent fever** based upon the frequency of the shaking chills. . . .

Some exact figures illustrate the medical situation. According to the Confederate medical returns, the Confederate forces in Mississippi in March 1863 numbered 53,542 men. A total of 21,970 soldiers, 41% of the fighting forces, were taken ill or were wounded during March. Of these, 2,851 were evacuated from the Department of Mississippi and East Louisiana to general hospitals in other departments. Malaria afflicted 4,903 soldiers and chronic diarrhea disabled 8,463. The remaining soldiers on the sick and wounded list suffered from a wide variety of diseases, but only 129 were wounded. During the same month of March, the opposing Union forces in the Department of the Tennessee numbered, according to the medical reports, 146,790. Of these, 35,376, or 24%, were ill. The major illnesses again were diarrhea, disabling 10,960 soldiers, and malaria, afflicting 6,995. Only 128 soldiers were wounded.

Despite the fact that illness disabled a greater proportion of Confederate than Union forces, the percentage of those afflicted who died was roughly similar. The overall death rate (percentage of those on the sick list who died) for the North was 2.15% and for the South 2.48%: In other words, the chance of a person on the disabled list dying was between 1 in 50 and 1 in 40. . . . The high case fatality rate from pneumonia, smallpox, and typhoid fever was not as severe a problem as one might think because of the few number of soldiers, less than 1% of the force, afflicted with these disorders.

The Trans-Mississippi Campaign

After the fall of Vicksburg and the opening of the Mississippi in the summer of 1863, the great Union war-idea of the West had been accomplished. The Confederate Secretary of War, in his official report, claimed that the unhealthy nature of the Mississippi Valley now became a Southern advantage. The fall of Vicksburg, he said, "requires the enemy to maintain, cooped up, inactive, in positions insalubrious to their soldiers, considerable detachments from their forces." While he was obviously trying to make the best of a bad situation, his prediction that the insalubrious climate would inhibit Union activities in the Mississippi Valley proved correct. The percentage of the troops of the Army of the Tennessee disabled by malaria increased after the fall of Vicksburg on July 4:

May:	3.9% of all Union troops
June:	8.5%
July:	14.5% (after the surrender)
August:	16.6%
September:	15.5%

. . . The Union goal for the Mississippi Valley in the last two years of the war involved the military occupation of the Confederate states along the river. President Lincoln hoped that the presence of a strong military force would swell union sentiment and induce the states of Arkansas and Louisiana to rejoin the Union. Despite the occupation of Little Rock, the southern half of the state of Arkansas remained in rebel hands and much of the northern half was disrupted by guerrilla activity. Union forces abandoned the goal of occupying Louisiana after their failure to advance up the Red River. The inability of the Union to accomplish its goals for the Mississippi Valley were caused, in part, by the deteriorating health of the Trans-Mississippi Union armies during the final 2 years of the war.

The Union forces in Arkansas and Louisiana were, in fact, virtually paralyzed by illness in summer and early fall. During this sickly season, over 40% of the troops were disabled; many sick soldiers sent North were replaced by others who also soon fell ill. During a typical sickly month, July 1864, in the Department of Arkansas, 13,994 soldiers were too sick for duty out of a total command of 36,109. The two great debilitating illnesses, malaria and diarrhea, were responsible for 72% of these sick soldiers. Combat injuries produced only an infinitesimal effect on the battle readiness of the Army of Arkansas; only 69 of the nearly 14,000 disabled soldiers were in the hospital because of gunshot wounds. The Confederate statistics are not known. . . .

Review of an individual with the debilitating symptom of diarrhea shows how a sick soldier had difficulty performing his military duties despite the best intentions and, furthermore, shows how convalescence at home can deplete the army of troops. Charles B. Johnson was a hospital steward with the 130th Illinois Infantry Regiment. In July 1863, he suffered a fit of vomiting and diarrhea that he attributed to drinking water directly from the Mississippi River. He expressed the feeling that he was as weak as "the classical dishrag." The vomiting stopped but he experienced loose bowel movements. He lost so much weight and became so listless that the regimental physician sent him to a nearby convalescent camp. After a few hours among strangers who all looked as thin and sallow as he did, Johnson became lonely for his friends and rejoined his regiment. His diarrhea worsened, however, and he obtained a medical furlough. From New Orleans, he traveled by riverboat to Cairo, Illinois, by train to Vandalia, Illinois, and then by wagon to his home in nearby Greenville. He spent almost 6 months enjoying the healthful conditions of his home and his mother's cooking. Upon his own initiative, he returned downriver and found his regiment in Baton Rouge, Louisiana. He estimated that he did not fully recover from his debilitating illness until 1871.

Malaria as well as chronic diarrhea took the vigor out of fighting troops. This disease was characterized by a terrible fever that shook the body, then disappeared for a day or two, then returned. This intermittent fever, accompanied by sweating, prostration, and sometimes delirium, was so characteristic that the diagnosis was not difficult. The soldiers of the 33rd Iowa Infantry Regiment, stationed in Arkansas, could tell when their bugler had malaria by the quivering of the notes. Every day a new bugler replaced the one sent to the hospital; the shaking of the bugle call at taps, however, indicated that the new bugler had contracted the disorder. The soldiers joked that the bugle was itself the source of the malaria.

Since the occurrence of malaria was known to be related to climate, physicians believed that it was beneficial to move the sick soldier to a region where the disorder was not established. The Massachusetts physician in charge of the Union army hospital in Baton Rouge felt that the southern climate was so unhealthy that medical science was almost helpless. . . . He sent his malaria patients to the North as frequently and as far as he could, even to New England. While this transfer of sick soldiers to the North may have been helpful in individual cases, a continuous hemorrhage of the sick and the convalescent sapped the military strength of the Union army in Louisiana and Arkansas during the final 2 years of the war.

Analysis

The study of military medicine in the Mississippi Valley during the American Civil War allows a double comparison. One can compare Union and Confederate medical efforts during the Vicksburg campaign of 1863. The Union force was, in general, more healthy. A second analysis compares the Union forces during the Vicksburg campaign with the Union forces during the subsequent

Trans-Mississippi campaign. The Union force became more sickly and failed to fulfill the mission of the second campaign.

Why was the Union army in the Vicksburg campaign the most healthy army in the Mississippi Valley? The two diseases responsible for the majority of illness, malaria and diarrhea, were preventable by knowledge then in existence. While the number of sick was great in both armies, it is reasonable to assume that the number would have been even greater without efforts at prevention. Of course, these efforts involved line as well as medical officers, but the stimulus to action to prevent disease was medical knowledge.

The medical science of the era had just concluded that a person in a malarious region who took quinine every day was less likely to develop malaria than one who did not. During the Vicksburg campaign, the Surgeon-General of the Union Army, William Hammond, ordered that every soldier in the Army of the Tennessee was to take quinine every day. While the medication was so bitter that it is doubtful that this order was fully carried out, perhaps enough quinine was taken to decrease the incidence of malaria. The Confederate Surgeon General ordered that quinine was not to be taken by healthy troops as a preventative but was to be reserved for the treatment of soldiers who were ill. Because of the naval blockade, quinine was in short supply throughout the Confederacy.

During the Trans-Mississippi campaign, however, the North also found quinine in short supply. Joseph Smith, the Medical Director of the Department of Arkansas, complained about his inability to obtain quinine. . . . In July 1864, Smith ordered his medical officers to husband their quinine, reserving it for those soldiers already stricken with malaria.

Chronic diarrhea, like malaria, could also be prevented. Contemporary physicians had sketchy ideas about the cause of diarrhea. . . . Today, it is clear that while diarrhea during the Civil War was undoubtedly a symptom of many different diseases, most chronic cases resulted from drinking impure water, water tainted by human waste. Contemporaries, physicians and ordinary soldiers alike, knew that fecal contamination of the water supply was

bad. . . . But the effort to separate latrines from the water supply was dissipated by the lack of bacterial knowledge that would explain how very small amounts of contamination could produce sickness.

While malaria and chronic diarrhea were disorders that might have been decreased in incidence by medical actions, the total absence of yellow fever was the great medical victory of the Mississippi Valley. The quarantine was probably of importance in preventing the outbreak of yellow fever in New Orleans and possibly its spread upriver. In 1864, there were 19 deaths from yellow fever in the New Orleans quarantine station; 3 of the victims were sailors of the U.S. Navy. If the ships carrying these sailors had been allowed to enter New Orleans, yellow fever would have spread throughout the city, and perhaps throughout the Mississippi Valley, rather than being restricted to the quarantine station.

In 1868, former Confederate physician Edwin Gaillard concluded that the greatest medical lesson of the war was to end the argument about quarantine. He thought that the experience at New Orleans and other ports proved unequivocally that ruthless quarantine could prevent yellow fever. Within a few years, however, this "lesson" was forgotten; commercial interests in New Orleans had produced a lapse of the quarantine system. The most ferocious yellow fever epidemic in American history swept up the Mississippi Valley in 1878, killing several thousand people. If this epidemic had occurred during the Vicksburg campaign, Grant's army would have been seriously crippled and the course of the war might well have been different.

Summary

In summary, sickness seriously depleted the fighting strength of the armies in the Mississippi Valley. This is not surprising: disease was common in many, even most, military campaigns prior to the development of bacteriology, although malaria added a factor to the Mississippi campaigns not present in most European wars. Analysis of military activities in the valley of the Mississippi allows a double comparison. The Northern army at the siege of Vicksburg was healthier than the

Southern one. If the Southern army had decreased its sickness rate from the measured value of 50% to the Northern rate of 25%, an additional 10,000 healthy combat soldiers would have been available. This additional manpower might have made a difference in the outcome of key combat actions such as the battle of Champion's Hill.

The second analysis compares two Union armies. The Union force during the Vicksburg campaign in 1863 was much healthier than the Union force in the Trans-Mississippi theater in 1864. The medical authorities in Washington concentrated upon the more important campaigns in Georgia and in Virginia. The supply of quinine

fell so low in the Trans-Mississippi theater that Union medical officers were forced to restrict their supply to treat rather than to prevent malaria. The medical evacuation system in 1864 shipped sick soldiers to distant departments, as far away as New England, while the commanding general in 1863 had restricted evacuation only as far north as Memphis, allowing better control of recuperating soldiers. While there is little doubt that the Confederates enjoyed superior military leadership in the Trans-Mississippi theater, additional combat forces at such key points as the battles of Mansfield or Blair's Landing might have made up for poor Union generalship.

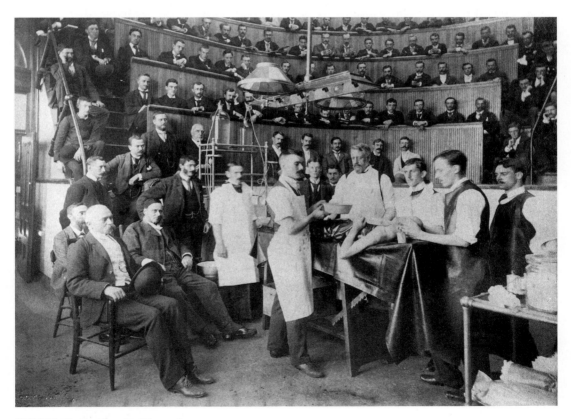

FIGURE 10–2 Surgical Procedure
Revolutionary changes in the field of surgery in the nineteenth century were due to advances in the use of anesthesia and sterile technique (antisepsis) and the control of shock and blood loss. As a result, myriad new surgical techniques were developed to correct organic defects and deal with the effects of trauma and disease. In this 1898 photo of a surgical procedure in a teaching hospital, the new principles of anesthesia and antisepsis are being taught to a new generation of physicians.

⚊

Doctors of the American Frontier

RICHARD DUNLOP

The hardy individuals who trekked west to California and Oregon faced a number of daily dangers. Attacks by hostile Native Americans constituted only one risk, and not the most common. Far more dangerous to the pioneers were the ever-present infectious diseases, most notably cholera. Any kind of accident—whether a broken bone, a knife cut, or a burn from a campfire—could cause death. It was a risk-intensive situation at best.

Few wagon trains had a physician among their members. The groups who did were expected to share their medical provider with nearby trains. More often, the wagon master kept a box with some basic remedies and instruments. The wagons could not stop to let the ill and injured recuperate, a fact that probably increased the number of fatalities. Remedies, most of which were patent medicines, were generally ineffective, and surgery in an era before anesthesia or antisepsis was a last resort.

Despite such setbacks, most of the pioneers, including the doctors, reached their destinations. They certainly had no question about what profession they would pursue in their new homes.

⚊

CHAPTER X

Physicians of the Wagon Trains

. . . Only a few wagon trains were lucky enough to have a doctor along. Men and women placed their faith in their own skill and the medical books and emergency kits they had with them. Dr. C. M. Clark, who accompanied a wagon train in 1860 in the Pikes Peak gold rush, observed: "Every man had a package of drugs and nostrums, with written directions for use, sometimes consisting of blue pills, a little ipecac and opium, together with a bottle of peppermint, pain killer and somebody's 'sovereign remedy for all ills.'"

Dr. Clark testily advised pioneers to leave their medicines at home and "pay more attention to the quality and quantity of food used, and be more careful in the matter of exposure."

Sometimes a wagon master became noted for his medical acumen, and families would join his train to be safeguarded from the diseases that infested the trails. Sol Tetherow was such a wagon master on the Oregon Trail. He relied heavily on wild ginger tea to effect his cures. How much should a patient take?

"Always git all you can but youse what you can git," he said. . . .

Sometimes the afflictions of the trail were cured by a stray mountain man, hunter, or Indian medicine man. Sometimes a granny or midwife was along. One Oregon-bound wagon train was fortunate to include Elizabeth Perry, a seventeen-year-old bride from Iowa, who showed a talent for healing. Although she had never received medical training, she delivered babies on the journey and lost only one mother and child. She scoured the country for herbs and tended the sick. When she reached Oregon, she raised a family of her own

Reprinted by permission of Joan Dunlop, from Richard Dunlop, *Doctors of the American Frontier* (Garden City, NY: Doubleday, 1965), 97–104.

and hung out a sign at her homestead which read: MRS. E. PERRY, DOCTRESS.

Typhoid fever, scurvy, smallpox, cholera, tuberculosis, and wounds inflicted by the Indians all took their toll. "Sickness often visited the emigrant," wrote Dr. Clark in Colorado. "The prevailing diseases were bilious fever, which often assumed a typhoid character, pleurisy, pneumonia and scurvy, and besides there were many other incidental ailments which were excited into action by exposure, insufficient and improper food and overexertion. Many were suffering from rheumatism, ophthalmia. I mentioned scurvy as one of the prevailing diseases but do not remember having seen a pure case; it was often, however, a complication, and I neglected to state that diarrhoea and dysentery were prevalent."

The sick were carried in the wagon resting atop the load. Exposed to weather and the jolting action, they usually got sicker instead of better. Nostalgia, according to Dr. Clark, also "exercised a most baneful influence, seemingly paralyzing all life and hope, filling the mind with corroding fears and frustrating every vital energy."

J. Goldsborough Bruff in his *Gold Rush Journals* describes a pioneer family on the trail in the Far West. An old man, sick with **flux** and scurvy, rode a horse. Beneath him was a mattress to cushion his aching bones from the jaded mount's gait. Around him was a coverlet. Pale and haggard, he stayed on the horse by holding to its neck. Another man sick with fever and ague plodded by on a mule. Women in the wagons chocked the wheels on the hills, and ten-year-old boys led the animals.

With each party of pioneers running a wilderness gauntlet of disease, accidents and wounds, a wagon train which had a doctor along was expected to share him with all others in the vicinity. Dr. John Powell on the Oregon Trail in 1852 not only cared for the sick of his own train, but rode fifty miles to care for patients with other trains. He delivered babies and fought typhoid and cholera, which he came to believe were spread by contaminated drinking water. He advised pioneers

to stay away from the water holes and organized teams of well diggers to go ahead and dig clean wells. He insisted that wagon trains keep the wells clean for pioneers still to come.

Cholera was the most fearful of the deaths that stalked the western trails. On the Overland Trail to the California gold fields 200 emigrants had already died of cholera as early as June 7, 1849, east of Fort Kearney, Nebraska, alone. By 1850 there were 40 cholera graves along the 60 miles of trail through Plum Creek Valley. Between the Missouri River and Fort Laramie there were 700 graves, the final resting places of the poor wretches who drank from the stagnant pools and water holes instead of from the Platte River. Dr. William R. Allen, who traveled overland to Oregon in 1850, reported that from 2000–3000 emigrants died of cholera on the Oregon Trail that year. He himself cared for 700 cases and claimed good success when treatment was begun early enough.

As J. Goldsborough Bruff pushed westward with a wagon train in 1849, he observed frequent graves of cholera victims. Then on July 8 cholera struck his own train. A man was stricken as they were hitching up the mules one morning. Bruff says he "drank of slew water." Mad with agony, he begged his friends to shoot him. The next day he was dead. . . .

Since fear of contagion kept even the Indians from robbing cholera graves, some wily travelers dug false graves and cached provisions or valuables in them. They erected crosses bearing their own name and the frightening legend, DIED OF CHOLERA. A St. Louis doctor on his way to the settlement on Great Salt Lake dug such a grave and hid five hundred dollars' worth of medicine in it. Later he sent a wagon out from Salt Lake to bring in his hoard. To his dismay someone had broken in and removed two hundred dollars' worth of drugs. The thief left a note giving his regrets and correctly estimating the worth of the medicine he took. He very likely was another doctor.

Cholera frightened pioneers even before they set out on the trail. Any digestive upset was imagined to be the dread killer. Army doctor William

Hammond, Jr., stationed at Fort Kearney, Nebraska, in June 1850 observed that California emigrants suffered a great deal from a disease which they called cholera. Actually it was acute diarrhea brought about by poor diet and the hardships of traveling across the high plains. He reported with disapproval the emigrants' nostrum of brandy and cayenne pepper and treated the sufferers with calomel and opium stringents.

A wagon-train doctor sometimes was also captain of the train. Dr. Elijah White led a train of 100 settlers to Oregon in 1842. Dr. Justin Millard led a party to the northwest from Keokuk, Iowa, in 1852. Hardships, exposure, and cholera destroyed Dr. Millard's health. He gave all the funds he had to the needy en route and arrived in Portland penniless and sick. Other doctors were more fortunate. In 1853 Dr. Thomas Flint of Maine, incredibly enough, drove 2000 sheep and a few oxen, horses and cows from Illinois to California through hostile Indians. He stood off the attacks of bear and wolves and brought his livestock across the Mohave Desert and through Cajon Pass. He settled down to practice at San Juan Bautista. That same year Dr. Jesse Scott Cunningham and a party brought a still greater herd of 4000 sheep overland from the Midwest. En route 375 sheep died. Dr. Cunningham paid seventy-five cents a head for them and sold them for eleven dollars a head in Sacramento.

Doctors who took the trails west did so for reasons as varied as were those of other pioneers. They looked for an adventurous release from humdrum practices in the East; they traveled west for their health; they sought gold or land; they wished to save lives. In 1852 Dr. Anson Henry, who had cared for Abraham Lincoln when he suffered his emotional disturbance, treated cholera on the western trails. When the Stephen Meek party was lost in the mountains of central Oregon in 1845 while seeking a short cut to the Willamette River, Dr. Ralph Wilcox was with them. He tended the dying as the food and water ran out. Cheerful and rotund Dr. Theophilus Degen, known to his wagon train as the "Dutch doctor," looked out for the Sager children after their father died in Wyoming, and

brought them safely over the Oregon Trail to Dr. Whitman's mission on the Walla Walla.

Forty-two-year-old Dr. David Maynard was a fugitive from a sharp-tongued wife and $30,000 in debts back home in Ohio. When he joined a westering wagon train his sole possessions were his mule, a buffalo robe, a gun, a few books, and his surgical instruments. Dr. Maynard tended cholera cases until he contracted cholera himself. He recovered because, as he observed in his diary, nobody meddled with him. Ninety miles west of Fort Kearney he stopped one afternoon to care for an emigrant family which was down with the cholera. Before morning the husband, son, and mother of comely Mrs. Israel Brashears were dead. The doctor put his scanty belongings into the tearful widow's wagon, and they started down the trail. When they reached the west coast, the doctor married the widow.

Between one winter and the next, emigrants to California and Oregon had to cover 2000 miles. The mountains were high; the deserts were wide. Pioneers traveled in a wooden box on wheels, nine to ten feet long and four feet wide with a canvas top supported by bent hickory bows. Wagon tongues and front axles snapped but could sometimes be replaced. Wheels broke, and the wagon had to be abandoned. Heat, dust, and mosquitoes plagued the emigrants. Always the wagon trains raced against the winter's first snowfall in the high mountain passes. Isaac Jones Wistar, later to be a Union general in the Civil War, traveled west with a wagon train and kept a diary which offers laconic testimony to the inexorable nature of the contest with the advancing season. Sickness could not be allowed to stay the wagons.

"May 8th. Waiting in camp on J.'s illness. If it should be small pox, we will be in a bad way, as we could neither carry him on nor expect Lipscombe to keep him in his one-roomed log cabin. To empty a wagon and haul him back to Independence would cause delay that might have serious results, in case we should arrive at the Sierra too late to cross this year."

The wagon train pressed on when J. was slightly improved. J. grew worse again. At the insistence of the train doctor the pioneers paused again so that J. could die in peace. Then they were off again on their journey that must lead over the mountains before winter.

In the evening by the trailside the life of the pioneering families went on. Children played and were disciplined. Women cooked the meals while men watered the stock and repaired the wagons. There was time in the evening for love and friendship, talk, the strumming of a banjo, and the songs of home. The campfires glowed within the circle of wagons. After a hard day's march a doctor still had to go from wagon to wagon to take care of his patients. He dispensed such medicines as Dover's powder, dragon's blood, Peruvian bark, and calomel. He bled, cupped, and leeched. He used carbolic acid for antisepsis and employed knife and saw to amputate and probe. He set broken bones and patched up heads of brawling men. He carried a small supply of candy to cure the evening misery of a homesick child. When all but the guards bedded down, he too crawled into his blankets and was thankful for the rest at the end of the day.

▲

Imperial Health in British India, 1857–1900

Radhika Ramasubban

In the last part of the nineteenth century, the British proudly boasted, "The sun never sets on the British Empire." The French touted the "civilizing mission" of their acquisition of colonies. The Russians pushed eastward into Siberia; the Americans pushed westward to the Pacific. It was the Age of Imperialism.

One of the strongest excuses for the unbridled European collection of colonial possessions was their ability to bring the advances of Western medicine to parts of the world that had never had access to it. As Europeans moved into the tropics in Asia and Africa, a new medical specialty emerged: tropical medicine. However, the primary goal of organizations such as the Indian Medical Service was not to dispense medical care to the native peoples, but to care for the British soldiers and their families stationed abroad. Only when the local epidemiology posed a massive threat to the European colonial elite did the colonial governments consider medical care and sanitary reforms for the local populations.

In fact, the coming of the Europeans worsened the disease profile of Africa, India, and other areas. In Africa, penetration of the interior spread sleeping sickness into areas where it had never been. Demanding more cash cropping for export from Egypt meant greater exposure to schistosomiasis and other water-related diseases. In India, building railroads into the interior meant that people could flood into already-overcrowded cities like Calcutta—and that any outbreak of cholera, plague, or any other infectious disease could travel much faster and farther than before. In short, the European rush for colonies was generally a medical disaster, not a benefit, for the native peoples.

▲

Reprinted by permission of Taylor & Francis Books Ltd., from Radhika Ramasubban, "Imperial Health in British India, 1857–1900," in *Disease, Medicine, and Empire: Perspectives on Western Medicine and the Experience of European Expansion,* ed. Roy M. MacLeod and Milton James Lewis (London: Routledge, 1988), 38–39, 48–55.

. . . Among the more important instruments of the British presence in India were those policies of the imperial and colonial governments concerning the investigation, prevention and cure of epidemic diseases. Periodic outbreaks of cholera, enteric fever, malaria, dystentery and diarrhoea, influenza and kala azar endangered the health of European officials—civilian and military—and their families. . . . To the extent that large-scale epidemics affected Britain's international trade, the living conditions of the general population assumed increasing importance too. . . .

. . . Death and invaliding from epidemic diseases haunted the East India Company's European troops in India from the early nineteenth century. In the 1860s, when the British made their first significant health intervention, the death-rate in the British army on the subcontinent was 69 per mille [thousand], while an estimated 84 per mille were constantly in hospital. . . . Of the total number of British deaths in the army in the first half of the nineteenth century, only 6 per cent were due to military conflict. . . . The diseases which killed European soldiers were endemic to the country. The general population, too, died from them in large numbers, although . . . what . . . had . . . been only occasional localized outbreaks now took the form of regular and widespread epidemics. This was particularly the case with cholera which, spread by marching troops, seemed to have 'engrafted itself on the soil', and with epidemic malaria, which accompanied the creation of large-scale irrigation, road and railway building works. . . .

. . . Cholera, which had spurred sanitary reform in the British army, was also the focus for extending medical administration to the general population. The international pronouncement on Indian pilgrim congregations turned the government's attention towards pilgrim centres and pilgrim routes, and the annual sanitary reports began to carry features on the major fairs and festivals in different parts of the country. . . .

. . . The puzzling mode of cholera transmission and the fear of invasion by the disease into army and European enclaves led the government to resort to sanitary cordons around pilgrim encampments, land quarantine along pilgrim routes, and the prohibition of pilgrims from entering the neighbourhood of military stations. Notwithstanding the policy of segregation of the enclave population and containment of the disease within 'native areas', the anti-contagionist stand of the Indian sanitary establishment raised for the government the unpalatable option of providing for an extensive public health machinery on an enduring basis, not only for pilgrim centres but also for the general population. The officials who sought Indian opinion on the matter of sanitary measures at pilgrim centres found that people were willing to submit to any measures calculated to promote their health. . . .

Even as the question of finding the resources for curative and preventive measures at fair sites was being posed, doubts were expressed as to whether improving the salubrity of these centres might not actually have the effect of attracting greater numbers, and thus aggravating the problem of pilgrim control. The railways added a dimension to the public health problem well beyond the confines of the pilgrim centres. The absence of rapid communications had hitherto kept disease strains localized. With the railways, this isolation broke down. The conditions of railway travel also facilitated the spread of disease. Pilgrims were stuffed into overcrowded third-class carriages and dirty goods wagons with no ventilation, lighting, drinking water or sanitary arrangements. Because allowing pilgrims to climb in and out at stations would cause delays, doors were fastened from the outside and not opened for hours at a stretch. For years, no provision existed for clean accommodation, drinking water or meals at halting stations. Death from suffocation and disease, cholera, smallpox, malaria, dysentery, and diarrhoea, and conditions conducive to tuberculosis, became more frequent as pilgrim traffic increased. The spread of communications also meant that pilgrims now poured into holy places in much larger numbers and in constant streams, overburdening local accommodation. All this further aggravated the problems of sanitation.

The pilgrim question continued to fester through the late nineteenth century. Cholera in the army had almost disappeared, and the spread of cholera beyond the country's borders was being kept in check through port health regulations. But epidemics continued to rage among the general population. It was only in the second decade of the twentieth century that the Government of India ordered an exhaustive review of the pilgrim situation. The Pilgrim Enquiry Committees found that even fifty years after the introduction of the railway system into India, the facilities were appalling. The *ad hoc* arrangements made by the government at the large pilgrim centres were inadequate. Hospital care, where it existed, was unsatisfactory and did not reflect recent advances in knowledge about cholera, or the use of bacteriological examination to prevent 'carriers' spreading the disease. Nor was there any organization for the compulsory notification of infection. Detailed and carefully investigated reports of the origin and spread of epidemics and of measures taken to combat them were lacking. Whatever limited recording and reporting was done was 'inaccurate and careless'. . . . In the absence of accumulation of accurate knowledge, remedial measures could only be based on surmise. If this was the case with the largest festivals, the smaller ones escaped attention altogether, and these constituted as great a danger as the large ones as *foci* for the spread of epidemics.

There were clearly identifiable areas where effective government intervention was essential if the complex linkages between disease at pilgrim centres and in the country at large were to be snapped. Apart from checking the worst abuses of railway travel, these included the compulsory notification of cholera; the enforcement of legal power to ensure the treatment of cases; compulsory vaccination against smallpox; more skilled sanitary and scientific officers to tour the provinces for a steady accumulation of information; [and] the provision of filtered and piped water supplies to overcome the pollution of irrigation canals and rivers. . . .

But sanitary reforms were expensive where they concerned a large and complex population. Further, such reforms and their administration required personnel qualified in medicine and sanitation to be intensively deployed among the

general population, as well as effective legislation backed by enforcing agencies. Such a huge commitment of funds and personnel was not the brief of a colonial government. The focus on pilgrims and pilgrim centres permitted the assertion that compulsory measures would offend people's religious sensibilities and be construed as interference in their customs. . . .

The bogey of interference in the religion and customs of the people was not new, but was more self-consciously applied after the Mutiny. Eighteenth-century East India Company officials, many of whom recognized in India a superior civilization, had been replaced in the early nineteenth century by administrators who saw their mission as 'civilizing' and 'modernizing' Indian society. Indian society was seen as a *tabula rasa,* waiting to be impressed in a western mould. The civilizing influence would be western social and economic institutions, especially education, and western religion, i.e. Christianity. After the Mutiny, however, the enthusiasm for remaking Indian society declined. Theories of racial exclusiveness came to the fore as Britain established itself as the governing power and as the European establishment in the country perfected the mechanisms of physical and social segregation.

Outside the feeble intervention represented by the pilgrim problem, the actual exercise of responsibility for public health was left entirely to the concerned local bodies in the various administrative units. . . . In addition to other developmental responsibilities for the areas under their jurisdiction, these bodies were expected to provide for drainage, water supply and general sanitation and maintenance of hospitals and dispensaries. . . .

These local bodies made no impact on sanitation. There was no regulation compelling municipalities to employ medical officers of health, with the result that they largely employed only Sanitary Inspectors, who, too, were untrained. The District Local Boards employed no public health staff at all, apart from vaccinators who were poorly paid and ill-educated. . . . Their ineffectiveness led, between 1888 and 1893, to the formation of a Sanitary Board for each province. . . .

But the weakness of the basic investigative and executive structures was a fundamental one. The district-level fulcrum on which the Sanitary Boards rested was the Civil Surgeon (an Indian Medical Service officer). In addition to his primary responsibilities—which included his regular medical duties, the medico-legal work of the district, medical charge of the jails and, more perfunctorily, inspection of outlying dispensaries—he was expected to be the adviser on sanitation in the municipalities of the district. His own lack of experience or of any formal training in sanitation was compounded by a lack of authority to enforce his recommendations. Overseeing several districts were the Deputy Sanitary Commissioners of each province. . . . Upon them rested the entire burden of investigating the province. But they . . . had no executive or disciplinary authority over the civil surgeons or local governments. The Deputy Sanitary Commissioners were a hopelessly small number even for their investigative functions. In Bengal, for instance, one temporary and four permanent officials were expected to oversee a population of about 71 million. Madras, with a population of 35.5 million, had three Deputy Sanitary Commissioners. . . .

At the other end of the scale were the executive agencies described earlier with their meagre and generally untrained public health staff, where the onus of registration of deaths by cause rested with the village *chowkidar* (watchman), and the tackling of epidemics was the responsibility of the district revenue subordinate officials.

In the wake of the Pilgrim Enquiry Committees in the second decade of the twentieth century, some remedial measures came to be focused on the pilgrim problem. The conditions of pilgrim movements were regulated. Conveying pilgrims in closed airtight wagons meant for goods was discouraged, eating houses at railway stations were licensed, and provision was made for drinking water and toilets at stations. At pilgrim centres, special efforts were made to check and periodically cleanse water sources (wells, tanks) and ensure general cleanliness. But the neglect of public health measures among the general population, accompanied by an intensification of trade and commerce and the growth of population in

seaport towns, as well as repeated famines, the increasing impoverishment of the rural areas and the flow of migrants into the cities in search of work, produced a plague epidemic in 1896. This was followed by successive epidemics which spread the disease to large parts of the country and which by 1918 had taken a toll of almost 10.5 million lives. . . . The absence of accurate vital statistics made it difficult to estimate the death-rates among the Indian population, but 70 per cent of the cases admitted into hospital died in the immediate aftermath of the first outbreak.

The plague, like cholera before it, invited international condemnation of the British government in India. But, unlike cholera, it prompted quick and decisive action. An epidemic of such proportions in an important commercial seaport town which caused the flight of skilled labour from the city and held out the possibility of considerable trade dislocation if the disease spread to other Indian ports by railway, was quite a different problem to the cholera outbreaks in pilgrim centres. Two pieces of legislation were passed—the Births, Deaths and Marriages Registration Act of 1896 and the Epidemic Diseases Act of 1897. The granting of legal status to vital registration and the notification of three diseases—plague, cholera and smallpox—was long overdue. . . .

Backed by the Epidemic Diseases Act, a plague committee, set up and charged with 'keep[ing] down the death rate while preventing panic and trade dislocation and lessen[ing] the risk of a third epidemic', undertook compulsory measures to combat the plague. This followed the new medical policy of the Indian government. The irrefutability of contagion, reinforced by germ theory advances, had come to be accepted in India from about the last decade of the nineteenth century. The old enthusiasm for fumigation and isolation . . . now came to be revived where the public health was concerned, in the belief that all sorts of bacteria could be destroyed in this manner. Police cordons conducted house-to-house searches, deaths were reported, the sick were isolated, dilapidated houses were vacated and disinfected and the occupants removed to camps, rural migrants were detained, and at railway stations passengers and their luggage were disinfected. Check points were instituted at major railway stations and at entry points on the borders of provinces and regions. And precautions were particularly stringent to prevent infected persons from entering the vicinity of large ports like Calcutta.

This first direct intervention in public health . . . was not only violent and insensitive but . . . was also to prove scientifically inaccurate. The single most important factor contributing to bubonic plague was insanitation, which created conditions for rats and rat fleas. And overcrowding and squalor among the teeming poor in cities like Bombay were appalling. Deliverance from the public protests generated in Bombay by the plague measures, and from the panic among rulers and ruled alike, came from the new bacteriological science. Waldemar Haffkine, a Russian emigré research worker from the Pasteur Institute in Paris. . . . was called upon for help, and by January 1897 he had developed an anti-plague vaccine which proved to have a success rate of 80–90 percent. Haffkine personally conducted the inoculation programmes and made efforts to popularize vaccination. . . . After 1898 the politically unwise compulsory measures were given up. But public health policy continued to vacillate.

Although Haffkine had been formally taken into government service in a nonpensionable capacity since 1897, he was still regarded as an outsider, and his initiative was resented by the authorities who saw it as an undue concern for their Indian subjects and as an interference in their public health policy. The growing popularity of inoculation also required more money, men, and technical and administrative facilities to be put into the anti-plague measures. . . . The British Army Medical Department on its part saw his authoritative handling of the epidemic and his apparent command over the new scientific knowledge as a threat to their professional monopoly in India. . . .

The Government of India at this time was not sufficiently aware of the importance of the new scientific advances. . . . In an era when scientific rivalry was an integral part of the national rivalries among the European powers, the leadership of the new science could not be left in the hands of a foreigner, nor applied to civilian ends. Its role in relation to the army had to be worked out first. The sponsoring of a research institute—even if fully funded—by Indian princes clashed with the prevailing attitude towards Indian princes and Indians in general which had strong racist overtones. . . . The Government of India suspended Haffkine from all research and administrative responsibilities on trumped-up charges of negligence and administrative ineffectiveness. . . . The undermining of Haffkine's contribution found its ultimate expression in the end of the inoculation drives. The efficacy of his vaccine was not given proper testing; inoculation, being 'only a personal prophylactic measure', no longer remained at the centre of the anti-epidemic campaign. Deaths from plague continued unabated, at an average of 500,000 every year from the beginning of 1898 until 1918. In fact, in the ten years from 1898 to 1908, there were an estimated 20,000 deaths a week. In 1904 alone, about 1.5 million deaths from plague were recorded.

The plague epidemic, which precipitated the deterioration in public health conditions that was to continue through the early decades of the twentieth century . . . demonstrated the continuing reluctance of the government to move in the direction of extended public health measures. Like smallpox vaccination before it, plague inoculation foundered on the rocks of inaction, justified as caution in reducing the pace of sanitary reform for fear of pressurising public opinion.

This was, in fact, quite contrary to the native Indian response. The result of the inoculation drives—the first major attempt at epidemic control—was a growing desire for sanitary reform among the general population. Representations were made by Indians requesting the government to take the initiative in maintaining the struggle against plague, and in widening the scope of sanitary reform.

But the prospect of a large-scale and expensive intervention was an alarming one for a colonial government. In the opinion of the Sanitary Department, the living conditions of the general population had gone 'beyond the influence of sanitary effort', and the government followed the route of leaving the field to the curative efforts of the private medical profession.

In a despatch of 1900, the Secretary of State for India reiterated that it was in the best interests of the people of India that the spread of an independent Indian medical profession be encouraged 'which alone can adequately supply the needs of the people'. The historical option of tackling the problem of public health through wide-ranging and enduring preventive sanitary measures—as was done in western countries—was thus lost.

KEY TERMS

African sleeping sickness, 205 • Elephantiasis, 205 • Flux, 221 • Intermittent fever, 216 • Leishmaniasis, 205 • Nosologic, 216 • Puerperal fever, 204 • Schistosomiasis, 205

QUESTIONS TO CONSIDER

1. Florence Nightingale's success in breaking through the gender barrier surrounding health care was a major advance for women who wanted to enter the profession. Nursing rapidly became an "acceptable" profession for women, largely because of the efforts of women like Nightingale, Clara Barton, and Dorothea Dix. Yet, breaking the barrier to become physicians remained exceedingly difficult for women, a fact that has changed only relatively recently. Why do you think this was so? What was more "acceptable" about the nurse, but not the physician, in the nineteenth-century mind? Why has most of the history of medicine been so strongly male dominated?

2. Wars and epidemics have been close partners throughout history. Consider the Peloponnesian War, the Hundred Years' War, and the U.S. Civil War. All had an intimate connection with major outbreaks of disease, and, to some extent, they were influenced by epidemics. What wars in the twentieth century do you think had the same connection? Why did this connection exist in the first place? Has the paradigm shift to the germ theory of medicine made any difference in the symbiosis of war and pestilence?

3. Another close relationship involving infectious disease is that with exploration and colonization. Consider the impact of the westward expansion in the United States. How did it change the epidemiological map of the continent? Why was disease so common in the wagon trains? What was the impact of these imported pathogens on the Native Americans? Have similar patterns occurred in other places that had a frontier experience, such as Australia?

4. As can be seen from the interview with Louis Pasteur, the reporter was fascinated with Pasteur's laboratory and the animals in it. Modern-day researchers routinely run experiments on animals before moving to clinical trials on human beings. From what the reporter saw, how would Pasteur's setup and methods have adhered to modern guidelines on animal research?

5. Consider the various ways that women in all cultures throughout history have nursed family members; then look carefully at the nurse in Figure 10–1. How has her role changed as a caregiver, and how has it *not* changed? How does her role appear different from that of the modern nursing professional?

6. The surgical suite shown in Figure 10–2 looks dramatically different from its twenty-first-century counterpart. Find a picture of a modern surgical suite in a book or on the Internet, then place it side by side with Figure 10–2. How many contrasts can you find? Are any similarities apparent?

RECOMMENDED READINGS

(Note: The nineteenth century is probably the most-studied period in the history of medicine. This list represents only a smattering of the scholarship for this time frame.)

Berlin, Jean V. *A Confederate Nurse: The Diary of Ada W. Bacot, 1860–1863.* Columbia: University of South Carolina Press, 1994.

Bynum, W. F. *Science and the Practice of Medicine in the Nineteenth Century.* Cambridge: Cambridge University Press, 1994.

Cunningham, Andrew. *The Laboratory Revolution in Medicine.* Cambridge: Cambridge University Press, 1992.

Denney, Robert E. *Civil War Medicine: Care and Comfort of the Wounded.* New York: Sterling, 1994.

Farley, John. *Bilharzia: A History of Imperial Tropical Medicine.* Cambridge: Cambridge University Press, 1991.

Fenster, Julie M. *Ether Day: The Strange Tale of America's Greatest Medical Discovery and the Haunted Men Who Made It.* New York: Harper Collins, 2001.

Freemon, Frank E. *Gangrene and Glory: Medical Care During the American Civil War.* Madison, NJ: Associated University Presses, 1998.

Furst, Lilian R. *Women Healers and Physicians: Climbing a Long Hill.* Lexington: University Press of Kentucky, 1997.

Humphreys, Margaret. *Yellow Fever and the South.* Baltimore: Johns Hopkins University, 1992.

Nelson, Sioban. *Say Little, Do Much: Nurses, Nuns, and Hospitals in the Nineteenth Century.* Philadelphia: University of Pennsylvania Press, 2001.

Pati, Biswamoy, and Mark Harrison, eds. *Health, Medicine, and Empire: Perspectives on Colonial India.* New Delhi, India: Orient Longman, 2001.

Peard, Julyan G. *Race, Place and Medicine: The Idea of the Tropics in Nineteenth Century Brazilian Medicine.* Durham, NC: Duke University Press, 1999.

Pernick, Martin S. *A Calculus of Suffering: Pain, Professionalism, and Anesthesia in 19th Century America.* New York: Columbia University Press, 1985.

Rutkow, Ira M. *American Surgery: An Illustrated History.* Philadelphia: Lippincott-Raven, 1998.

Simmons, John G. *Doctors and Discoveries: Lives That Created Today's Medicine.* Boston: Houghton Mifflin, 2002.

Straubing, Harold E. *In Hospital and Camp: The Civil War Through the Eyes of Its Doctors and Nurses.* Harrisburg, PA: Stackpole Books, 1993.

Valencius, Conevery B. *The Health of the Country: How American Settlers Understood Themselves and Their Land.* New York: Basic Books, 2002.

Watts, Sheldon. *Epidemics and History: Disease, Power, and Imperialism.* New Haven, CT: Yale University Press, 1997.

Chapter Eleven

The Nineteenth Century
Change and Upheaval

INTRODUCTION

A number of themes run through the social history of nineteenth-century medicine. Women moved into the ranks of professional health-care providers. A wide variety of popular remedies and alternative systems of medicine appeared in the marketplace. Local and national governments were forced to deal with public health concerns greatly worsened by industrialization and urbanization. Hospitals and clinics became more numerous in the cities, although rural health care remained nearly nonexistent. New diseases appeared, some of them sweeping around the world in repeated **pandemics.** In part because of better medical care, the life expectancy in Europe and the United States began to increase, and infant and maternal mortality rates declined. New vaccines allowed some diseases, such as rabies, to be avoided altogether. In short, the nineteenth century was the most dynamic period of change in the history of medicine to that time.

The increased importance of public health greatly affected individual families, neighborhoods, cities, and ultimately entire nations and societies. Much of the need for attention to public health can be traced to the industrialization of the Western world and the urbanization that accompanied it. Europe and the United States had been overwhelmingly rural societies at the beginning of the century, but by 1900 a significant portion of the population of many countries lived in cities. As workers and their families flooded into cities in search of jobs and housing, urban areas exploded in size, which put an enormous strain on the available food and water supplies, sewage removal, housing, and services such as police and fire protection. The working class lived in abject poverty, amid filth in the homes and streets, with polluted water and nearly unbreathable air.

Although the upper middle class, which increasingly controlled political power, was not particularly known for its altruism or humanitarian concerns, city and national governments had to deal with the growing problem. A healthy workforce was a productive workforce, and industrial growth depended on productive workers. Although affluent neighborhoods were certainly cleaner than the slums, disease associated with pollution and filth, such as cholera, knew no boundaries. Thus, albeit grudgingly, bodies such as the British House of Commons began to fund studies such as James Kay-Shuttleworth's *The Moral and Physical Condition of the Working Class Employed in the Cotton Manufacture* (1832) and Edwin Chadwick's *Report on the Sanitary Condition of the Labouring Population of Great Britain* (1842). As a result of their findings, public health acts were passed, which began the process of urban cleanup. Events such as London's Great Stink in 1858 forced the funding and construction of new sewers. Vaccination for diseases such as smallpox became mandatory in most industrialized countries. In time, legislators addressed the problems of child labor and the adulteration of food and drugs. In the 1880s, health and accident insurance became available for workers in Germany. In short, developments in public health made a significant difference in ordinary people's lives.

Public health was not the only area that evolved. Nearly everything about medicine changed. Medical education improved as new schools opened, and hospitals such as Johns Hopkins University were established as research and teaching institutions. Anatomy classes no longer had to depend on grave robbers for a supply of cadavers. Curriculum changed as new research results were published, and new textbooks were written. Women were finally admitted into medical schools by midcentury, although they could not join professional organizations such as the American Medical Association and the British Medical Association until somewhat later. Schools of nursing were established as that ancient role became a licensed profession. The list of changes goes on, but the point is made: Because of the advances in medicine—largely a result of the Bacteriological Revolution—the picture of health care in Europe and the United States had changed drastically. Increasingly, a new trend became visible: For some people, in some places, at certain income levels, health care improved. For others, who did not fit within these parameters, it did not.

TIME LINE

(Note: The following time line is by no means complete, but is rather a sampling of the hundreds of advances in this period.)

1796–1815	Napoleonic Wars—treatment of the wounded leads to advances in surgery and the use of "flying ambulances" to take the wounded from the battlefield; during the retreat from Moscow, which is largely forced by a typhus epidemic, Dr. Larrey performs surgery with the first local anesthetic: freezing limbs before amputation
1802–1887	Dorothea Dix—the Union's Superintendent of Female Nurses during the U.S. Civil War—lives; to fight skepticism, she accepts applications from only plain-looking women older than age 30; more than three thousand women serve during the war
1804	Haiti becomes independent from France, largely because of the decimation of French troops by yellow fever

1812	Disguised as a man, Miranda Stewart Barry receives a doctor of medicine (MD) degree at age 15 from Edinburgh University, serves at Waterloo, and becomes Inspector General in 1858; only at her death is her gender discovered
1817–1821	First cholera pandemic; begins in India, travels to West Africa, Asia, and the Philippines
1821–1912	Clara Barton lives—volunteers during the U.S. Civil War; becomes Superintendent of Female Nurses in 1864; in 1881 becomes the first president of the U.S. Red Cross and makes it into a peacetime as well as a wartime relief agency
1827–1833	Second cholera pandemic; first time it reaches Europe
1829	Louis Braille (1809–1852) introduces printing for the blind
1830–1831	Pandemic of influenza; other pandemics follow in 1833, 1889–1890
1830s	Sylvester Graham travels lecture circuits promoting his "health through diet" regimen, based on whole wheat bread and no meat or fats; now primarily remembered for the graham cracker
1832	In England, the Warburton Anatomy Act legalizes the sale of human bodies for dissection, which ends body snatching, even murder, to procure bodies
1839–1854	Third cholera pandemic
1840	Medical missionaries begin work in China
1842	Edwin Chadwick's *Report on the Sanitary Condition of the Labouring Population of Great Britain* is published
1846–1850	Irish Potato Famine—estimated one million deaths from crop failure, famine, and epidemics
1848	Scurvy outbreak in California gold fields
1850s	Repeated yellow fever epidemics in New Orleans
1854	Florence Nightingale arrives in Scutari, Crimea, during the Crimean War (1853–1856) and slashes the death rate from 40 percent to 2 percent in 6 months; her experiences there solidify her desire to develop nursing as a profession for women
1855	Third known pandemic of bubonic plague, starts in China
1858	London's Great Stink; results in design of new sewer system
1859–1869	Building of Suez Canal; thousands of local workers die of malaria and other fevers

1861	Prince Albert (UK) dies from typhoid—the disease becomes a matter of national interest
1861–1865	U.S. Civil War—last major conflict before germ theory is widely accepted
1862	Henry Dunant (Switzerland) makes an appeal to create a relief society that becomes known as the International Red Cross, founded in 1863
1863–1874	Fourth cholera pandemic
1865	Hawaiian government creates leper colony on Molokai; Father Damien arrives there in 1873, contracts leprosy, and dies there in 1889
1869–1872	Women are accepted into medical schools throughout Europe
1873	Lydia Pinkham (U.S.) begins marketing her famous "Remedy," probably the best-known **patent medicine**
1874	Andrew Taylor Still (U.S.; 1828–1917) pioneers the field of osteopathy—the idea that disease can be cured through manipulating joints
1875	Measles outbreak in the Fiji Islands; kills at least a quarter of the population
1878	Red crescent symbol is adopted unofficially to relieve the religious symbolism of the Red Cross movement; the International Federation of Red Cross and Red Crescent Societies is founded as the League of Red Cross Societies in 1919
1878, 1879	Yellow fever epidemics in Memphis, Tennessee
1881–1896	Fifth cholera pandemic
1882	British control Egypt—more cash crops and irrigation leads to more cases of waterborne diseases like schistosomiasis; United States signs The Geneva Convention for the Amelioration of the Wounded in Armies in the Field
1883	German Chancellor Otto von Bismarck introduces compulsory health insurance for factory workers; the following year, he introduces legislation for accident insurance to help families of workers injured on the job
1886	Spelman Seminary in Atlanta, Georgia, opens the first school for African American nurses; Coca-Cola is created—containing small amounts of cocaine, it is advertised as a "brain tonic and intellectual beverage"

1889	First osteopathic college is founded, in Kirksville, Missouri
1891	Keeley Institute opens in Illinois—one of the first **sanitaria** for treating alcoholism and drug addiction
1892	Ellis Island immigration station opens officially, having received immigrants since 1847; begins medical inspections of immigrants, primarily to interdict infectious diseases
1894	Plague in China; in Bombay, 1896; San Francisco, 1900; Sydney, 1902; John Kellogg (U.S.) invents the world's first precooked flaked cereal as health food, which revolutionizes breakfast
1898	Daniel Palmer (U.S.) establishes the study of chiropractic at the Palmer School; a new German cough suppressant has an opium derivative with the brand name "Heroin," patented by Bayer Pharmaceuticals, which also patents aspirin in 1899
1898–1899	Spanish-American War—85 percent of all deaths are due to disease, one of the worst records in U.S. military history
1899–1923	Sixth cholera pandemic
1900	Measles and influenza outbreaks occur during the Alaskan gold rush
1906	Pure Food and Drug Act is passed, especially to stop the worst frauds and to prohibit dangerous ingredients from being used in patent medicines

▲

Report on the Sanitary Condition of the Labouring Population of Great Britain

Edwin Chadwick

The first few decades of the Industrial Revolution in England brought enormous hardship for the working classes. Forced from the countryside and crowded into slums and newly constructed substandard housing, they were exposed to all the dangers of urban life. In time, even the middle

Reprinted from Edwin Chadwick, *Report on the Sanitary Condition of the Labouring Population of Great Britain* (Edinburgh, UK: Edinburgh University Press, 1965), 88–90, 138–39, 141, 224–25, 258–59.

class and the government became concerned about the squalor and filth in working-class neighborhoods. In 1842, sanitarian Edwin Chadwick published an official report that graphically described the horrors of working-class living conditions. As a result of his report, plus the repeated cholera epidemics that afflicted all classes, the Public Health Act of 1848 was passed, and increasing attention began to be paid to the need to clean up England's cities.

The Report *provided a new approach to public health. Much of the* Report *comprised information from field research reports by an army of individual investigators. Such reports provided a much more detailed picture than before. The* Report *also used statistics in the form of lists and tables. As a result, tabulating raw data to substantiate information found in the anecdotal evidence became a permanent part of public health reporting.*

▲

General Conditions of the Residences

Mr. Harding, medical officer of the Epping union, states:

> The state of some of the dwellings of the poor is most deplorable as it regards their health, and also in a moral point of view. As it relates to the former, many of their cottages are neither wind nor water tight. . . . As it relates to the latter, in my opinion a great want of accommodation for bedrooms often occurs, so that you may frequently find the father, mother, and children all sleeping in the same apartment, and in some instances the children having attained the age of 16 or 17 years, and of both sexes; and if a death occurs in the house, lest the person die of the most contagious disease, they must either sleep in the same room, or take their repose in the room they live in. . . .

. . . The following extract from *Mr. Hodgkins,* the medical officer of Bilston, in the Wolverhampton Union, describes the condition of the population of a colliery district:

> Bilston, like Wolverhampton, has not been visited by fever to any extent since the cholera in 1832. . . . The occupations of the poorer classes are chiefly colliers, labourers, &c., great members of the latter being Irish. The houses of those applying for parochial medical relief which I have visited have been dirty and crowded, the habits of the working classes here being generally improv-

ident and dirty, many parties forming heaps of filth close to their doors; and here, as in Wolverhampton, I am afraid it would require the interference of the law to effect any permanent good. . . .

Dr. Edward Knight gives the following description of the sanitary condition of the town of Stafford:

> During the year ending September 29th, 1839, there have been in the fever-wards connected with the Stafford County General Infirmary 76 cases of fever. . . . The far greater part of these cases commenced in the town of Stafford, some being brought to the infirmary in a dying state, which gives a greater rate of mortality. Although the fever-wards are well arranged, and every comfort and attention provided for the patients, there is a general dislike on the part of the poor to be removed to them from their own houses, except in cases of actual necessity. . . .
>
> These parts of the town are without drainage, the houses, which are private property, are built without any regard to situation or ventilation, and constructed in a manner to ensure the greatest return at the least possible outlay. The accommodation in them does not extend beyond two rooms; these are small, and, for the most part, the families work in the day-time in the same room in which they sleep, to save fuel.
>
> There is not any provision made for refuse dirt, which, as the least trouble, is thrown down in front of the houses, and there left to putrefy. The back entrances to the houses in the principal

streets are generally into these, the stabling and cow-houses, &c., belonging to them, forming one side of the street, and the manure, refuse vegetable matter, &c., carried into the street, and placed opposite to the poorer houses. . . .

The sedentary occupation of the working classes (shoemaking being the staple trade of the town), their own want of cleanliness and general intemperance, form, also, a fruitful source of disease. One-half of the week is usually spent in the public-houses, and the other half they work night and day to procure the necessary subsistence for their families. There is a great want of improvement in the moral character of the poor; they can obtain sufficient wages to support their families respectably, but they are improvident and never make any provision against illness. . . . The situation of Stafford also offers every facility for an efficient drainage; it is nearly surrounded by a large ditch, in which there might be a running stream of water, well calculated to remove all impurities; but it is always choked up, and in a stagnant state. . . .

Supplies of Water

. . . *Mr. Forrest,* in his report on the sanitary condition of the population of Stirling, states that in that town:

The supply of water is often very deficient. There is no water-company, and the water is not conveyed into the houses even of the wealthy inhabitants. In times of scarcity it is no uncommon occurrence to see from 80 to 100 persons waiting at each public well for water; and the scarcity of it is often made an excuse by servants for the neglect of domestic duties. I may therefore with propriety say, that the poor of Stirling are often not properly supplied with water for the purposes stated in the query.

. . . In answer to the question, whether the residences of the population amidst which contagious febrile diseases arise are properly supplied with water for the purposes of cleanliness of the houses, person, and clothing? *Dr. John Macintyre,* of Greenock, states that:

Their proprietors or landlords, with a few exceptions, have not properly supplied them with water, although an ample supply of that necessary aid to cleanliness can be cheaply obtained by means of pipes from the Shaws' Water Company.

. . . Supplies of water obtained from wells by the labour of fetching and carrying it in buckets or vessels do not answer the purpose of regular supplies of water brought into the house without such labour, and kept ready in cisterns for the various purposes of cleanliness. The interposition of the labour of going out and bringing home water from a distance acts as an obstacle to the formation of better habits; and I deem it an important principle to be borne in mind, that in the actual condition of the lower classes, conveniences of this description must precede and form the habits. It is in vain to expect of the great majority of them that the disposition, still less the habits, will precede or anticipate and create the conveniences. . . . The whole family of the labouring man in the manufacturing towns rise early, before daylight in winter time, to go to their work; they toil hard, and they return to their homes late at night. It is a serious inconvenience, as well as discomfort to them to have to fetch water at a distance out of doors from the pump or the river on every occasion that it may be wanted, whether it may be in cold, in rain, or in snow. The minor comforts of cleanliness are of course forgone, to avoid the immediate and greater discomforts of having to fetch the water. . . .

Comparative Chances of Life in Different Cases

No. of Deaths	Bethnal Green	Average Age of Deceased
101	Gentlemen and persons engaged in professions, and their families . .	45 years
273	Tradesmen and their families	26

1,258   Mechanics, servants, and
         labourers, and their
         families 16
                        .
                        .
                        .

3,395   Operatives, labourers,
         and their families . . 19
                        .
                        .
                        .

No. of Deaths	LEEDS BOROUGH	Average Age of Deceased
79	Gentlemen and persons engaged in professions, and their families . .	44 years
824	Tradesmen, farmers, and their families . . .	27

No. of Deaths	LIVERPOOL, 1840	Average Age of Deceased
137	Gentry and professional persons, &c. . . .	35 years
1,738	Tradesmen and their families	22
5,597	Labourers, mechanics, and servants, &c. . .	15

Widowhood and the Pecuniary Burdens Created by Neglect

ALSTON WITH GARRIGILL PARISH
Number of Widows, and Children dependent upon them, in receipt of Relief in the above Parish; Age of Husband at death; and the alleged Cause of Death

Initials of Widows	Number of Children Dependent at the Time of Husband's Death	Occupation of Deceased Husband	Age at Death	Years' Loss by Premature Death	Alleged Cause of Death
R. W.	—	Miner	83	—	Decay of nature.
M. S.	—	Tailor	78	—	Natural decay.
M. B.	—	Miner	73	—	Not stated.
M. R.	—	Miner	72	—	Decay of nature.
S. M.	—	Miner	72	—	Decay of nature.
M. T.	—	Mason	72	—	Asthma produced from age.
A. V.	—	Miner	67	—	Asthma produced from working in mines.
M. L.	—	Miner	64	—	Influenza.
A. M.	—	Miner	63	—	Asthma produced from working in the lead-mines.
M. S.	—	Miner	63	—	Natural decline.
J. P.	—	Labourer	62	—	**Consumption.**

(continued)

Initials of Widows	Number of Children Dependent at the Time of Husband's Death	Occupation of Deceased Husband	Age at Death	Years' Loss by Premature Death	Alleged Cause of Death
H. T.	2	Mason	62	—	Asthma.
S. H.	2	Miner	60	—	Rupture of blood-vessel.
J. R.	—	Miner	60	—	Asthma produced from working in the mines.
H. L.	—	Miner	60	—	Asthma.
J. P.	—	Miner	60	—	Consumption.
M. T.	2	Miner	60	—	Bursting blood-vessel.
A. C.	—	Joiner	60	—	Jaundice.
E. K.	—	Miner	60	—	Asthma produced from working in the mines.
E. H.	—	Miner	60	—	Cholera.
D. J.	—	Glazier	59	1	Affection of the liver.
N. D.	4	Butcher	59	1	**Apoplexy.**
M. T.	—	Miner	59	1	Inflammation of the lungs.
H. A.	—	Miner	59	1	Asthma produced from working in the lead-mines, which terminated in consumption.
J. B.	—	Miner	59	1	Asthma ditto.
E. T.	—	Labourer	58	2	Accident by a coal-waggon.
M. P.	—	Miner	58	2	Asthma produced from working in the lead-mines, which terminated in consumption.
H. T.	—	Miner	57	3	Consumption accelerated by working in the lead-mines.
M. P.	1	Turner	57	3	Consumption.

Initials of Widows	Number of Children Dependent at the Time of Husband's Death	Occupation of Deceased Husband	Age at Death	Years' Loss by Premature Death	Alleged Cause of Death
H. S.	3	Miner	57	3	Influenza, terminating in dropsy.
M. J.	3	Blacksmith	55	5	Asthma.
S. M.	—	Miner	55	5	Inflammation of lungs from cold.
R. W.	—	Miner	55	5	Asthma produced from working in lead-mines.
M. R.	—	Miner	55	5	Asthma from working in the mines.
J. W.	2	Miner	54	6	**Pleurisy.**
A. F.	—	Miner	54	6	Asthma and rupture of blood-vessel.
J. L.	2	Miner	53	7	Chronic disease of rheumatism.
N. H.	2	Miner	53	7	Asthma produced from working in the lead-mines.
A. S.	—	Miner	52	8	Asthma and bursting blood-vessel.
M. W.	6	Miner	52	8	Asthma produced from working in the mines.
E. W.	5	Miner	52	8	Asthma produced from working in the mines, which terminated in consumption.
J. S.	6	Miner	51	9	Paralysis.
H. P.	9	Quarryman	49	11	Asthma by working in the lead-mines.
H. P.	5	Miner	48	12	Typhus fever.
E. H.	6	Miner	48	12	Killed in lead-mines.
M. A.	7	Miner	48	12	Consumption by bad air in the pit.

(continued)

Initials of Widows	Number of Children Dependent at the Time of Husband's Death	Occupation of Deceased Husband	Age at Death	Years' Loss by Premature Death	Alleged Cause of Death
J. C.	8	Miner	47	13	Asthma produced by working in the lead-mines.
S. E.	6	Miner	47	13	Consumption produced from a continuance of influenza.
M. T.	8	Miner	47	13	Consumption and asthma.
E. B.	3	Miner	47	13	Affection of the head, caused from an accident received in the mine.
D. R.	—	Miner	46	14	Asthma produced from working in the lead-mines.
E. B.	5	Miner	46	14	**Rheumatic fever**, which produced inflammation of the brain.
M. S.	5	Miner	46	14	Killed in lead-mine.
M. R.	1	Joiner	46	14	Dropsy.
M. F.	7	Coal Miner	46	14	Explosion of fire-damp in a coal-mine.
L. T.	3	Miner	45	15	Asthma, which terminated with dropsy.

'Report by James Mitchell on the Lead Mines, etc. in Durham, Northumberland, and Cumberland', Appendix to *First Report of Children's Employment Commission, P.P.* 1842, XVII.

▲

Public Health and Public Healthiness, São Paulo, Brazil, 1876–1893

Robin L. Anderson

The nineteenth century was a time of significant emigration from Europe. Factors compelling people to leave included political unrest and the desire for better economic opportunities. As a result,

Reprinted from Robin L. Anderson, "Public Health and Public Healthiness in São Paulo, Brazil, 1876–1893," *Journal of the History of Medicine and Allied Sciences,* 1986, vol. 41, no. 3, pp. 293–296, 302–307, by permission of Oxford University Press.

countries such as the United States, Argentina, and Brazil became the target of a huge influx of immigrants. As they flooded into the New World cities, urban expansion required attention to problems of housing, sanitation, and provision of essential services such as medical care. The city of São Paulo, Brazil, is a case in point. Until the 1880s, Brazil had a reputation of being extremely unhealthy because of yellow fever and cholera, smallpox, malaria, and tuberculosis epidemics; but even with new attention to public health matters, the expanding São Paulo population remained distinctly underserved in medical care. As this article demonstrates, the majority of working-class and poor people had to survive with little more than a charity hospital and native healers. While medical care was available to individuals who could afford it, and the new germ theory of disease was being taught in the medical schools, São Paulo was still only the most healthy in a list of extremely unhealthy cities in Brazil.

▲

Between 1876 and 1893, the city of São Paulo was undergoing considerable and often stressful change as it matured rapidly from a relatively small interior city to a thriving metropolis. The coffee planters, whose income provided most local and national revenue, were having to accept the fact that slavery was a rapidly fading institution, and that new sources of cheap labor were essential for their economic survival. The solution they devised involved importation of thousands of European immigrants, principally from Italy, a mass immigration well underway by the mid 1880s. . . .

With the influx of new people, the city of São Paulo had to deal with such urban problems as provision of utilities, sanitation and clean water, maintenance of streets and city property, and above all, public health care. During the first half of the nineteenth century, São Paulo had shared in Brazil's image as a relatively healthful country, but as in other large cities, by the 1870s that image was hopelessly shattered. The return of yellow fever in 1850 after an apparent absence of 150 years, followed immediately by the outbreak of cholera in 1855–56 dealt a heavy blow to that image. These diseases appeared periodically in Brazil during the rest of the century, claiming roughly a quarter of a million lives.

Those two diseases, which caused great consternation among all elements of the population and demands for government action to deal with them, were by no means the only infectious diseases present. Smallpox claimed hundreds of lives every year, in spite of an official policy of vacci-

nation. Malaria was endemic, even as far south as the state of São Paulo. Tuberculosis, the universal bane of nineteenth century urban existence, killed more people in almost any given year than all other diseases combined.

The Brazilian imperial government began taking an active role in public health care to attack these problems, but until 1889 little constructive work was done. . . .

In São Paulo itself, the local government had no real decision-making power in health care delivery, but was expected to handle emergencies with little financial or technical aid, and without real authority. In the late 1880s the provincial president, Francisco de Paula Rodrigues Alves, later president of Brazil, put more emphasis than ever before on the need for attention to public health, starting several important programs and financing them with money from immigration credits. His attempts to improve health care for the public represented the first step toward creation of a local public health service. . . .

After the Revolution of 1889 which replaced the Brazilian Empire with a Republican government, public health at national and state levels began to receive considerably more attention in São Paulo and elsewhere. The state of São Paulo created and financed a public health system founded on the best medical knowledge of the time, and *paulista* legislators passed a large number of laws designed to enforce compliance with new regulations. The new State Sanitary Service was officially begun in 1892, and within weeks was trying to enforce regulations on smallpox vaccinations. While relatively little was as yet known about the transmission of many infectious diseases, serious attempts were being made to limit, and indeed to prevent, some of the most spectacular contagious diseases. . . .

Medical care of any sort was difficult to obtain in São Paulo during the late nineteenth and early twentieth centuries. For those who could afford private care by licensed doctors, there were some private clinics available. Some doctors even advertised their clinic's services in the newspaper. One Dr. Carlos Botelho, who operated the Instituto Cirúrgico Hydrotherápico e Orthopédico de São Paulo even occasionally published lists in the major paper *Estado de São Paulo,* showing operations he had performed as well as the outcome of those treatments. He noted in his advertisement that he was a diplomate of the Faculty of Medicine in Paris, with specialties in eye, gynecological and genito-urinary problems, and went on to describe his rates and terms for treatment.

The only true hospital in the city of São Paulo was the Santa Casa de Misericordia, founded in 1715, which provided the only medical care facility for the poor. The Santa Casa was primarily funded through subscription membership in the Brotherhood (*Irmandade*), and the facilities were available to all, regardless of ability to pay. According to the regulations, the only people refused admission were the insane, chronic invalids, and those suffering from elephantiasis. Slaves used the Santa Casa as virtually their only source of medical care, and the mortality rate was quite high among slave admissions. The slaveowners usually waited until the slaves were incurably ill, then allowed them to enter the Santa Casa to die, thereupon being buried at no expense to the owners. Another major source of patients was the foreign population, primarily the immigrants. During the frequent bouts of yellow fever in Santos, the port city to São Paulo, the United States consular reports made constant mention of sailors and others who were taken to the Santa Casa in that city.

As was common throughout Latin America, the Santa Casa also assumed the task of caring for abandoned children. In 1824 the "roda" or wheel was built, so that parents could leave their infants to be abandoned without embarrassment of being seen. Female infants were far more likely to be abandoned than males. The Santa Casa was supposed to raise these children educate them, and care for their health, but the mortality among those abandoned was extremely high, as much as 60%. Since the hospital did not have facilities to handle the large number of foundlings, most were farmed out to nurses until they reached school age. The Santa Casa served as a foundling hospital until 1927.

Staffing the Santa Casa was a constant problem. Nursing care before 1872 was minimal, but that year funding was put on a more regular basis, making it possible to hire more people. Most patient care was done, however, by family members. Also in 1872 the French order of the Sisters of St. Joseph of Chamberg began sending nuns to serve as nurses, their maintenance being paid partly by the order and partly by the *Irmandade.* Until that time, the entire staff consisted of two nurses and four slaves. The physician staff in the clinics and wards was composed of doctors in private practice who offered their services gratis. The Santas Casas in Rio de Janeiro and Bahia were also used as a teaching facility for the medical schools there, but not in São Paulo where no such school existed.

Facilities for the Santa Casa were apparently perennially inadequate. Three moves to new sites were made to enlarge the hospital, and renovations were made periodically. In 1872 piped water and gas were added, but three years later the annual report of the physician-in-charge noted the lack of modern facilities. Numerous recommendations were made to install showers and toilets, acquire surgical equipment, and build an operating theatre, pharmacy, and pediatric ward, but were not put into practice until the final move in 1884.

Aside from the Santa Casa there were few if any places where the poor could get medical treatment. The private clinics were too expensive, and the only other hospital was the Hospital de Beneficéncia Portuguesa, which was originally intended primarily to aid those of Portuguese extraction who subscribed to the organization. The regulations were amended to permit any destitute persons to receive care, but the Santa Casa remained the principal care facility for the poor.

In the late 1870s and again in the late 1880s monthly reports from the Santa Casa were published in the *Estado de São Paulo*. The reports gave numbers of admissions, releases, and deaths, and showed the volume of care being given to the poor of the city. The poor definitely outnumbered those who could afford to pay, being roughly 97% of all admissions of non-slaves. In general the division between foreigner and Brazilian was nearly even, but of the foreigners the men outnumbered the women by nearly three to one. Few slaves appeared on the early reports, being outnumbered ten to one by the non-slave admissions, but the mortality rate was significantly higher among slaves admitted.

Outpatient care was also the responsibility of the Santa Casa. In the published reports of 1889/90, an average of nearly 500 cases came through the clinics monthly, with occasional months reaching peaks of 800 to 1,000 cases. Prescriptions from the pharmacy for the same period, which included hospital and outpatient treatment, averaged about 1,500 a month. The monthly totals increased steadily during the period and occasionally were as high as 2,200 per month.

Even considering the contribution of the Santa Casa, the population of São Paulo had only limited recourse to professional medical care. There were few trained doctors, surgeons, or pharmacists. Those who were professionals came largely from French universities until roughly the 1870s when the medical schools in Rio de Janeiro and Bahia began to graduate an increasing number of diplomates. Even so, Brazil as a whole was woefully short of doctors, particularly away from the large metropolitan centers. São Paulo before the 1880s was a provincial backwater, medically as well as economically. Doctors practicing there did not have access to current research and publication, they had no scientific societies, medical journals or the like. The situation remained static through most of the nineteenth century until the coffee boom brought new wealth to the re-

gion, and the Italian immigration brought large numbers of new people. *Paulista* medicine and medical research began to flower after 1890 under the guidance of a few men such as Drs. Adolfo Lutz, Evandro Chagas, and Emilio Ribas. Yet even by the turn of the century, the city's population was still not adequately served in matters of health care.

For the bulk of the population, cost factors often prevented the use of either prescribed drugs or patent medicines advertised in the local paper. For those who could afford only inexpensive remedies, an entire pharmacoepia of native herbal lore provided a tremendous variety of drugs. In fact, many people simply preferred to use Indian and African remedies rather than drugs prescribed by doctors in whom they placed little trust. Using roots, leaves, and fruits of an array of plants available regionally, herbalists mixed concoctions in teas, infusions, and poultices to deal with every symptom imaginable. While many such remedies were only marginally effective in dealing with symptoms, leaving aside the actual cause of the disease itself, some at least contained elements which were useful agents. In any case they were probably no more detrimental to recovery than some of the drugs prescribed by doctors and were certainly more readily available and cheaper.

Homeopathic medicine was practiced in Brazil, but did not achieve nearly the popularity among patients nor the hostility among allopaths that characterized North American medical history. Based on the principle that the smallest dose was the best dose, homeopathic remedies were available in pharmacies and enjoyed a fair degree of popularity. They were advertised in the newspapers and often used comparatively innocuous ingredients such as pepsin, glycerine, cod liver oil, and quinine. Homeopaths advertised their services openly, offering the best in French, English, and native homeopathic remedies.

While allopaths did not remonstrate vitriolically against the homeopaths, many licensed doctors did speak out against the local *curandeiros* or curers. A very large segment of the population depended on curers, particularly in situations where medical practitioners were ineffectual. In fact, people often went to the *curandeiros* until they were virtually at death's door, thereupon seeking professional advice which usually came too late. According to reports from the Santa Casa, the victims of curers accounted for a large number of those who died shortly after admission. In 1890 the Academia Nacional de Medicina heard a petition signed by several São Paulo doctors requesting that the new republican government do something to rid the city of the *curandeiros,* but in the ensuing debate over centralization versus decentralization of government services, the real issue was forgotten. Nothing was done about the curers. In fact, it is unlikely that much could have been done. Relying on a mixture of magical rites and traditional medicine, the curers attracted a large and loyal following among the poor and ignorant. Given the state of the art of medicine and the availability of doctors, hospitals, and public health care, the *curandeiros* could depend on keeping their clientele.

For the resident of São Paulo in the late nineteenth century, the prognosis for a long life of the Biblical "fourscore and ten" years was decidedly poor. If individuals could survive the first year of life, they could expect to be constantly exposed to a range of health hazards from epidemics to dietary deficiencies, all compounded by inadequate public care, medical knowledge, and sanitation. The magnitude of urban growth of São Paulo from a population of 27,557 in 1872 to 130,005 in 1894 is paralleled by the high morbidity and mortality rates of a host of diseases. Despite improvements in sanitation and availability of health care, and a substantial increase in the number of medical personnel relative to the population, health hazards continued to present a grave threat to urban life. According to statistics accumulated in 1895, the city of São Paulo had a higher mortality rate than any other major Brazilian city. . . . Thus, the stress on the rapidly expanding *paulista* capital was clearly more burdensome than in other urbanizing areas. The residents of São Paulo had to depend on the Santa Casa for most of their care, on various remedies to cure their ills, and on faith in mystical medicine when all else failed. At least in matters of health, the working class paid a heavy price for urban development.

▲

Some Account of the Yellow Fever Epidemy by Which Brazil Was Invaded in the Latter Part of the Year 1849

Br J. O. McWilliam, M.D., F.R.S., R.N.

Yellow fever was one of the most feared diseases of the nineteenth-century world. Probably African in origin, yellow fever spread throughout the tropics and temperate zones on both sides of the Atlantic, striking particularly viciously at individuals who were new to the areas where it appeared. As the British physician J. O. McWilliam's report from Brazil in 1849 shows, no one knew how the epidemic spread. Some people thought it was due to miasma—bad air and physical conditions such as decomposing organic materials that caused disease to appear. Other people followed the contagionist model of disease etiology: the idea that disease was caused by some

Reprinted from J. O. McWilliam, "Some Account of the Yellow Fever Epidemy by Which Brazil Was Invaded in the Latter Part of the Year 1849," *Medical Times (London)* 2 (1851): 423–26, 448–49, 452.

sort of harmful matter somehow transmitted either directly or indirectly between individuals. The two theories were not mutually exclusive, and each had some element of truth. However, in 1851, scientists had not yet learned that disease could be spread by a vector—a third party—in this case, the Aedes aegypti *mosquito.*

The McWilliam report was typical of the new attention being paid to epidemics throughout the nineteenth-century world. The author described the physical environment, weather, geography, and rainfall, then tracked the spread of the epidemic. Patient by patient—starting with "patient zero," the original case—was discussed. He looked for connections between them, then, based on these data, concluded with his analysis of the nature of the outbreak.

▲

. . . Notwithstanding the geographical position of Brazil, its great variety of climate, and its abounding in those elements which theoretically are supposed to induce the more aggravated forms of tropical disease, endemic disease, except in a mild form, is little known; from sweeping epidemic disease, of any kind, with the exception of small-pox—introduced by slavers—the country has, until lately, been generally considered as wholly exempt.

It was, therefore, with astonishment not unmixed with doubt, that information of the existence of yellow fever in the city of Bahia, in the month of November, 1849, was received in the other parts of the empire; and it was not until the disease had extended to Pernambuco and Rio de Janeiro, that the people in general could be led to believe that so formidable an invader had arrived among them.

I shall now endeavour to trace the origin and progress of the yellow fever epidemy of Brazil, commencing with Bahia, and then taking up the other ports of the empire in the order, so far as my information enables me, according to which they were respectively invaded by the disease, prefacing the account of the fever at each place by some brief topographical remarks.

Bahia.—The town is situated in lat. 13° south, within the north-eastern boundary of the magnificent Bay of All Saints. The shore rises high, and is richly wooded. The lower town, the resort of the shipping and the great mart of trade, consists of long narrow streets, filthy, and badly paved. The upper town rises abruptly behind, is beautifully situated, and contains some fine buildings and private residences.

The population of Bahia is about 140,000; of whom one-third are whites; the same number are mulattoes, and the rest negroes. . . .

Bahia had for several months enjoyed an immunity from all diseases except those common ailments incident to every such community, when, on the 30th September, 1849, the American brig Brazil arrived at that port, her papers said from New Orleans, but, as was afterwards ascertained, actually last from the Havannah. She had lost two men on the passage from fever, attended with black vomit; but, as their deaths were not reported to the authorities, the vessel was not placed in quarantine. The circumstance of admitting to immediate pratique a vessel from New Orleans, the very focus, as it was said, of yellow fever, while quarantine was being rigorously enforced upon all vessels coming from European ports where cholera prevailed, was much discussed by the people in the town, and even became the subject of comment in the public prints.

. . . On [the 3rd of November], Dr. Paterson, one of the chief medical men of the place, was called to his first two cases of yellow fever. "One of them was a Brazilian boy, living over the American store, frequented by the captain of the Brazil. He had been ill," says the Doctor, "for some days prior to my visit, and on the afternoon of the 3rd he had black vomit, and died within a few hours." On the same day, Dr. Paterson was also called to an Englishman who had long resided in the country, and who had frequent communication with the captain of the Brazil. During the convalescence of this, the second patient, fell ill the third case,—a young man, recently from Europe, living in the same house, and still more intimate with the captain. At the end of nine days he died of black vomit. Dr. Paterson adds: "One of the first fatal cases, and immediately succeeding those of my own, was the American Consul, also not long in the Brazils, and who constantly associated with the captain of the Brazil, and with him frequented the house of my second and third patients." . . .

Up to the 18th of November, no recorded case had occurred afloat. In a day or two, however, two deaths were reported in a Swedish brig, which was the next vessel to the Brazil, and, being consigned to the same house, had frequent intercourse with that ship. And two other deaths, as it afterwards appeared, had already occurred on board the Swede without any medical man having been called. In a few days, every man on board the Swedish vessel had caught the disease, and the greater number of them died. . . . From this time, however, there was scarcely a vessel in port that escaped. Once the disease had established itself on board of a vessel, says Dr. Paterson, "it was the rarest thing possible for the fever again to quit it until every one capable of catching it had caught it." Meanwhile the disease had extended over the town and immediate suburbs, and ceased not to rage until it had "burnt itself out for want of fuel." . . . By the end of February, it had attacked not less than 96 per cent of the inhabitants. Out of 700 seamen (English) in port, between the 1st December, 1849, and the 28th February, 1850, 223 were attacked, and 72 died. Among the native Brazilians, "and those long resident in a tropical climate, the disease was comparatively mild; not fatal, certainly, in 1 per cent. Among the African blacks it was still milder. The native coloured population suffered as numerously, but, perhaps, less severely than the whites." In those recently arrived from extra-tropical climates, the fever assumed a more intense and malignant character, the mortality amongst such having exceeded 25 per cent. . . .

Rio de Janeiro. . . . The city is built on an undulating plain, which is said to have been a swamp, and is scarcely elevated above the sea level. There still exists a considerable marsh in the immediate vicinity of the city, to the westward. The salt water passes freely through a small creek, and mingles with the waters of this marsh. Although this source of malarial exhalation is . . . not less than fifteen hundred paces long, and nearly five hundred paces wide, the inhabitants of its neighbourhood are said to be not more liable to fever than those in other parts of the city.

The mountains which encircle Rio consist of granitic rocks, and the soil is composed of disintegrated granite, with a variety of clays in beds of considerable depth.

The city itself occupies about three miles along the shore. There are some fine squares, but the streets in general are long and narrow. Sewerage and public cleanliness are matters of little concern. There are a few drains, but they seem to be little attended to, and, from the flat situation of the city, there is no run of water through them. The town is well supplied with good fresh water. The large aqueduct which conveys it from the Corcovado Mountain, is one of the most remarkable buildings in the city. . . . The population may be estimated at about 100,000 whites, 200,000 negroes and mulattoes. . . .

Intelligence that a malignant fever was raging at Bahia reached Rio by the Portuguese steam-vessel, Don Alphonso, on the 13th December, 1849. On the following day, the Portuguese ship Don João arrived from Bahia, five of her crew having sickened, and two having died, during the passage. . . .

The first known case of yellow fever in the city of Rio de Janeiro was seen on the 28th December; on which day, says Dr. Lallemand, "On entering Fergusson Ward in the large city hospital, 'Misericordia,' to which I have been physician for seven years, I found two new patients whose appearance greatly struck me, and who presented a complication of morbid phenomena, especially a 'yellow colour of the skin, black vomitings, suppression of urine, hæmorrhage from the mouth and bowels;' and, in the case of one of them, great disturbance in the mental faculties, which led me to suppose something peculiar in these cases." . . .

The Navarre sailed from Bahia . . . and arrived at Rio de Janeiro on the 3rd December. As we have already seen, yellow fever was raging at Bahia at the time the Navarre left that port. The Navarre's crew were, to appearance, in good health; the vessel was sold, and the men were paid off. Some of them went into other vessels, and were no more heard of; others went on shore at Rio, and took up their abode in the Rua da Misericordia, at a lodging-house kept by a man named Frank. . . . [There] were two other lodging-houses, the one kept by an Englishman named Wood, and the other by a Frenchman called Auguste Flourde. The lodgers of these houses very frequently visited each other. . . .

By the 10th of January ten cases of yellow fever, of which seven proved fatal, had been admitted into the Misericordia Hospital; all of them were either from the lodging-house of Frank or Wood. . . .

By the 19th of January, Dr. Lallemand had seen and treated twenty cases of yellow fever, all them belonging to the houses of Frank, of Wood, or of Flourde. Of these, fourteen were admitted to the hospital in a hopeless state, and ten died. . . .

. . . [According to Dr. Lallemand], "In the Rua da Misericordia, between the lodging houses of Flourde and Wood, separated from each by a few intervening dwellings, and exactly opposite Frank's, (the street being about twenty-four feet wide,) in the mercantile house of a German coffee merchant, whose eldest daughter had arrived from Hamburg . . . in the middle of December, bringing with her a strong healthy girl. This girl went frequently to the merchant's house, was taken ill on the 8th of January, and died on the 18th . . . of fully developed yellow fever."

The sailors of the Maria Christina frequented the merchant's house, and in the course of a few days the fever broke out on board that vessel. The crew of the now infected ship purchased their fresh meat at a Danish butcher's in the Praga da Don Manoel. The apprentice, a German, who sold them the meat, was seized with a violent attack of yellow fever on the 8th; but he recovered in three weeks.

In consequence of the grent influx of patients into the hospital from the vessels, on or about the 18th January Dr. Lallemand was ordered to take all his yellow fever patients in the hospital to an uninhabited convent on the "Ilha da Bon Jesus," distant about six miles from the city. It was not until now that Dr. Lallemand's diagnosis, given on the 30th of December, and hitherto severely combated, that the disease was yellow fever, was considered incontestably true.

"From this period," says Dr. Lallemand, "it was impossible for me to take cognizance of all the cases of yellow fever that occurred. The disease fixed itself in the Rua de Misericordia, proceeding from the house above mentioned, running almost without interruption from house to house, though with milder symptoms, and even passed into the narrow or cross streets, until that entire quarter had sickened, while, during that and the following days, not a single suspicious case occurred in any other part of the city." . . .

"In the harbour," continues Dr. Lallemand, "the disease did not take any sudden leaps, but went slowly from ship to ship. There then were lying alongside each other, the Norna, Niord, Scandia, Alfbild, Elizabeth, Maria, Helrenford, Louisa, Vestalinden, Adam, Brave, Frodo, and also another Niord, all carrying different amicable flags, so that the captains and crews visited each other; whereas the American and English vessels, which had less intercourse with the above-named ships, were not attacked by the fever till afterwards."

Subsequently the crews of the Brazilian men-of-war were affected by the fever; and now the far-spreading epidemic raged in and around Rio de Janeiro and in the harbour. . . .

I have not been able to ascertain with any degree of accuracy the number of deaths from the epidemy at Rio Janeiro and the other provinces of the empire; but it is probable that at Rio Janeiro alone not less than 14,000 or 15,000 persons perished.

At Rio Janeiro, and indeed everywhere else, the disease dealt its fury upon the natives of extra-tropical climates, and more especially upon new comers from the more northern latitudes. . . . The men of the most colossal stature died most rapidly. Of 299 northern patients treated at the hospital of Bon Jesus, 154 died, and only 145 recovered.

The mortality among the newly-arrived Portuguese was also very remarkable. . . . Next to the Portuguese, the Italians suffered most. Of the company composing the Italian opera, seventeen died; as did also nearly every member of an equestrian company. For a long time not a single image-vender, rag-merchant, or umbrella-seller, (who are almost without exception Italians) was to be seen in the streets of Rio. In many instances, half the passengers who arrived by vessels from Havre de Grace,—nay, sometimes even three-fourths of them, died within three weeks after their arrival. . . .

I consider, then, that the whole tenor of the evidence adduced bears out the following conclusions:—

1. That the Brazilian yellow fever epidemy did not arise from endemial causes. . . .

2. That the epidemy did not depend upon any general morbific agency, either stagnant in or travelling through the atmosphere. . . .

3. That the evidence of the importation of yellow fever into Bahia, Pernambuco, and Rio de Janeiro, although not of so absolute and positive a nature as there was in the case of Boa Vista, in the Cape de Verds, is still sufficiently presumptive to warrant the belief that disease was a foreign introduction into these and other ports of Brazil. . . .

▲

Hydropathy, or the Water-Cure

Marshall Scott Legan

During the nineteenth century, a considerable consumer backlash to the so-called heroic medicine that developed in the previous century took place. In Europe and the United States, people who had access both geographically and financially to medical care by licensed physicians began to reject taking massive doses of medicine to the point of toxicity and losing massive amounts of blood from bloodletting. Looking for less-drastic and less-invasive cures, medical consumers turned to a variety of alternatives, and in response to this demand, a number of new methods appeared. Osteopathy and **chiropractic** *offered cures for many ills besides those of bones and joints. Homeopathy presented a minimalist approach to medication levels. Christian Science turned to a more spiritual approach to illness.*

Hydropathy, or the "water cure," was another of these alternative systems, a mode of treatment involving the copious and frequent applications of water, usually cold, externally and internally. Clinics and sanitaria opened throughout the United States and Europe, catering to the wealthy who could afford their services, and "taking the waters" became a fashionable form of vacation. Although little evidence suggests that the concentrated application and ingestion of water cured anything, at least hydropathy was far less apt to kill its patients than was resorting to bloodletting and overdoses of medications.

▲

Reprinted by permission of The University Press of Kentucky, from Marshall Scott Legan, "Hydropathy, or the Water-Cure," in *Pseudo-Science and Society in 19th Century America*, ed. Arthur Wrobel (Lexington: University of Kentucky Press, 1987), 74–77, 79–92.

The principles of hydrotherapy have occupied a time-honored position in man's arsenal against disease and infirmity. Hydropathic remedies have enjoyed a continuum in the annals of medical practice from antiquity to the present. But never has so much emphasis been placed on the value of hydrotherapeutics as in the period 1820-60, when its practitioners developed their own unique "system," known as Hydropathy or the Water-Cure. To persuade the uninitiated of the soundness and legitimacy of their new "discovery," the hydropaths produced an elaborate structure of methodology and a vast panoply of "scientific" literature. Negatively, hydropathy, like Thomsonianism, homoeopathy, and other single-theory cures came to reject many of the valid practices in the pantheon of regular medicine. However, as a system devoted to the improvement of health, the water-cure deserves analysis as one of the least harmful, at least in its regimen, of the pseudo-sciences.

The originator of the hydropathic or water-cure system which enjoyed such vogue in the "age of the common man" was the Silesian peasant Vincent Priessnitz. Born October 4, 1799, in the vicinity of Gräfenberg, Silesia, Priessnitz, while aiding his father with farm chores, observed the efficacious effects of cold water compacts in sprains, bruises, and tumors on horses' hoofs. . . . But it was not until 1816 when Priessnitz was injured while baling hay that he became an unconditional convert to the therapeutic merits of cold water for human ailments. Kicked in the face by the horse and run over by the wagon, Priessnitz suffered two broken ribs and a severely bruised left arm. . . . Applying wet cloths as bandages an his ribs and face, he drank plenty of cold water, ate sparingly, and observed perfect repose. Within ten days, Priessnitz was able to go out, and at the end of a year, he had resumed working in the fields.

The success of his self-cure stimulated Priessnitz's imagination, and he began to broaden his investigations. . . . Ultimately, he devised a hydropathic system which employed at least three modes of treatment: (1) general application of water to the external body by either a bath or douche; (2) local application of water to particular parts of the body through the method of ablution, and (3) internal use of water by drinking, lavements, and injections. As his therapeutic reputation spread locally, especially his success in relieving gout and rheumatism, Priessnitz established a hydropathic institute in Gräfenberg in 1826. . . . A close viewer of the hydropathic scene, R.T. Claridge, reported the number of individuals treated by Priessnitz at his establishment. Starting with only 45 patients in 1829, the numbers had increased to 469 by 1836, and in 1840 1,576 took the cure. Between 1829 and 1841, Claridge calculated, over 7,298 patients followed the regimen of the Silesian hydropath.

Even more remarkable than the numbers was the geographic diversity of the clientele attracted to Gräfenberg, which included patients from "St. Petersburg, Moscow, and Paris, London and Philadelphia, Astrakhan and Constantinople, Vienna, Berlin, and Warsaw; and all Germany, Hungary, and Italy furnish their several contingents." Indeed, the inmates had a decidedly "upper crust" tinge; for example, in 1841 there resided for treatment an archduchess, ten princes and princesses, at least a hundred counts and barons, military men of all grades, several medical men, professors, lawyers, and other notables. . . .

As the evolving panacea had its adherents, it also had its critics, and considerable print and paper were devoted to the fallacies, evils, and potential harms inherent in the hydropathic regimen. The British *Lancet* condemned the itinerant physicians of hydropathy and began to report unsuccessful cures and even deaths in the fallacious attempts to cure every malady with water. . . . American periodicals especially delighted in repeating the experience of Jean-Jacques Rousseau with the cure back in 1736. Adopting the cold-water system with little discretion, Rousseau recalled that "it nearly relieved me, not only of my ills, but of my life." . . .

In spite of its critics, the water-cure system developed by Priessnitz soon spread with major impact into England. The English people had not been unaware of the benefits of cold water in the treatment of disease. In the early 1700s works had appeared in England . . . but especially a work by the British novelist and surgeon Tobias George Smollett, entitled *An Essay on the External Use of Water* (1752). . . . With the hydropathic craze infecting England, a London hydropathic institute was organized in 1842, and water-cure centers were hastily established in other localities. A published monograph described English spas, and Malvern, England's leading hydropathic institution, became a center of English society. Older health spas like Bath and Brighton were refurbished and adopted the Priessnitzian regimen. Rules for the bath were minutely prescribed for the decorum-conscious. . . .

As in England, the general tenets of hydrotherapy had been described in America long before the time of Priessnitz. . . . Americans, quite early, had discovered the delights of mineral and natural springs. Travelers had long extolled the merits of particular locations, two of the more popular being Saratoga Springs, New York, and Hot Springs, Virginia. However, other local promoters published reports of miraculous cures as they undertook to gain similar reputations for their own regional health spas. . . . It was not until the beginning of the 1840s that the brand of therapy advanced by Priessnitz began to spread to the United States.

In the 1820s the American nation had entered the period known as the "age of the common man," when little credence was given to professional credentials. Consequently, the mood of the nation was ripe for the spread of the pseudo-sciences, in part because of reaction against the excessive practices of regular medicos who often depended on the radical use of phlebotomy, vomiting, blistering, sweating, purging, and intemperate medication. It is little wonder that Americans, observing the debilitating effects that eclectic physicians had on patients, would seek cures that promised less shock to the body and seemed, at least initially, just as effective in their curative powers. Americans had always taken water with their meals—a habit which Europeans tolerated only in the interest of international goodwill. Under these conditions the water-cure would blossom full-blown as the handmaiden of health in the egalitarian American society.

The spread of hydropathy became another example of the readiness of the American public to accept anything new. The "system" devised by Priessnitz had scarcely reached the United States before several water-cure journals began to be published, two medical schools of hydropathy opened, and in a few years a hundred or more practitioners, male and female, were dispensing therapy with positive hygienic results. . . . No section of the nation enjoyed a monopoly on the "system," and hydropathic institutes were erected in all sections. The Northeast, however, by virtue of its more diverse society, often looking for leisure as well as relief, both real and perceived, proved most amenable to the panacea. . . .

The professional's and layman's Bible of the hydropathic panacea became the *Water-Cure Journal and Herald of Reform,* which under various titles survived from 1845 until the eve of the twentieth century. Initially edited by Dr. Joel Shew, the periodical enjoyed remarkable success, claiming a circulation of fifty thousand shortly after 1850. Its prospectus in 1845 claimed that the journal would be devoted to "explaining in a way the new system . . . to provide information on Bathing, Cleanliness, Clothing, Ventilation, Food, Drinks, and in general the prevention of disease." . . . Essentially, the hydropathic journal lasted, in its original form, from 1845 until 1862, when it became the *Hygienic Teacher and Water-Cure Journal,* and under other titles such as the *Herald of Health* and *Journal of Hygiene and Herald of Health* until 1897. . . .

As the definitive authority on the new pseudo-science, the *Water-Cure Journal* became the principal butt of the critics' scorn. . . . Condemning the one-idea system, the *{Boston Medical and Surgical Journal}* argued that "all the while water is still water." . . .

Indeed, it was the proposed mild regimen of the hydropaths that proved most attractive to the public's desires. Although refinements in cures might differ from locale to locale and practitioner to practitioner, they generally followed the pattern of Dr. Shew in his New York establishment. . . . The wet sheet became the approved technique, although other hydropaths might employ alternative methods for administering such treatment. Generally, a sheet of cotton or linen dipped in cold water was spread on several thick woolen blankets. The patient would then be wound in the sheet and blankets by an attendant who would secure the wrap with large pins and tape. Over the encased patient was thrown a feather bed, and the patient would remain in his cocoon for twenty-five minutes to several hours, depending upon the seriousness of his condition and his ability to work up a good perspiration. As soon as he was sweating freely, the victim was unswathed and cold water poured over him, or he was plunged into a cold bath, finally being briskly rubbed dry.

For patients with weak constitutions, the shock of the wet sheet treatment was determined to be too radical. An alternative was the wet dress, a gown with extra wide sleeves which was dipped in cold water before being put on. . . . The wet dress became the model of the so-called bloomer costume, designed in one of the hydropathic institutions, which would add zest to the dress reform movement. . . . Because of frequent bathing, wearers usually cut their hair short for easy drying, and felt themselves emancipated from the prevailing dress codes of trailing skirts, petticoats, corsets, and corkscrew curls. . . .

Another therapeutic variation was the water girdle, made of toweling three yards long and soaked every three hours in cold water. Prescribed for varying periods in the day, in extreme cases the girdle might be kept on continuously for twenty-four hours. Treatment

by these methods was made even more effectual by the baths. Baths of every kind were utilized, foot, head, finger, elbow, and arm, but the most popular was the sitz bath which employed cold water just deep enough to cover the abdomen. Only the part of the patient actually immersed was bare; otherwise, he was clothed. With his head, arms, trunk, and legs at strange angles, the patient remained in the sitz for twenty to thirty minutes, or as long as his acrobatic talents permitted. The most powerful dousing stimulant employed was the shower bath, but even the milder douche was used with greatest caution, for water falling on the head from an extended height or for an extended period was deemed extremely dangerous.

Another essential ingredient of the hydropathic cure was water drinking for internal cleansing. Most patients were directed to drink copious amounts of water, the quantity varying from five to forty tumblers in twenty-four hours. The *Water-Cure Journal* extolled water drinking and advised that twelve to twenty-four tumblers should be the minimum and maximum doses. . . . The process when sufficiently repeated for a significant time would "evacuate anything acid, acrid, irritating, effete; and without the forced, unnatural, and exhausting efforts of the organism which drugs induce." . . . Enemas were prescribed for constipation and in certain cases of diarrhea, with two pints, enough to produce distension of the colon, the recommended dose. In treatment of diseases, however, the warning was given that such techniques must be administered under professional direction. Cold injections into the urethra and vagina were of "indispensable necessity in all chronic or acute mucous or muco-purulent discharges of those passages." . . .

Dietetic regimen was also an important ingredient of the Priessnitzian cure, for he believed that the intake of hot food was injurious to all men. His remedy was to eat cold food, use water for drink, and regulate the patient's diet. Every stimulant was taboo, from brandy and claret to mustard and pepper. Luxuries imported from foreign ports, such as coffee, tea, and every kind of spice, were deemed harmful. No warm beverage whatever was permitted throughout the day, and most of the food served in the hydropathic establishments was considerably cooled, although those inmates slightly affected were allowed to consume warm meats. The caloric value of the dietetic regimen may not have been as nourishing as promised, though most patients bore their reduction in weight willingly. . . . A patient in a cold water asylum in Massachusetts joyously proclaimed after five months' treatment that he had weighed 127 pounds when he entered the asylum but had been relieved of 33 pounds of bad flesh and now felt that he had been made over. . . .

A final significant element in the hydropathic therapy was exercise, which was generally prescribed at the time of water drinking. Patients were expected to take large amounts of exercise periodically through the day, but especially after the cold baths, which would stimulate the proper therapeutic reactions. The most popular form was walking in the open air. . . . In case of inclement weather or lameness, gymnastics, dancing, and sawing or chopping wood were utilized. In an age when fainting and frailty were considered desirable for young females of the better classes, the use of dumbbells, skipping rope, and other forms of exercise must have helped the ladies. . . .

The growing army of hydropathic practitioners and the proliferation of hydropathic establishments soon found Americans of all backgrounds actively seeking the water-cure. Water for drinking, bathing, compresses, and every other purpose imaginable became the great panacea, and persons high and low, north, south, and west, extolled its benefits. . . .

In nearly all water-cure establishments miraculous cures were claimed and testimonials appeared frequently in the popular press. The experience of three members of the William S. Hamilton family may be taken as indicative of the system's success. Spending time in a Biloxi, Mississippi, institution run by Dr. Alexander Byrenheit in 1851, Kitty Hamilton wrote of the institution's proprietor: "I have never had to deal with a Physician possessed of the same delicacy and consideration for female modesty. He is a perfect gentleman." . . . John Knight, a successful Mississippi merchant who suffered from a throat infection and dyspepsia, wrote his wife from a water-cure in Pennsylvania that his health was good, and that he was eating stale brown bread, rice, and either boiled mutton or roast beef. . . . Indeed, he claimed chat his whole system was now under the full force and effect of the water treatment. He wrote that the treatment left none of the terrible after-effects of mercury and other medicines.

While the *Water-Cure Journal* is the most useful source of testimonials for hydropathy as well as other sectarian cures, no tabloid was immune from extolling cures wrought by water. The Vicksburg, Mississippi, *Weekly Sentinel* joyously reprinted a letter from the New Orleans *Delta* describing how cold water could cure the most dreaded malady in the South, yellow fever. The Vidalia, Louisiana, *Concordia Intelligencer* extracted the following from a New Jersey paper in support of hydropathy: "The watercure treatment of the various diseases to which civilized humanity is subject, is assuming an importance of which those who take [but] slight notice of passing events, can have but one conception . . . it is crowned by a success unparalleled in the history of the healing art." . . .

The paper's editor may well have had mercenary motives, for in the same issue as this glowing review there appeared under "Hydropathy Advertisement" the notice of a Dr. Gray, who had moved his water-cure location to "Wild Wood Springs," twenty-three miles east of Natchez. Gray claimed success in such acute diseases as fevers, inflammation, measles, smallpox, scarlet fever, whooping cough, as well as the following chronic diseases: debility, obesity, nervousness, neuralgia, epilepsy, insanity, gout, rheumatism, dysentery, diarrhea, headache, **dyspepsia,** disease of the spine, liver, and spleen, all skin diseases, all female diseases, scrofula and consumption in the first stages, hemorrhages, dropsy, white swelling and hip joint disease, and all other minor diseases "too tedious to name." . . .

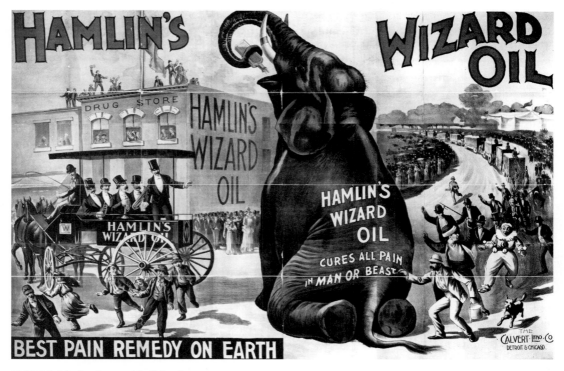

FIGURE 11–1   Patent Medicine Poster
As the consumer public in the United States and Europe became increasingly literate and sophisticated, they turned to over-the-counter preparations known as *patent medicines*. Throughout the U.S. West, such concoctions were often peddled in traveling medicine shows such as the Hamlin Company's. Their "Wizard Oil," with its trademark elephant, was claimed to be a cure-all for any ailment, but such remedies were completely unregulated by the government until the early 1900s.

In spite of the widespread popularity of water-cure therapy, pessimistic reports concerning the validity of the single cure system continued to appear in print, especially in American medical journals, which took great delight in pointing out the weaknesses or hazards of the system. . . . John Townsend Trowbridge, who spent some time in a water-cure institute, complained of little benefit from the douching, soaking, or skin friction to which he was subjected. While praising the restful conditions provided by the institution, he bitterly denounced the society of people inhabiting the water-cure whose invalidism was their chief interest in life and topic of conversation. At Brattleboro, Vermont, the prominent abolitionist Thomas Wentworth Higginson, decrying the inclement weather, wrote that "we thought it best to take all the moisture together and so we had a party of Hydropaths. Some came in tubs, other paddled in punts, and the most desperate invalids came in douches through the ceiling. We had large pails of water for supper." . . .

By the mid-1850s the water-cure mania had reached its crest. The *Boston Medical and Surgical Journal* printed an article in 1850 on its downfall and reported that water was proving unsuccessful in the most thorough hydropathic institutes.

However, this does not indicate that hydropathy disappeared, for the vogue of the water-cure system lasted until the Civil War. . . . The fate of hydropathy was not its collapse or disappearance, but rather its sublimation into the general hygienic cult. Its claim to exclusiveness as a single cure system would be lost as it merged into other health reforms. . . . Dietetic regimen, exercise, and hydrotherapeutic principles continue to be extolled as proper ingredients in maintaining holistic health even today. Not a physical fitness center, health and beauty spa, or athletic training room fails to provide its patrons with some form of hydrotherapeutic agent, be it a whirlpool bath, a swimming pool, or a steam room. . . . The availability of bottled mineral water, spring water, or jugs of distilled water which line the grocer's shelves, often at outlandish prices, gives continuing testimony to the public's faith in the efficacy of water (and distrust of public water supplies). . . . The conclusion to be drawn is that certain aspects of the pseudo-science of water-cure have found an honored place in the mind-set of the American public, and will remain. Some of the perceptions are medically and scientifically valid, but those that are not will continue to flourish because of the deep taproots of American egalitarianism best embodied in the phrase "Physician, heal thyself."

▲

Remedies for a Society's Debilities

Medicines for Neurasthenia in Victorian America

John Stea, MD, and William Fried, PhD

The nineteenth century saw its share of fad diagnoses based on cultural stereotypes, primarily of women's complaints. **Chlorosis,** *or the "green disease," was a frequent diagnosis for many young women who presented with symptoms of anorexia and* **pica,** *exhaustion, pallor, and irregular menstruation. Primarily reported among young women of well-to-do urban backgrounds, it carried a certain air of refinement and gentility, although it was also common among working-class women. In retrospect, the symptoms may have been caused by iron-deficiency anemia, physical damage due to the fashion of tight corseting, or perhaps even anorexia nervosa.*

Women were considered frail, irritable, moody, and prone to nervous disorders. The most common diagnosis, which reflected this attitude, was neurasthenia, or "nervous exhaustion," a diagnosis primarily of Victorian America. General weakness, fatigue, poor nutrition, depression and mania, and impaired intellectual function were the most common symptoms. Physicians prescribed a variety of medications and treatments ranging from electrical stimulus and bed rest, to cocaine, opium, chloral hydrate, and cod liver oil. Patients also self-prescribed the numerous patent medicines of the time, many of them primarily composed of alcohol. The most famous of these was Lydia Pinkham's "Remedy." However, this ailment affecting women who were caught in the socially acceptable explanation of simply being a member of the "weaker sex" had no true cure.

▲

Reprinted by permission of the *New York State Journal of Medicine,* from John Stea and William Fried, "Remedies for a Society's Debilities: Medicines for Neurasthenia in Victorian America," *Journal of the New York State Medical Association* 93, no. 2 (1993): 120–26.

. . . Neurasthenia, commonly termed nervous exhaustion in Victorian America, was viewed by George Beard, a New York City neurologist and prolific writer on the topic, as predominantly an American phenomenon that had arisen from the "fatiguing" effects of an increasingly urbanized society. Encompassing a wide range of symptoms, including malaise, depression, insomnia, and indigestion or dyspepsia, the diagnosis gained in popularity with both physicians and the general public as the 19th century unfolded. Those professionals who were diagnosing and treating neurasthenia . . . offered an almost endless variety of treatment regimens, including "rest cures," special diets, "electrotherapy," and medicines. The medicines used for neurasthenia between the years 1869, when George Beard's first paper on the topic appeared, and the first decade of the 20th century, were a broad range of substances, from atropine to zinc oxide. Medical journals became replete with advertisements for commercial medicines that were said to be of benefit for neurasthenia or nervous exhaustion. In their endless quest for alleviation of the Debilitating symptoms, however, many individuals placed their trust in the inexhaustible supply of patent medications. In an era of minimal regulation, there was no clear distinction between standard medicines for treatment and the patent medicines. . . . The wide gamut of substances available for neurasthenias throughout the latter decades of the 19th century was used to fill a therapeutic vacuum created by the dearth of effective, scientifically proven psychopharmacological and psychological therapies.

. . . Nineteenth century writers on neurasthenia ascribed psychological symptoms to somatic causes. Allusions to neurasthenia appeared in a number of popular journals, household "medical advisors" and medical advertisements, encouraging the Victorian public to biologize aspects of mental disorders. The importance of neurasthenia lies in its timelessness, as modern conditions such as chronic fatigue syndrome are comparable. These diagnostic labels confer respectability on sufferers by imputing a biological rather than psychological origin to their complaints. . . .

Among the myriad symptoms that were observed by physicians treating these disorders, the central feature was prostration or general weakness. . . . Beard, who had worked with Thomas A. Edison, evoked the analogy of dimmed lights, resulting from an overloaded dynamo, to explain the diminution of energy described in neurasthenia. . . . Beard postulated that the nervous system itself underwent molecular changes, becoming "dephosphoralized" from its use, resulting in changes that inevitably impaired the brain in those who were vulnerable. Undoubtedly influenced by the works of Charles Darwin, Beard also stressed the role of heredity in the etiology of neurasthenia. He described the "nervous **diathesis**," or "tendency of the constitution for nervous disease," including "nervous debility." Characterized as "strongly heredit[ar]y," Beard suggested that these conditions "may run in families for many generations." Abbey and Garfinkel attribute Beard's argument that the higher classes were predisposed to neurasthenia because of their presumably more highly evolved nervous system to his belief in social Darwinism. This presumably advanced nervous system was thought to be vulnerable to the stressful conditions of modern civilization. . . .

The role of diet and nutrition was often a central concern of physicians whose treatment of neurasthenia took into consideration the production of toxic substances that they thought were deleterious to the nervous network. . . .

. . . Many writers on neurasthenia, including George Beard, believed that women were especially vulnerable to this condition, a view that was also held by many physicians during the era. Many thought that nervous prostration in women arose from "female weakness" or uterine abnormalities. . . . In her article, *The Fashionable Discuss: Women's Complains and their Treatment in Nineteenth Century America,* Anne Douglas Wood concluded that the general ill health of women described by many practitioners during the Victorian age had become "positively fashionable." . . .

Although physicians ascribed neurasthenia primarily to an enfeebled constitution resulting from a loss of nerve force and a pathological condition of the internal organs, they also conceded the importance of environmental factors in its etiology. A common motif was that the business activity of the urban professional or "brain-worker" consumed the nerve force with which he had been endowed. In addition to "domestic trouble," "prolonged anxiety," and "pecuniary embarrassment, leading to nervous exhaustion," Van Deusen's list of predisposing factors also included "prolonged exposure to a malarial region." During the years before the infectiousness and transmissible nature of malaria were elucidated, the disease was often associated with nervous prostration both in etiology and treatment. Beard wrote, for example: "one of the great afflictions of America—malaria, often complicates neurasthenia; . . . and the two diseases not only exist together, but may be mistaken for each other."

. . . Therefore, the treatment of neurasthenia by 19th century physicians was designed to restore the depleted nerve force and help buttress the body's natural healing processes. Rest cures, special diets, and medications that would stimulate the "system," rid the body of "auto-toxic" substances, and procure rest through sedation were used. Devices were constructed for the application of static electricity, thought to "recharge" the body's lost nerve force. Retreats were established in the outskirts of urban centers, serving as institutions of rest and relaxation. McComb, of the Emanuel Movement of Boston, offered relief for female sufferers of neurasthenia, through work in the ministry. . . . Other physicians, who treated neurasthenia included the homeopaths who generally prescribed smaller doses of medications, and the botanies, who shunned mineral therapeutics such as mercury, and used compounds derived from plants. . . . Of the different treatments, medications played a major role in the treatment of neurasthenia during

the years after the appearance of Beard's first paper on the subject in 1869.

Prescription Medicine for Neurasthenia

The long list of drugs used in physicians' prescriptions for the disorder included strychnine, phosphates, bromides, chloral hydrate, alcohol, cocaine, opium, cannabis, and cod liver oil. These were listed in the *United States Dispensatory* which, published since the 1830s, provided physicians with instructions for the preparation and administration of standard therapeutics. Prescriptions were either prepared by physicians themselves or at the pharmacy. Strychnine and its derivative, *nux vomica,* were recognized as stimulants in small doses and poisons in larger ones. . . . Commonly known as Peruvian Bark, quinine was derived from several species of the cinchona tree on the western coast of south America and had been used since 1688 for intermittent fevers or agues. This medicine was ranked "first as a nerve tonic" by Van Deusen, who . . . found it especially useful in "cases marked by considerable irritability with emaciation." Tonics were considered substances that fortified the system with a cumulative physiological effect. . . . Arsenic was widely used as a tonic and alternative for the treatment of nervous prostration. It was one ingredient of a prescription for a "nerve tonic and sedative" for neurasthenia, along with "coco and citric acid" in 1900. . . . Two other important tonics for neurasthenia were iron and zinc. . . . Phosphorus, the element that was observed to be a major component of the nerve cell, was ubiquitous in regimens for the treatment of neurasthenia. . . .

Other stimulants in the physicians' armamentarium for neurasthenia included cocaine, cannabis, and caffeine. The 1870 *Dispensatory* described how the South American natives obtained energy for a several days' journey by chewing the coca leaves, alleged to "support the strength for a considerable time in the absence of food." George Beard employed cocaine as a stimulant. . . . He also described *Cannabis indica* as "one of the most trustworthy, most reliable and valuable of remedies," adding that it was beneficial in headache. Caffeine was often used in conjunction with ergot and belladonna to abate the headache of the neurasthenic. Alcohol . . . served as an ingredient in many prescriptions for neurasthenia, and Beard recommended wine, particularly claret and burgundy. . . .

Insomnia was a major consideration in treating the neurasthenic and bromides, chloral hydrate and narcotics were among the popular sedatives employed. In this *Treatise on Nervous Prostration,* Bread compared the qualities of the bromides to those of "electricity and massage." He claimed that both "give rest by slowing down the nerve activity." Physicians treating neurasthenia employed a number of bromides, including salts of sodium, potassium, zinc ammonia, and lithium, often blending them with chloral hydrate. . . .

Regulating the patient's nutrition was considered important in restoring his depleted energy reserve. Cod liver oil, alone or combined with phosphorus, was a common nutritive supplement. . . . Koumiss, or conjugated milk products, and beef tea were commonly given to neurasthenics. "Oils and fats like cream and butter," according to Bread. "were nerve food." Foods were often combined with stimulants and tonics in an endless assortment of prescriptions for neurasthenia. . . .

Commercial Medications for Neurasthenia

After the Civil War, medical journals were replete with an ever growing number and variety of commercial medicines, and by the 1870s, may were advertised for the treatment of neurasthenia. They ranged from the crude drugs to mixtures of various substances. "Phosphorus as a remedy" headed a full page promotion in one medical journal in 1883, proclaiming the usefulness of a pill that contained ". . . unoxidized phosphorus, strychnine and reduced iron" for the ". . . loss of nerve power, neuralgia and hysteria." . . . The manufacturer of

this pill claimed that another product. Warner's Effervescing Caffeine and Bromide of Potassium, was useful for "sleeplessness, overexertion of the brain, overstudy and nervous debility.". . . The ingredients of this product consisted of "nerve-given principles of the ox brain," amalgamated with the embryo of the wheat and oat and would benefit "sleeplessness, irritation, nervous exhaustion and inability to work or study." . . . Several products that manufactures claimed to be advantageous in the treatment of neurasthenia illustrated a belief in strengthening the blood among 19th century physicians. Maltine, described as an extract of malted barley, wheat and oats, was purported to contain "nitrogenous constituents," with "a composition identical to the chief constituents of blood," in one 1879 advertisement. . . .

Patent Medicines for Neurasthenia

Many medicines that were available for direct sale to the public, commonly called patent medicines, carried claims for the cure of neurasthenia and nervous debility. . . . Popular patent medicines that rarely appeared in the medical journals but were widely consumed included Ayers' Sarsaparilla and Lydia Pinkham's Vegetable compound. Derived from the plant *Smilax officinasus,* Sarsaparilla was regarded for many decades as a panacea, and a tonic. . . . Dr Ayers, of Lynn, Massachusetts, boasted in one advertisement, complete with a picture of a forceful lion, that this product would cure "Thin blood, Anemia, Poverty of the blood, Weakness, General Debility, Nervousness, Nerve Exhaustion, Nervous Prostration, Nervous Dyspepsia, Indigestion, Dyspepsia, Skin Diseases, etc." Another native of Lynn, Massachusetts, Lydia Pinkham, developed a very popular patent medicine in 1876. Her vegetable compound contained the ubiquitous alcohol and herbs, including black cohosh. . . . Designed for the "worst form of female complaints," the panacea also promised to cure nervous prostration.

Some preparations for neurasthenia, such as Cherry Malt Phosphites, were presented directly to the public as well as to the medical profession. "A combination of wild cherry, the condensed extract of the important cereals and the elixirs of the hypophosphites of lime and soda," the malt drink occupied an entire page in an 1887 edition of *The Boston Medical and Surgical Journal.* An advertisement for the same product appeared on a card that same year for distribution to the public. . . .

Public consumption of the various over-the-counter medicines that were purported to benefit sufferers from neurasthenia and other illnesses was catalyzed by the availability of almanacs, books and other literature issued by their producers that described their attributes and by advertisements in catalogues and popular journals. In the drug section of one department store catalogue, there were references to 14 patent medicines that claimed to ameliorate nerve weakness, prostration, or debility. . . .

Concerns for the Use of Medication for Neurasthenia

The demand for relief from the 19th century disorder called neurasthenia paralleled the increase and availability of remedies for the illness. The relationship between the neurasthenic's quest for relief and his faith in available medicines was recognized by Cecil MacCoy, a Brooklyn, New York, neurologist, when he wrote. " . . . neurasthenies are peculiarly liable to suggestion, and the physician who fails to avail himself of its use drops one of the most important articles out of his list of remedial agents." . . . The use of addictive medications within the expanding realm of substances for the relief of neurasthenia, from the standard preparations to the patent medicines, elicited the concerns of many physicians by the late 1800s. . . . Chloroform, opium, or alcohol were [sic] among the substances that, according to Beard, "may be reported at first an incident, and finally a habit." F. M. Hamlin of Auburn, New York, estimated that the number of opium addicts in the United States stood at 500,000 in 1885. . . .

Other concerns emerged over the medications used to treat neurasthenia. Reports of side effects and toxicity increasingly surfaced. William Krauss of Buffalo, New York, commented on toxic doses of medicines for nervous disorders in 1900, including strychnine, and urged that the assignment of maximum dosages be given in their application.

The net effect of all these concerns, coupled with the growing disquietude with other medications that were addictive, inadequately labeled and sold directly to the public, was to precipitate action by the American Pharmaceutical Association, the AMA and the general public, who demanded regulation. . . . In 1881 the state of Illinois moved to regulate the sale of poisons, including substances used commonly to treat neurasthenia, specifying morphine, strychnine, chloral hydrate, belladonna, and zinc sulfate. . . .

Conclusions

The common denominator of the various descriptions of neurasthenia was the presence of fatigue or lack of nervous force. The advertisements of medicines for neurasthenia also revealed an emphasis on the alleviation of exhaustion. In a society that placed great emphasis on strength, industry, and productivity, these symptoms received priority over other features of the disease such as anxiety, depression, and somatic complaints. Victorian physicians recognized that fatigue arose from a number of medical conditions including malaria and consumption or tuberculosis. In addition, 19th century writers on neurasthenia felt that women were endowed with less nerve force, and that the female reproductive system further taxed the nerves, leading to nervous prostration. In the medical and social atmosphere of Victorian America, the subjective experience of exhaustion and malaise were probably related to conditions that we would now categorize under the headings of depression and possibly, such physiological afflictions as premenstrual syndrome or anemia. The higher prevalence of depression among women, together with premenstrual syndrome, may account for the frequency with which neurasthenia was diagnosed in the female population. . . .

Many popular and creative people were diagnosed as having neurasthenia during the Victorian era. They included William James, Jane Addams, and Theodore Roosevelt. . . . Lutz points out that the disease became a marker of status and respectability. By the turn of the century, it permeated every aspect of society. Men and women of distinction who were described as neurasthenic served as role models for people with anxiety, depression, and other psychological conditions, who could identify with their afflicted heroes.

The diagnosis of nervous exhaustion must have proven a dilemma for women in the Victorian Era, whose willingness to accept the condition of weakness imposed by the predominantly male physicians of the period contrasted with their increasing desire to participate in an industrial society. The prevailing attitude among these men was a reflection of the prevalent cultural view that women were the weaker sex. Accordingly most in the medical profession thought women to have weaker nerves. Gossling points out that the causes for neurasthenia most commonly reported for women were genital and reproductive disturbances. Even female physicians such as Margaret Cleaves found women particularly prone to neurasthenia. Many physicians also believed that neurasthenia would be induced in women by emotional stress such as accidents. It was easier, nevertheless, for female as well as male sufferers from neurasthenia to accept an affliction that was attributable to a physical condition rather than to mental illness. Manufacturers of medicines took advantage of this preference and in their advertising promised the abatement of exhaustion. These ads promised relief from derangements that exhausted the nerves of energy, as well as the reenergizing of weakened nerves to strengthen the body. In Victorian society, these remedies served as a staple for those who were labeled or considered themselves weak and languid, stemming from a condition that was thought to afflict the best and the brightest. Although psychiatrists today employ efficacious medications that are aggressively advertised by drug companies, many individuals continue to self medicate with various street drugs, including cannabis, cocaine, opiates and alcohol, substances used as medicines by 19th century physicians treating neurasthenia. . . .

KEY TERMS

Apoplexy, 238 • Chiropractic, 248 • Chlorosis, 254 • Consumption, 237 • Diathesis, 255 • Dyspepsia, 252 • Pandemics, 230 • Patent medicine, 233 • Pica, 254 • Pleurisy, 239 • Rheumatic fever, 240 • Sanitaria, 234

QUESTIONS TO CONSIDER

1. Diagnoses such as chlorosis and neurasthenia appear suspect to the modern medical mind, yet they were frequently found in nineteenth-century medical records. Have certain modern diagnoses become popular? Why do some diseases or syndromes seem to appear, become common, then disappear? What diagnoses that we often see do you think a physician fifty years from now will scorn?

2. Medical consumers of the early twenty-first century seem to have some misgivings about modern medical practices and medications, just as our nineteenth-century fore-bears did. How has this attitude manifested today? What similarities do you see between our interest in alternative medicine and that of earlier people who went to spas for the "cure" or believed that the shape of a person's head could predict personality and intellectual ability?

3. Edwin Chadwick's *Report on the Sanitary Condition of the Labouring Population of England* made extensive use of the new so-called political arithmetic—statistics. It is full of ta-bles and charts with considerable information, a way of presenting data that was new to the nineteenth century. Look at the table at the end of the *Report*. Mine this table for information. What conclusions can you reach as a result of analysis of these data?

4. In his presentation on yellow fever in Brazil, Dr. McWilliam went to some lengths to in-clude objective data about the outbreak, without imposing his conclusions until the end. On the basis of the evidence he presented, what conclusions would you draw about the origin and spread of the epidemic? How do your conclusions differ from his? (*Remember:* You must set aside any knowledge about "germs," because the germ the-ory of disease had not yet been published in 1849.)

5. Modern-day readers looking at the dangerous and totally unregulated ingredients in the nineteenth-century patent medicines are horrified at the potential risks of consuming such substances as opium, alcohol, and cocaine. However, do any parallels exist to to-day's billion-dollar business of over-the-counter remedies? These medicines are also not regulated in terms of their claims or quality control. What are the risks inherent in modern "natural" remedies?

Recommended Readings

(Note: The nineteenth century is probably the most-studied period in the history of medicine. This list rep-resents only a smattering of the scholarship for this time frame.)

American Medical Society. *Pamphlets on Medical Fakes and Fakers.* Chicago: n.p., 1912–1922.

Beizer, Janet L. *Ventriloquized Bodies: Narratives of Hysteria in Nineteenth Century France.* Ithaca, NY: Cornell University Press, 1994.

Bingham, A. Walker. *The Snake-Oil Syndrome: Patent Medicine Advertising.* Hanover, MA: Christopher Publishing House, 1994.

Cooley, Thomas. *The Ivory Leg in the Ebony Cabinet: Madness, Race, and Gender in Victorian America.* Amherst: University of Massachusetts Press, 2001.

Frawley, Maria H. *Invalidism and Identity in Nineteenth Century Britain.* Chicago: University of Chicago Press, 2004.

Metaxas Quiroga, Virginia A. *Poor Mothers and Babies: A Social History of Childbirth and Child Care Hospitals in Nineteenth Century New York City.* New York: Garland, 1989.

Ott, Katherine. *Fevered Lives: Tuberculosis in American Culture Since 1870.* Cambridge, MA: Harvard University Press, 1996.

Preston, Samuel H., and Michael R. Haines. *Fatal Years: Child Mortality in Late Nineteenth Century America.* Princeton, NJ: Princeton University Press, 1991.

Rosenberg, Charles E. *The Cholera Years: The United States in 1832, 1849, and 1866.* Chicago: University of Chicago Press, 1987.

Rosenkrantz, Barbara G. *From Consumption to Tuberculosis: A Documentary History.* New York: Garland, 1994.

Rosner, David. *Hives of Sickness: Public Health and Epidemics in New York City.* New Brunswick, NJ: Rutgers University Press, 1995.

Whorton, James C. *Nature Cures: The History of Alternative Medicine in America.* New York: Oxford University Press, 2002.

Woods, Robert, and John Woodward. *Urban Disease and Mortality in Nineteenth Century England.* New York: St. Martin's Press, 1984.

Chapter Twelve

The Twentieth Century
Advances and Challenges

INTRODUCTION

More so than any other century in history, the twentieth century was a period of change in the field of medicine. Medical advances came at an exponential rate, constantly building on previous inventions, procedures, and discoveries. Nevertheless, these innovations carried a price, sometimes a heavy one. For instance, diagnosing any given disease or syndrome was easier than ever, but being sued for malpractice if the diagnosis was incorrect or the surgical procedure had a poor outcome was also far easier. Likewise, premature babies and neonates born with birth defects had much higher survival rates, but, at the same time, parents of such children often faced bankruptcy because of the exorbitant medical bills incurred for their children's care. Discovery and mass production of sulfa drugs and antibiotics lowered death rates from infection significantly, but the disease-causing microbes adapted rapidly, and many became resistant to most, if not all, of the previous "wonder drugs." The list went on; every modern medical advance seemed to be accompanied by a new problem.

Medical care consumed a larger share of personal expenditure in the developed countries than any other single expense did. Previously in such countries, the solution to this problem had been found through the creation of health insurance plans. With time, these plans underwent change as companies adapted to the transformed medical marketplace. Managed care; the HMO; social programs such as Medicare, Medicaid, and the National Health Service; and use of diagnostic-related groups (or DRGs) all emerged as ways to try to restrain medical costs to some degree. Yet, even in these cases, a price had to be paid—for example, a patient could be denied treatment because an insurance plan administrator would not authorize payment for it.

The technological innovations, improved surgical techniques, and revolution in drug therapies presented another problem: The field of medical ethics, or *bioethics* as it is now called, had to undergo radical change to keep pace with the improvements in diagnosis and patient care. Serious questions about experimentation involving human subjects, allocation of scarce resources such as organs for transplantation, and the physician's role in the doctor-patient relationship needed to be answered. However, for most such issues, no perfect solution existed. End-of-life questions, such as whether physician-assisted suicide should be legalized, became another topic of controversy, as did many issues in the emotion-laden field of reproductive medicine. Practitioners in the field of ethics had to adapt and respond to questions that were unthinkable only seventy-five years prior.

Overall, for one contingent of the world's population, improved medical care significantly lengthened life spans. For example, a patient who sustained trauma and arrived in a modern emergency department within the so-called Golden Hour after injury had better chances of recovery than ever. The infant mortality rate decreased, as did the neonatal death rate, and children were no longer expected to die of childhood diseases. Persons who were elderly could get care to ameliorate the plethora of ailments associated with aging. Likewise, the soldier no longer needed to expect the lack of sanitation and prevalence of infectious disease present in military camps only a century before.

The problem that finally became obvious in the twentieth century was not so much the need for the cure of a disease or the relief of suffering. Rather, the problem was the inequitable distribution of medical care, primarily in less-developed countries, where limitations in transportation and communication, lack of education, and, most of all, poverty had worked to prevent progress. In these countries, the ratio of doctors and nurses to one thousand inhabitants was extremely low, as was the number of hospital beds. Infant mortality and childhood death rates remained high, life expectancy was extremely low in comparison with that in the developed countries, and basic sanitation, clean water, and a safe food supply were often absent. The challenge to the entire medical community moving into the twenty-first century was not how to diagnose and cure another disease, but how to make basic health care available to more people everywhere.

TIME LINE

1901	Alfred Adler and Sigmund Freud (both from Austria) establish the first psychoanalytic society; Army Nurse Corps is established
1902	Pan American Sanitary Bureau is established—first international health organization
1903	George Perthes (Germany) discovers that x-rays inhibit tumor growth; proposes their use in cancer therapy
1905	George Crile (U.S.) performs the first successful direct blood transfusion; German Society for Racial Hygiene is founded
1910	Havelock Ellis (UK) publishes *Studies in the Psychology of Sex*
1911	United Kingdom—National Health Insurance Act is passed
1913	John Abel (U.S.) develops the first artificial kidney
1915	American Medical Association (AMA) admits women to full status
1917	Margaret Sanger (U.S.) writes about birth control

1914–1918	World War I—medical advances include multistation evacuation plans and surgical blood transfusions; better sanitation and use of vaccines make this war the first in which battlefield injuries outnumber cases of disease; an estimated eight million are dead and twenty-two million are wounded
1919	AMA officially opposes any compulsory health insurance plans and any plans organized around restrictions to group practice
1925	Geneva Protocol for the Prohibition of the Use in War of Asphyxiating, Poisonous or Other Gases, and of Bacteriological Methods of Warfare is adopted
1927	Philip Drinker and Louis Shaw (both from the U.S.) develop the iron lung
1928	Alexander Fleming (UK) discovers penicillin; it is not mass-produced until 1941
1929	Iowa State Board of Eugenics is established
1932	Tuskegee syphilis study begins; lasts until 1972
1935	First sulfa drug, Prontosil, is used on strep throat—hailed as a "wonder drug"
1939	National Cancer Institute is founded; Germany's T-4 program of "mercy killings" is implemented—first euthanasia center opens at Brandenburg and an estimated eighty thousand to one hundred thousand people are killed there by 1941
1939–1945	World War II—medical advances include the first use of plasma, new drugs (penicillin, sulfa, atabrine), new surgical techniques, new treatments for surgical shock, and increased speed at which wounded are moved to medical attention; an estimated twenty-five million military persons and twenty million civilians are dead
1943	Selman Waksman (U.S.) discovers streptomycin
1945	Fluoridation of the water supply begins in the United States
1947	Nuremberg Code is written
1948	United Kingdom—National Health Service is established; World Health Organization (WHO) is established
1950–1953	Korean War—medical advances include the use of mobile army surgical hospital (MASH) units, the use of helicopters in medevac operations, and new surgical techniques; an estimated 33,700 are dead and 103,000 are wounded
1951	John Gibbons (U.S.) invents the first heart-lung machine—it is first used in 1953; acetaminophen (Tylenol) is marketed as an alternative to aspirin
1952	Jonas Salk (U.S.) develops the killed-virus polio vaccine; first successful kidney transplant from a relative is performed
1953	James Watson and Francis Crick (both from the UK) publish the first model of DNA structure

1957	Albert Sabin (U.S.) develops the oral live-virus polio vaccine
1959	Two thousand to three thousand children in West Germany and another five hundred in the United Kingdom are born severely deformed to mothers who took thalidomide during pregnancy
1965	Measles vaccine is developed; Medicare and Medicaid legislation is passed
1965–1975	Vietnam War—evacuation methods are streamlined; despite no frontline units (since there are no front lines), transport times and mortality rates are significantly reduced; an estimated 58,000 Americans are dead and 153,000 are wounded
1966	French Academy of Medicine is the first group to define death by lack of brain activity
1967	Christiaan Barnard (South Africa) performs the first successful heart transplant
1971	Prescription of the synthetic estrogen DES is ordered stopped for pregnant women
1972	First successful CAT (computerized axial tomography) scan is done
1975	Indian government legalizes abortion; launches campaigns advocating sterilization to deal with the exploding population
1978	First extrauterine "test tube" baby is conceived
1981	Best-seller Jane Fonda's *Workout Book* is published—starts the "get-fit" book and video market, which becomes increasingly important as the U.S. population becomes more overweight; Bruce Reitz (U.S.) performs the first successful heart-lung transplant
1982	Tylenol poisoning scare—leads to tamperproof packaging for medications and many other items
1983	Robert Gallo (U.S.) and Luc Montagnier (France) isolate HIV
1985	Ethics Committee of The Transplantation Society sets guidelines and prohibits buying and selling organs
1987	Prozac is marketed
1990	United States—gene therapy is used on the first human
1991	Human Genome Project begins
1994	First trials of artificial blood; breast cancer gene is discovered—1995 first treatment trials using gene therapy
1996	Dolly the sheep is cloned; dies in 2003
1997	Oregon is the first state to allow physician-assisted suicide
1998	UK scientists report the discovery of a bacterium that is resistant to all known antibiotics
1999	Jack Kevorkian (U.S.) is sentenced to ten- to twenty-five years in prison for murder in a physician-assisted suicide case

▲

The Care of Strangers

The Rise of America's Hospital System

Charles E. Rosenberg

The first hospitals date to the Roman and Muslim Empires. Until relatively recently, the hospital was a place to avoid, a place to go to die. As antiseptic methods became more commonplace in the early twentieth century, though, the much-improved hospital came to be seen in a more positive light. It had become a combination of many elements: clinics, inpatient treatment, sophisticated diagnostic units, laboratories, emergency departments and intensive care units, offices, and much more. In addition, hospitals and medical schools had partnered to make the hospital as much a teaching institution as a place of healing. As a result, the twentieth-century hospital bore little resemblance to that in which Roman legionnaires obtained care.

It also faced new challenges. Expenses continued to increase sharply, and hospitals had to care for individuals who could not pay. **Nosocomial** *infections plagued hospitals as the resistance of germs to antibiotics strengthened. The public continued to demand more services, and hospital administrators were constantly trying to provide them while staying within restrictive budgets. The principal question, as the author of this selection points out, was this: "Is the hospital an institution of the marketplace, subject to the laws of supply and demand, or does it answer instead to the issues of common need?" The answer remains unclear.*

▲

The Past in the Present

If the hospital in Thomas Jefferson's or Andrew Jackson's America had been a microcosm of the community that nurtured it, so is the hospital of the 1980s. Although we live in a very different sort of world, the hospital remains both product and prisoner of its own history and of the more general trends that have characterized our society. Class, ethnicity, and gender have, for example, all shaped and continue to shape medical care, and the hospital has become a specialized, bureaucratic entity of a kind that has come to dominate so many other aspects of contemporary life. National policies and priorities have come to play a significant role in affairs that had been long thought of as entirely and appropri-

ately local. The origins of America's hospitals are hardly recognizable in their quaint forerunners in a handful of early nineteenth-century port cities.

The hospital is a necessary community institution strangely insulated from the community; it is instead a symbiotically allied group of subcommunities bound together by social location and the logic of history. This insulated character is typical of a good number of social institutions: the schools, the federal civil service, the large corporations. But there are some special aspects of the hospital that have facilitated its ability to look inward, to pursue its own vision of social good. This institutional **solipsism** developed in ironic if logical conjunction with the hospital's defining function of dealing with the most intimate and fundamental of human realities.

Like the U.S. Defense Department, the hospital system has grown in response to perceived social need—in comparison with which normal budgetary constraints and compromises have come to seem niggling and inappropriate. Security, like any absolute and immeasurable good, legitimates enormous demands on society's resources. Both health and defense have, moreover, become captives of high technology and worst-case justifications. In both instances, the gradient of technical feasibility becomes a moral imperative. That which might be done, should be done. In both cases, cost-cutting could be equated with penny-pinching—inappropriate to the gravity of the social goals involved. Absolute ends do not lend themselves to compromise, and the bottom line is that there has been no bottom line.

In both areas, material interests obviously play a role; hospitals, doctors, and medical suppliers like defense contractors and the military have interests expressed in and through the political process. But ideas are significant as well. It is impossible to understand our defense budget without factoring in the power of ideology; it is impossible to understand the scale and style of America's health care expenditures without an understanding of the allure of scientific medicine and the promise of healing. Both the Massachusetts General Hospital and the General Dynamics Corporation operate in the market, but they are not entirely bound by its discipline; both also mock the categorical distinction between public and private that indiscriminately places each in the private domain.

This analogy can, of course, be carried too far. The hospital has, as we have emphasized, a special history incorporating and reflecting the evolution of medicine and nursing, and the parallel development of our social welfare system. The high status of medicine has been built into the hospital, not only in the form of an undifferentiated social authority, but in the shape of particular, historically determined techniques and career choices. The ideas that rule the world-view of medicine and its system of education and research have very practical connections with the pragmatic world of medical care and medical costs.

An increasingly subdifferentiated specialization, an emphasis on laboratory research and acute care, for example, have all played an important role in the profession and thus, in the hospital. So complex and intertwined are these interrelationships that changes in any one sphere inevitably impinge on other areas. Some aspects of modern medicine seemed at first unrelated to the marketplace. One, for example, was the increasing ability of physicians to disentangle specific disease entities. This was an intellectual achievement of the first magnitude and not unrelated to the increasingly scientific and prestigious public image of the medical profession. Yet, we have seen a complex and inexorably bureaucratic reimbursement system grow up around these diagnostic entities; disease does not exist if it cannot be coded. It was equally inevitable that efforts to control medical costs should have turned on these same diagnostic categories. Thus the 1980s controversy surrounding Diagnosis Related Groups can be seen in part as a natural outcome of the intellectual and institutional history of the medical profession—and of the hospital as well.

To most contemporary Americans, rising costs have been the key element in transforming the hospital into a highly visible social problem. And it is true that an apparent crisis in hospital finance may well be creating the conditions for fundamental changes. After all, it was not until after the Second World War that the hospital gradually emerged from the world of paternalism. Unions and a more assertive nursing profession, ever-increasing capital costs, a growing dependence on federal support, and rising insurance rates, even the need to pay house staff in dollars have moved the hospital system into the market—and exposed hospitals to the prospect of increasing external control. Still clothed with the public interest and promising immeasurable equities, the hospital remains a rigid and intractable institution.

As we contemplate its contentious present and problematic future, we remain prisoners of its past. The economic and organizational problems that loom so prominently today should not make us lose sight of fundamental contradictions in the hospital's history, contradictions that have fueled two decades of critical debate.

Scientific medicine has raised expectations and costs, but has failed to confront the social consequences of its own success. We are still wedded to acute care and episodic, specialized contacts with physicians. There is a great deal of evidence that indicates widespread dissatisfaction with the quality of care as it is experienced by Americans. Changes in reimbursement mechanisms will not necessarily alter that felt reality. Chronic and geriatric care still constitute a problem—as they always did. We cannot seem to live without high-technology medicine; we cannot seem to live amicably with it. Yet, for the great majority of Americans, divorce is unthinkable. Medical perceptions and careers still proscribe or reward behaviors that may or may not be consistent with the most humane and cost-effective provision of care. And despite much recent hand-wringing, it

still remains to be seen whether physicians will be edged aside from their positions of institutional authority.

There are many equities to be maximized in the hospital, many interests to be served, but the collective interest does not always have effective advocates. The discipline of the marketplace will not necessarily speak to that interest; the most vulnerable will inevitably suffer. In any case, I see little prospect of hospitals in general becoming monolithic cost minimizers and profit maximizers. Social expectations and well-established interests are both inconsistent with such a state of things. We will support research and education, we will feel uncomfortable with a medical system that does not provide a plausible (if not exactly equal) level of care to the poor and socially isolated. Health care policy will continue to reflect the special character of our attitudes toward sickness and society.

▲

Doctors and Discoveries
Willem J. Kolff

JOHN G. SIMMONS

Many of the most important improvements in twentieth-century medicine involved the invention of a vast number of technologies and medical equipment for diagnosis and treatment. New devices could be found in nearly every medical specialty—from the fetal heart monitor, the heart-lung machine, the ventilator, MRI (magnetic resonance imaging) and CAT scanners, electrocardiograms and electroencephalograms, and on and on. Constant inventions and improvements allowed physicians to diagnose disease and trauma with less-invasive methods, less patient suffering and recuperation time, and a better ability to discern pathological conditions that were previously invisible. Unfortunately, the trend also caused staggering increases in the cost of medical care and a high degree of depersonalization of the patient.

One of the most widely used of the new technologies was kidney dialysis, a procedure that significantly lengthened the survival times of patients with kidney disease and individuals waiting for kidney transplants. Its inventor, Dutch physician Dr. Willem J. Kolff, developed the prototype during World War II and perfected it in the 1950s. It is still widely available in the United States and Europe, although its expense makes it somewhat a rarity in less-developed nations.

All this innovative technology created a new set of problems: scarce resources. When such equipment is not readily available in sufficient numbers, or when the cost of treatment is prohibitive to persons without medical insurance, the question arises "How do we determine who will get treatment and who will be denied?" Such life-and-death decisions are currently debated in medical ethics committees and can be extremely difficult to make.

Furthermore, because of the expense of the new health care, a global paradigm has emerged in which patients live in one of two medical worlds: that in which people have health insurance and access to the technology and that in which they do not. The majority of the world's population belongs to the latter group. Unless a patient lives in the United States or Europe and has insurance to pay the high costs of care, or has the money to go to such treatment centers, the new technological health care remains a myth, unattainable and unbelievable.

Spare Parts Medicine

The pioneer of "spare parts" medicine is the Dutch physician Willem Kolff. During World War II, in occupied Holland, he invented the first successful kidney dialysis machine. In the United States after the war, Kolff went on to become the world's foremost bionics engineer. He headed teams that invented a wide variety of prosthetic devices, including machines to substitute for the kidney and the lungs. Although his role was not much publicized, he was one of the principal figures behind creation of the first artificial human heart. Kolff, who once asserted, "If man can grow a heart, he can build one," would live to see the first operation to replace a human heart with a fully implantable substitute, in 2001.

Kolff's landmark invention was the kidney dialysis machine, and this has, parenthetically, some nice ironies. For one thing, it took a Dutchman. The kidneys are nothing if not organs to maintain fluid balance throughout the body, and Holland's very existence depends on controlling sea level. In addition, the machine was developed during World War II, when the country was sorely afflicted by Nazi Germany. Indeed, the first patient to seriously benefit from

it was a collaborator, a Dutch National Socialist. People begged Kolff to let her die, but with characteristic humanity, he saved her life. With the help of his jerry-built machine, this despised and unpleasant woman emerged from a **uremic** coma, was heard to say, "I am going to divorce my husband," and entered the annals of medical history.

Willem Johan Kolff was born in Leiden, Netherlands, on February 14, 1911. His mother was Adriana de Jonge and his father, Jacob Kolff, was a physician who directed a tuberculosis sanatorium. Growing up, Kolff once said later, "For me, there was never anything else but being a doctor." In fact, as a child, Kolff was reluctant to follow in his father's footsteps "because I could not bear the thought of seeing patients die." But he was strongly and positively affected by his father's sensitivity to suffering and death. "He would agonize over his frustrations in treating [his patients], and I recall seeing him weep on several occasions." As a student, Kolff persisted despite dyslexia. He attended medical school at the University of Leiden. An assistant in the department of pathological anatomy from 1934 to 1936, he received his medical degree in 1938. For a short time afterward, Kolff worked as a teaching assistant, an unpaid position, at the University of

Groningen. In the medical service there, he became interested in treating kidney failure.

The basic science behind dialysis and the interest in building a machine to treat kidney disease dates to the mid-nineteenth century. Thomas Graham, a Scottish chemist, demonstrated liquid diffusion through a permeable membrane—a basic model of the kidneys at work. In the early twentieth century a small group of physicians developed what they called an "artificial kidney" and tested it on dogs with some success. World War I put an end to this research, however. Kolff's accomplishment was to develop—under adverse social circumstances—a machine that would work.

While at the university hospital at Leiden, Kolff first encountered a patient dying from a type of nephritis, or inflammation of the kidneys. The disease would be fatal if untreated, and the patient's death slow and painful. As his father had with tubercular patients, Kolff found renal conditions all the more distressing for being well understood. In principle, removing waste from the blood over a period of days or weeks would effect a cure. Kolff could seriously consider this prospect because a biochemistry professor at Groningen had recently discovered that the same cellophane used for sausage casing could be employed to determine osmotic pressure of various fluids and to concentrate blood plasma. Kolff soon performed experiments himself. He found that when cellophane casings were filled with blood and immersed in saline solution, the urea in the blood would leach through the permeable membrane. "I found that in five minutes," he explained, "nearly all the urea I had added to the blood sample, four hundred milligrams, had disappeared from the blood and entered the saline bath."

Kolff was already moving toward developing a machine when World War II interrupted. The Germans invaded the Netherlands in 1940, and the Nazi occupation proved a professional trauma, but also a fertile period of investigation and experimentation. In the wake of invasion, Kolff recognized that blood transfusions would be in demand, and he volunteered to establish one of Europe's first blood banks. But he could not remain at Groningen, especially after his mentor and head of the medical department, Polak Daniels, a Jew, took his own life. Kolff refused to work with his successor, a Dutch Nazi. Over the next five years, Kolff was consistently able to help and harbor fighters in the Dutch resistance. Toward the end of the war, at great personal risk, he directed a medical service that saved a large number of Jews and underground fighters from transport to Germany and certain death.

Kolff developed dialysis at a small municipal hospital in Kampen, an old town located on the Ijsel River, to which he moved after leaving Groningen. Solving a series of relatively uncomplicated problems, he constructed a machine that is easy to visualize. He wrapped about twenty meters of cellophane tubing around a slatted wooden drum that was suspended horizontally inside a tank filled with saline solution and connected to a motor. The tubing, snaked through the drum's hollow axle, shunted blood from and back to the patient. As the drum rotated, the blood was cleansed in the saline bath. Heparin, a naturally occurring substance, could be used to prevent clotting.

Kolff's cobbled-together machine, first put to use in March 1943, did cleanse the blood, but it was not immediately successful. Fourteen of the first fifteen patients died, and the survivor might have lived in any event. But Kolff was convinced the machine could be made to work. "I did not for one moment doubt that sooner or later a patient would come into our hands of whom it might be said, 'he is cured, and without the artificial kidney he would have died.'" A cure seemed especially possible for cases of acute reversible renal failure. Finally, at war's end in September 1945, the machine saved Maria Sophia Schafstadt. Imprisoned as a former Nazi collaborator, sixty-seven years old, she became the first person whose life was spared by dialysis.

Kolff consolidated his success in several ways. He had written articles for Scandinavian and French journals as early as 1944, and he soon wrote a book, *The Artificial Kidney,* that he published in both Dutch and English. In addition, after the war Kolff constructed and shipped kidney machines to researchers in England, Canada, and the United

States. (He did not patent the machine.) At the same time, he continued work on a Ph.D. in internal medicine and received that degree summa cum laude from the University of Groningen in 1946.

Kolff made several visits to the United States before he immigrated in 1950, taking a research position with the Cleveland Clinic. With some difficulty, over the course of a decade he assembled a team of researchers. One of his hopes was to develop improved dialysis techniques; he was much in favor of home dialysis and foresaw the possibility of small, portable versions. But he also wanted to continue work on a heart-lung machine, to be used during various types of **thoracic** surgery. Kolff built a "pump-oxygenator" that became an important factor in making open-heart surgery safer for many patients. He introduced this device, made from disposable polyethylene tubing, as early as 1955. Kolff and colleagues also created the first aortic balloon pump, introduced in 1961. An assist device for improving cardiac output in cases of cardiogenic shock, it became a widely used tool in emergency medicine.

The most ambitious project in Kolff's career, extending over a quarter century, was his work on the artificial heart. The possibility was broached in the mid-1950s by the American Society for Artificial Internal Organs, and within a decade it became a respectable area of research. As early as 1957, Kolff and his colleagues had tried to drive circulation in a dog using an air-driven pump, but the animal lived only ninety minutes. This gave a hint of the difficult task ahead. But with a workable heart-lung machine and with knowledge of the cardiovascular system expanding, the prospect for a bionic heart improved. Kolff tried several designs driven by electricity, including a self-cooling pendulum-driven model. But they were either weak or too heavy, and they often generated more heat than the body could stand. Kolff finally accepted the simpler concept of a silicone-rubber heart that operated with compressed air from an external power source.

Kolff was still at work on the artificial heart when, in 1967, he moved to the University of Utah, where he was professor of surgery as well as

professor of engineering and bioengineering. To his research team he soon added Robert Jarvik, an ambitious physician and inventor, and William DeVries, a cardiothoracic surgeon. Over the course of the next fifteen years, Jarvik designed a number of models of the artificial heart, while DeVries developed the techniques of the heart replacement operation in animals. In 1982, Barney Clark became the first patient to receive an artificial heart. Clark, a sixty-one-year-old retired dentist, was subjected to a media circus the likes of which had not been seen since the birth of the Dionne quintuplets in 1934. He survived the operation and lived for 112 days before dying of complications unrelated to the beating of his Jarvik-7 heart. Kolff, who remained largely in the background, lamented that Clark's funeral took place with newscast helicopters flying overhead.

Willem Kolff continued to work through his ninth decade. At the University of Utah he oversaw development of a number of increasingly sophisticated and lightweight artificial hearts. His institute also looked toward developing an artificial eye and artificial ear, and improved the prosthetic arm. From 1979 Kolff was distinguished professor of surgery at the university's College of Medicine and also, from 1981, research professor of engineering and professor of internal medicine.

From all appearances, Kolff has enjoyed a relatively tranquil personal life. He married Janke Cornelia Huidekoper in 1937, and they had five children, three of whom became physicians. Widely admired by colleagues, Kolff's strong personality, which mingles perseverance and considerable social skills, has always been in evidence. He belongs to a generation of physicians that has held a high measure of optimism about the prospects of modern medicine along with a strong social conscience. Responsibility for treating the sick, not a wish to garner encomiums for technological progress, has guided Kolff's choices on the kind of inventions he engineers. He has always aimed, he maintains, not at merely prolonging life, but at improving its quality and prospects for happiness. "These are honest and good goals," according to Kolff, "and deserve to be pushed."

▲

Interview with Four Survivors, Department of Health, Education and Welfare Study, 1973

SUSAN M. REVERBY

The twentieth-century emphasis on scientific medicine, with its requirements of laboratory re-search and drug trials, created a new challenge to existing ideas of medical ethics. A particu-larly controversial point became the use of human subjects in medical research, and two events stand out in the story of this issue.

First, in 1932 in Alabama, the U.S. Public Health Department began a forty-year study entitled the "Tuskegee Study of Untreated Syphilis in the Negro Male." The study involved 600 African American men, 399 with syphilis. Researchers told them that they had "bad blood," a local term for syphilis and a number of nonspecific symptoms. In return for their participation, the men received free medical examinations, free meals, and burial insurance. However, they were never told anything about the project or its purpose and were never given the choice to refuse treatment or quit the study. They received misinformation about the procedures, and, in fact, were never given proper treatments at all, at a time when the drug of choice, penicillin, achieved excellent results. They were simply human guinea pigs, deprived of anything approaching informed consent.

The Public Health Department was within legal boundaries in 1932 when the study began, because no guidelines or regulations existed regarding the use of human subjects. However, the study lasted until 1972, and in that interim, the law changed. Nevertheless, the study continued unaltered.

Second, in the aftermath of World War II and the discovery of the Nazi atrocities committed in the concentration camps, the Nuremberg trials of major war criminals were held in 1945–1946, followed by the famous Doctors' Trial in 1946–1947, in which Nazi doctors were tried and sen-tenced for their research on camp inmates. Various experiments, involving pure torture in most cases, had been performed on uninformed, unwilling, and totally vulnerable prisoners. At the end of the trial, twenty-one verdicts of life imprisonment or death were handed down, but another result of the trial focused on the future rather than the past of human experimentation.

The Nuremberg Code of 1947 established an entirely new code of ethical medical behav-ior based on the concept of voluntary informed patient consent. Such consent, designed to protect the individual's right to control his or her body, requires complete disclosure about the research, including hazards, and the opportunity to refuse treatment. The Nuremberg Code went on to become the foundation of all modern bioethics worldwide.

Yet, the Tuskegee experiments continued for decades after the Nuremberg Code was formu-lated. Not until 1972 was it ended in the face of public scrutiny and government investigation. In 1973, a nine-million-dollar lawsuit was settled in favor of the participants, but only in 1997 did the federal government officially claim responsibility—in President Clinton's apol-ogy to the survivors of Tuskegee.

▲

Reprinted from Susan M. Reverby, ed., *Tuskegee Truths: Rethinking the Tuskegee Syphilis Study* (Chapel Hill: University of North Carolina Press, 2000), 132–35.

Four subjects were interviewed in sequence.

Interview #1

Subject was asked what the study meant to the people involved, how it started, etc.

Subject—Started with a blood test. Clinic met at Shiloh Church. They gave us shots. Nurse (Rivers) came out and took us in (to John Andrews Hospital). One time I had a spinal puncture—had to stay in bed for 10 days afterward. Had headaches from that. Several others did too (and stayed in bed awhile). I wore a rubber belt for a long time afterward. Had ointment to run in under the belt.

Doctors came every year or so. After 25 years they gave everyone in the study $25.00 and a certificate. They told him he was in pretty good health.

At the beginning he thought he had "bad blood." They said that was syphilis. (He) just thought it was an "incurable disease." He was booked for Birmingham for "606" shots but "nurse stopped it." Some other doctor took blood that time and he was signed up to go to Birmingham. Nurse Rivers said he wasn't due to take the shots . . . he went to get on the bus to Birmingham and they turned him down. This was sometime between 1942–1947.

He did not know he was sick before 1932. They gave them a bunch of shots—about once a month. Then they did a spinal. Nurse would notify them about the blood tests and bring them down.

He had not talked to any of the other participants lately.

He had the shots in his arm. In 1961 he had a growth removed from his bladder. (He is 66.) Health insurance paid for it. He paid his bill and his insurance paid back all but $20.

Question—could all the people in the group afford hospitalization? What would others have done?

Subject—don't know. I asked the (government) doctors about it (the growth) and they sent me to my family doctor. The government people didn't know I had insurance.

He didn't know of any others in the study who had been in the hospital although one man had become blind after a while. He hadn't thought much about whether his disease had been cured. The doctor was seeing him every year, and he was feeling pretty good. He was not told what the disease might do to him. He stayed in the program because they asked him to. Nurse came and got him. He thought they all had the same disease. The blind man had been blind nearly 20 years—had worn glasses a while, then had become blind.

Question—Did anyone do anything about the blind man's eyes?

Subject—I think he told nurse. They talked one time about sending him somewhere. Wasn't treated that he knew of. He (the blind man) never went anywhere and he (subject) didn't know the details. The blind man is about 75 now.

He knew maybe 15–20 people in the study. The only time they got together as a group was when the government doctors came in.

Interview #2

(This subject was a control)

Subject had come into the program when "they were recruiting up people." Nurse got him in. He was never told what was wrong with him. He had rheumatism. He has (and had at the time) swollen fingers. He has heart disease—his heart "skips." When he says "they" he is referring to "that government affair."

He didn't always come up to the clinics. Sometimes he was away. He thought maybe Nurse Rivers came and got him because someone told her where he lived.

When asked if he had been sick, the subject said no—he had never been sick. Just slight rheumatism all his life. He really thought they were interested in his fingers. Then he thought they were interested in his heart.

Before Nurse Rivers came to see him no one had tested him. Then he was examined and his blood tested. Nothing was said about his blood although his peculiar heart was later commented on.

He had "never been in the hospital." But I was for my hernia. Had a pain in my side once. Doctor gave me pills. I'm a pretty unusual person. Two or three years ago I had a headache that lasted about three weeks. Slowed down all my work.

He had known several others in the program. All now dead. He is now 66.

Interview #3

Subject is 81 years old. Had farmed all his life (up to three years ago) and had gone through the third grade. When he got into the program he had been sick. Nurse Rivers said he could get treatments. He was told he had "some funny name thing." Main thing though was his cataracts. He had them out in 1953 at John Andrews Hospital.

Nurse Rivers had told him to be at the school and they would check them up. Every couple of years (they came). Nurse Rivers came to the plantation to get them. He first saw her at the hospital clinic (after she suggested that he go to the clinic).

Subject's wife interjected that the nurse had said government doctors were coming from the north and had suggested that he join the program. Later he got notices.

The doctors told him different things. They never said he had any diseases. Once they gave him shots in his back. He just got up and left.

They took blood every time. Said they sent it off. Never told him anything. Said the first test was good. Later said it was not so good. The doctors gave them pills and medicines and shots—hip and arm mostly. He didn't know why they were giving him shots. The doctor told him he had a bad heart, bad circulation, arthritis. He also had falling spells.

Lots of people went to the clinic with him. He didn't know them all. They all got the same medicine. Nobody ever said anything about his blood. They never told them what was wrong with them. They got a lot of pills. He took some of the pills, not all. He had never been hospitalized before his operation for cataracts. He took a lot of home remedies. Nurse would tell him to come in and get checked over. He saw different doctors over the years. Sometimes private doctors. When he went to private doctors, he had to pay. He didn't know if they knew he was in the program.

The doctor (he was seeing) now said his blood was good. He had had different shots over the years. Some hip shots. He didn't know if he had ever heard of penicillin or if he had ever had any. He said he had never heard of syphilis. He had heard of "bad blood" but didn't know what it meant.

Interview #4

Subject had gotten into the program when people were going around giving treatment. He didn't know what kind of treatment or what the treatment was for. They drew blood. Had them come up at different times. They never told him anything. Never said they tested the blood. Never said anything was wrong. Did not say why they were testing (the subjects).

The first contact he had with the study was in church. "Lady came down talking about what they would do." It was on a Sunday. Said go to city hall for blood tests. He went. Then he got a letter saying they wanted to see him. He got a letter each year.

Each year they took blood. Sat down and talked. Gave them some medicine. He went every time. No one said anything to him about his health. Nurse Rivers asked him how he was.

Asked about his health, subject said he'd been getting along o.k. He had had shots (sometime) in his arm. He had seen no private doctors. Nothing was said about his blood. He had no good friends in the program. Had known some—all dead and gone. He didn't know the causes of death (of his friends).

He didn't know why they wanted him to be in the program. He didn't think it was helping him. He just went along.

The subject is in his 70's. He had gone through the second grade.

▲

Trials of War Criminals Before the Nuremberg Military Tribunals Under Control Council Law #10

▲

Directives for Human Experimentation

Nuremberg Code

1. The voluntary consent of the human subject is absolutely essential. This means that the person involved should have legal capacity to give consent; should be so situated as to be able to exercise free power of choice, without the intervention of any element of force, fraud, deceit, duress, over-reaching, or other ulterior form of constraint or coercion; and should have sufficient knowledge and comprehension of the elements of the subject matter involved as to enable him to make an understanding and enlightened decision. This latter element requires that before the acceptance of an affirmative decision by the experimental subject there should be made known to him the nature, duration, and purpose of the experiment; the method and means by which it is to be conducted; all inconveniences and hazards reasonable to be expected; and the effects upon his health or person which may possibly come from his participation in the experiment.

    The duty and responsibility for ascertaining the quality of the consent rests upon each individual who initiates, directs or engages in the experiment. It is a personal duty and responsibility which may not be delegated to another with impunity.

2. The experiment should be such as to yield fruitful results for the good of society, unprocurable by other methods or means of study, and not random and unnecessary in nature.

3. The experiment should be so designed and based on the results of animal experimentation and a knowledge of the natural history of the disease or other problem under study that the anticipated results will justify the performance of the experiment.

4. The experiment should be so conducted as to avoid all unnecessary physical and mental suffering and injury.

5. No experiment should be conducted where there is an *a priori* reason to believe that death or disabling injury will occur; except, perhaps, in those experiments where the experimental physicians also serve as subjects.

6. The degree of risk to be taken should never exceed that determined by the humanitarian importance of the problem to be solved by the experiment.

7. Proper preparations should be made and adequate facilities provided to protect the experimental subject against even remote possibilities of injury, disability, or death.

8. The experiment should be conducted only by scientifically qualified persons. The highest degree of skill and care should be required through all stages of the experiment of those who conduct or engage in the experiment.

9. During the course of the experiment the human subject should be at liberty to bring the experiment to an end if he has reached the physical or mental state where continuation of the experiment seems to him to be impossible.

Reprinted from *Trials of War Criminals Before the Nuremberg Military Tribunals Under Control Council Law No. 10,* vol. 2 (Washington, DC: U.S. Government Printing Office, 1949), 181–82.

10. During the course of the experiment the scientist in charge must be prepared to terminate the experiment at any stage, if he has probable cause to believe, in the exercise of the good faith, superior skill and careful judgment required of him that a continuation of the experiment is likely to result in injury, disability, or death to the experimental subject.

▲

Baby and Child Care

DR. BENJAMIN SPOCK

One medical specialty established in the late nineteenth century was pediatrics, *or the care of children. Pediatrics is now a field with a number of subspecialties, from pediatric oncology to child psychiatry, which emerged as physicians came to understand that children are not simply small adults but present medical problems entirely unique to their age group.*

As parents began to consult their pediatricians on caring for their offspring, the physician often became a dispenser of advice on everything from breast-feeding and treating chicken pox to thumb sucking. Probably the most famous pediatrician to offer advice on child rearing was Dr. Benjamin Spock, author of Baby and Child Care, *first published in 1947. Dr. Spock emphasized a gentler model for child rearing, replacing an often harsh disciplinarian ideal and offering a parent the opportunity to understand child behavior rather than simply rewarding or punishing it.*

The book became an instant best seller, and more than fifty million copies of it had sold by 2000. Entire generations of children worldwide have been raised according to Dr. Spock's combination of sage advice, optimism, and Freudian psychology. As the book was translated into thirty-nine languages and progressed through seven editions, Dr. Spock revised the content to reflect changing mores in a modernizing society. In the fourth edition, from which this selection is taken, he made his advice gender sensitive, using inclusive references throughout. He also added considerable new advice about adolescent psychology, an increasingly complex issue for parents to understand. Baby and Child Care *is still a favorite source of advice, even though Dr. Spock died in 1998.*

▲

Psychological Changes

Self-Consciousness and Touchiness

As a result of all the physical and emotional changes, adolescents become much more self-conscious. They may exaggerate and worry about any defect. If a girl has freckles, she may think they make her look "horrible." A slight peculiarity in the body or how it functions easily convinces them that they are "abnormal."

They may not manage their new body with as much coordination as they used to, and the same applies to their new feelings. They are apt to be touchy, easily hurt when criticized. At one moment they feel like a grown-up and want to be treated as such. The next they feel like a child again and expect to be cared for.

Rivalry with Parents

It isn't often realized that the rebelliousness of adolescents is mainly an expression of rivalrousness with parents, particularly the rivalry of son with father and girl with mother, which first developed back in the 4-to-6-year-old period. This rivalrousness becomes much more intense in adolescents because they have stronger emotions and because they sense that as an almost adult person they are ready to compete in the parents' own league, you might say. It's now their turn to challenge the world, to fascinate the opposite sex, to be the heads of families. So they feel like elbowing the has-been parents off the seat of power. Subconsciously the parents sense this and, understandably, don't feel too gracious about it.

Rebellious rivalry takes many forms. A mountaineer's son may suddenly at the age of 16 become angry at his father in an argument and, without premeditation, knock him down. He then realizes that it's no longer dignified to stay on in his father's house, so he abruptly leaves home to look for a job. Another boy may continue to get along well enough on the surface with his father but he displaces his defiance onto the school authorities or the police.

In families with children in college parent and child are apt to be so self-disciplined that they keep their anger under control and deal with each other by reasonableness. A child from such a background, feeling angry rivalrousness underneath, may have difficulty finding a legitimate complaint against the considerate parent. In families like this, rivalry is sometimes expressed unconsciously through unexpected school failure—in high school or college or graduate school—even though the child has a high degree of intelligence, conscientiousness and an excellent previous school record. The student, more often a boy, is sincere in saying he has no idea why he can't study or hand in papers or take examinations, whichever the problem may be. When such a youth seeks help through psychoanalysis it may be discovered that, especially if he is planning to work in the same field as his father, he is afraid *unconsciously* either that he will ignominiously fail to come up to his father's level or, conversely, that he might

outstrip his father and make him very angry. (The failing girl student may have the same problem in relation to her mother's or father's field of work.) In either case the school failure is the worst kind of blow to the parents; but the child, who has no conscious control, doesn't have to feel responsible for it. (Some, not all, of the youths who leave school because of unexpected failure find that they regain their academic efficiency and a heightened ambitiousness after working at a job for a couple of years; i.e., they outgrow the unconscious fear. A more purposeful method is psychoanalysis.)

Other children may express their anxious competitiveness by steering very clear of their parent's occupation though some of them swing around to it later when they have matured enough to overcome the irrational fear.

Psychoanalysis has also revealed that many boys who feel overawed by their father suppress their resentment and antagonism toward him and displace it onto their mother, flaring up at her over quite reasonable requests or imagined slights.

An adolescent girl is, on the average, much less often over-awed by her mother than a boy is by his father, so her rivalrousness is more apt to be expressed openly around the house, not often in academic failure. A girl can even be flirtatious with her father right under her mother's nose or reproach her mother for not being nice enough to her father. Few boys would dare taunt their father in such ways.

If youths were not rebellious, they would lack the motive to leave home and make their own way in the world. Rivalrousness also provides the motive power for young people who try to improve the world, find new methods that will supersede the old, make discoveries, create new art forms, displace old tyrants, right wrongs. A surprising number of scientific advances have been made and masterpieces of various arts created by individuals just on the threshold of adulthood. They were not smarter than the older people in their fields and they were admittedly less experienced. But they were critical of traditional ways, biased in favor of the new and the untried, and that happened to be enough to do the trick. This is how the world makes progress.

Identity

A central problem for the adolescent and the young adult is to find out what kind of person she or he is going to be, doing what work, living by what principles. It's partly a conscious but even more an unconscious process. Erik Erikson has called this the identity crisis and exemplified it in his biography of Martin Luther.

Youths have got to separate themselves emotionally from their parents in order to find out who they are and what they want to be. Yet they are basically made from their parents—not just in the sense that they have inherited their genes from them but that they have been deliberately patterning themselves after them all their lives. So they must pry themselves apart. The eventual outcome will be influenced by 3 factors: the pull of their dependency, the intensity of their rebelliousness and the kind of outside world they find and what it seems to ask of them.

In groping to find this identity adolescents may try out a variety of roles: dreamer, cosmopolitan, cynic, leader of lost causes, ascetic.

As adolescents try to emancipate themselves from their parents, they are apt to have a great need to find compensation in intimate ties to friends of the same age; more often ties to those of the same sex at first, because of the residual taboos against the opposite sex. These friendships, within or across the sexes, help to lend the youths some external support—like the timbers that are sometimes used to prop a building up during alterations—while they are giving up their identity as their parents' child and before they have found their own.

A boy finds himself through finding something similar in his friend. He mentions that he loves a certain song or hates a certain teacher or craves to own a certain article of apparel. His friend exclaims with amazement that he has always had the very same attitude. Both are delighted and reassured. Each has lost a degree of his feeling of aloneness, of peculiarity, and gained a pleasurable sense of belonging.

Two girls talk fast all the way home from school, talk for another half hour in front of the house of one, finally separate. But as soon as the second reaches her home she telephones and they resume the mutual confidences.

A majority of adolescents help to overcome their feelings of aloneness by a sometimes slavish conformity to the styles of their classmates—in clothes, hairdos, language, reading matter, songs, entertainers. These styles have to be different from those of their parents' generation. And if their own styles irritate or shock their parents, so much the better. It is revealing, though, that even those youths who adopt extreme styles to differentiate themselves from their parents must still conform to the styles of at least a few of their friends.

A majority of adolescents become ashamed of their parents for a few years, particularly when their friends are present. This is partly related to their anxious search for their own identities. Partly it is the extreme self-consciousness of the age period. Most of all it is the intense need to be just like their friends and to be accepted totally by their friends. They fear that if their parents deviate in any way from the neighborhood pattern, they, themselves, might be rejected by their own friends. What youths choose to deplore in their parents is sometimes ludicrous. But the parents shouldn't accept discourtesy. Their best cue, when they find themselves with their children's friends, is to be agreeable but not talk too much. It's most important, from their children's point of view, that they not try to talk or act as if they are young themselves.

Youths in trying to achieve emotional independence are on the lookout for evidences of hypocrisy in their parents. To the extent that their parents are obviously sincere in their ideals, their children feel under obligation to continue to adhere to them. But if they can find hypocrisy, this relieves them of the moral duty to conform. It also gives them a welcome opportunity to reproach their parents.

Demands for Freedom and Fear of Freedom

A common reproach of adolescents is that their parents don't allow them enough freedom. It's natural for children nearing adulthood to insist on their rights, and their parents need to be reminded that they are changing. But parents don't have to take every claim at its face value. The fact is that adolescents are also scared of growing up. They are unsure about their capacity to be as knowledgeable, masterful, sophisticated, and charming as they would like. But their pride won't allow them to recognize this. When they're unconsciously in doubt about their ability to carry off some challenge or adventure, they're quick to find evidence that their parents are blocking their way. They reproach them indignantly, or blame them when talking with friends. Parents can particularly suspect this unconscious maneuver when their children suddenly announce a plan of their group for some escapade—like an evening at an unsavory roadhouse—which is way beyond anything they've done before. They may be asking to be stopped.

Withdrawal, Eccentricity, Radicalism

It sometimes takes youths 5 or 10 years to truly find their own positive identity. Meanwhile they may be stalled at a halfway stage characterized by a passive resistance to and withdrawal from ordinary society (which they equate with their parents) or by an excessively rebellious radicalism.

They may decline to take an ordinary job, and may emphasize unconventional dress, grooming, acquaintances, residence. These seem like evidence of vigorous independence to them. But these by themselves don't add up yet to a positive stand on life or a constructive contribution to the world. They are essentially a negative protest against the parents' conventions. Even when the striving to be independent shows up only in the form of eccentricities of appearance it should be recognized as an attempted step in the right direction, which may go on to a constructive, creative stage later. As a matter of fact, the young people who have to strain so visibly to be free are apt to come from families with unusually strong ties and high ideals.

Other youths, who are idealistic and altruistic in character, often take a sternly radical or purist view of things for a number of years—in politics or in the arts or in other fields. Various tendencies of this age period operate together to draw them into these extreme positions—heightened criticalness, cynicism about hypocrisy, intolerance of compromise, courageousness, willingness to sacrifice, in response to their first awareness of the shocking injustices—most of them unnecessary—of the society they live in. A few years later, having achieved a satisfactory degree of emotional independence from parents and having found out how to be useful in their chosen fields, they are more tolerant of the frailties of their fellow men and more ready to make constructive compromises. I don't mean that they all become complacent conservatives. Many remain progressive, some remain radical. But most become easier to live with, work with. . . .

▲

Doc: Platoon Medic

DANIEL E. EVANS, JR., AND CHARLES W. SASSER

The twentieth century was a period in which the most-destructive wars in history took place. During this time, peace existed throughout the world for only a few years. One challenge that military medical personnel faced was dealing with the effects of increasingly deadly weaponry—from poison gas and land mines, to radiation, and, ultimately, to biological and chemical weapons.

Reprinted by permission of Daniel E. Evans, Jr., from Daniel E. Evans, Jr., and Charles W. Sasser, *Doc: Platoon Medic* (New York: Pocket Books, 1998), 44–47, 70–77, 140–43.

Transportation of wounded soldiers from the battlefield to the hospital was another obstacle, and a particularly important issue because of the need to treat wounds quickly. From the horse-drawn ambulances of World War I, to the MASH units of the Korean war, to the highly mobile, self-contained surgical units put in use in later years, the military sought to get aid to the wounded in the fastest, most-effective way possible.

One indispensable part of this plan was the medic: a noncombatant individual assigned to units on the front lines. The medic's role had changed substantially from that of previous centuries—from litter bearer only, to supplier of immediate pain relief, to controller of blood loss and infection, to a highly trained, essential member of the medical team. The medics in Vietnam faced an unprecedented, and especially difficult, wartime challenge: being in the middle of a jungle war with no front lines. Nevertheless, in Vietnam, the speed with which a wounded soldier was evacuated from combat increased substantially. The medics in Vietnam, although technically noncombatants, performed some of the most dangerous tasks of the war, going in under fire to treat the wounded, and many received commendations for their bravery. Following is part of one such medic's autobiographical account.

▲

12

. . . The platoon moved cautiously along a trail bordered on one side by a thick forest and on the other side by a field that gradually disappeared as the last of the sun's memory faded. My imagination ran wild. I visualized man-eating tigers, bloodsucking insects, and VC crawling toward us on their bellies or waiting ahead, alerted by the mama-san on the buffalo. Deadly devices awaited our approach—trip wires attached to grenades or mines, shit-smeared punji stakes, spike-filled foot traps. Out of the darkness charged buzzing black clouds of mosquitoes, surrounding the outside of my head the way black clouds of impending evil filled the inside of my head.

The platoon entered the forest, then split into two squads. Sergeant Wallace and his squad veered to the right. . . . Sergeant Richardson moved the rest of us to a tiny grassy clearing next to a river. . . .

I ate canned turkey loaf and fruit cocktail in the dark. I was halfway through my meal when gunfire filled the air. . . . Men hit the ground and crawled into a hasty 360-degree perimeter. . . . This was the first time I had ever heard small arms being fired with deadly intent, but it sounded like M16s to me. . . .

[Sergeant Wallace] explained [over the radio] that his squad had been moving through a ceme-tery when it received fire and returned fire . . . [but] no WIAs—no wounded.

I let out a sigh of relief. . . .

It took a while for me to settle down after [Sergeant] Wallace's little firefight. I kept hearing the stealthy dipping of sampan paddles into the river, seeing shadows forming into human shapes. After a while, when nothing happened, my heart slowed to its normal rate. A full moon bloomed and turned the river into a silver pathway fringed by low undergrowth and nipa palms. It was such a lovely night that it reminded me of a Boy Scout camporee. Except that Boy Scouts never set up ambushes to slaughter other Boy Scouts. . . .

. . . The sun was already up and sucking steam out of the rice paddies around Vinh Kim by the time the platoon reconsolidated its two squads and straggled back through the gates at the fire support base. . . . Hot cocoa from my canteen cup, plus meatballs and beans heated over C4, tasted especially good this morning. I removed my jungle jacket and settled back to enjoy breakfast and the sunrise. I had survived my first combat mission. . . .

19

. . . An American-made claymore mine triggered the ambush. The world in front of the Jeep blew up suddenly in smoke and fire. A wall of supersonic steel balls blasted into the Jeep and its passengers, shredding metal and flesh.

RPG rockets hissed viciously from the foliage on either side of the road. Contrails of smoke ended in violent explosions that lifted the vehicle and trailer into the air in the center of an expanding fireball and shook mangled soldiers all over the road.

Automatic rifle fire stitched every square foot of macadam as those few GIs still able made a run for the water-filled ditch that bordered the road. Those left behind screamed and wailed and cried out. They crawled and pulled themselves around in the middle of the road like crushed bugs with limbs and pieces of their bodies missing. The hellish sounds of their terror and torment diminished even the staccato grinding of rifle fire.

"Mommy! Mommy!" someone shrieked.

Tall, lanky Teddy Creech used his elbows to claw his way across the road like a mangled worm. His hands were mutilated beyond recognition. His leg had been severed from his hip, except for a tether of bloody skin and flesh. . . .

Fletcher, Stevenson and Abrahamson, the supply sergeant, all made it to the ditch. The water was stagnant and about waist deep, turning red now from the blood of the wounded men tumbling into it. Fletcher's elbow was blown off. . . . Stevenson contorted to bring his belly wound out of the water, trying to get a look at it.

Steve Seid held on to Eugene Harvill to keep Harvill from drowning. One of the lenses in his glasses was shattered and smeared with blood. Mario Sotello splashed over to help. Blood from a nasty cut streamed down his brown cheek. The lid of the open can of peaches he had been eating had slashed his cheek open to the bone. . . .

Pandemonium erupted in the command bunker. Everyone wanted to go on the rescue. In spite of the laxness, the outfit was tight when it came to the platoon. Only Browner [a conscientious objector] remained sulking and afraid in his corner as men snatched up their M16s and fighting harnesses. Sergeant Richardson grabbed them and jerked them back.

"Goddamit, you *all* can't go!"

"It's my squad," Wallace cried. "I'm going out there!"

I had no choice; I was the Doc. "I'm going," I snapped. "I'm the medic."

I had known this day would come sooner or later. I remembered what we had been told in medic school about triage—the sorting of casualties to decide who was treated first. "In a mass casualty situation," the instructor had said, "it is your job to decide who will live and who will die." . . .

We could be running directly into a trap, a secondary ambush. Charlie wasn't stupid; he knew the round-eyes always sent help. But we charged on anyhow, like trying to break a four-minute mile, cross-country runners overdressed in green jungle fatigues, helmets, and combat boots. Shadows along the trail swelled with potential threat as we bounded over obstructions and over log bridges like a troupe of Flying Wallendas. . . .

. . . I shot out of the narrow road into a scene of unbelievable carnage. The high-pitched crack of a bullet passed near my head—rude awakening. . . . I subconsciously adjusted my horn-rimmed glasses, which had come loose during the heart-pumping run. That was my only hesitation. I lurched forward, combat-running across the violent field of death. . . .

. . . Total chaos. Carnage. It awed me. Sickened me. I was the medic trainee who couldn't watch the Vietnam casualty movies at Fort Sam. Giving a hypodermic injection nauseated me. But this was no longer training or a movie. It was real, and I was stuck square in the middle of it. . . .

Death. I had seen it neatly encased in body bags back at the morgue I helped build for the 9th Med. I had not seen it like this—waiting to strike in a blinding flash of light or the split-second impact of a bullet screaming into flesh. . . .

I switched into automatic mode, just like that. . . . Treatment on the fly. Everyone had some type of wound. I soon ran out of bandages. I ripped up my shirt and cut off my trouser legs to use as tourniquets and bandages. I treated the men in the ditch, then crawled out onto the road to make house calls on those too sick to come to me. . . .

When the medevac chopper arrived, it skimmed in low over the trees, dragged its tail, and sat down on the narrow road in an explosion of dust and sniper fire. Dust-off medics leaped out to assist with the evacuation while the crew chief knelt on the roadway with an M16 across his knees.

"Get 'em aboard! Goddammit, load 'em!" the pilot roared above the whumping of the blades and the engine that he kept revved at full rpm, ready to bolt. An AK-47 round bored a hole through the chopper's thin skin. . . .

We medics were feeding torn bodies into the chopper's belly as fast as we could. The bird's floor was slippery with blood. The chopper kicked in even more rpm. Its skids bounced lightly on the road, kissing it, like a racehorse trying to bolt from the starting gate. The pilot was going frantic on us. . . .

Afterward, stunned and emotionally spent, I stood wearily in the middle of the road and stared without seeing the splotches and puddles of thick blood left around the smoldering Jeep. . . .

"What happened to your clothes, soldier?" one of the battalion leaders demanded.

I wore only my boots and the remains of my jungle trousers. I had ripped off the legs for bandages and tourniquets.

"Where's your helmet and weapon, GI?" . . .

As if from a distance at the end of a pipe, I overheard someone explaining to the officer that I was the medic and I had used my clothing in treating WIAs.

Someone nudged me. A gentle voice. "Doc? Doc, here. You can have my shirt." . . .

36

Little James "Billy" Scott was nineteen years old and weighed about 100 pounds after being soaked by a monsoon all night. His oversize helmet banged on his head like a loose hubcap. His big dark eyes were those of a young deer caught in the open away from its forest home. Billy was a conscientious objector, like Rick Hudson, but not the Browner type. He was a kid of deep religious convictions who simply could

not carry a weapon. Conscientious objectors, when drafted into the military, were traditionally assigned to the medical corps. Billy was given to Charlie Company of Hackworth's Hardcore Battalion.

. . . I first picked up the thread of Billy Scott's story late one night in the aid tent when shrill screaming jarred me awake: "Watch out! *Watch out!*"

I rolled out of my bunk and hit the ground before I realized Billy was having one of his nightmares. I jumped up. "It's okay, Billy. Nothing's happening."

"Watch out!"

"Billy! Wake up."

His eyes bounced around like a wild pool shot. After a moment he calmed down and apologized. . . . Billy had similar nightmares every time he closed his eyes.

"I keep trying to ward them off," he explained shyly. "It's gotten where I'm afraid to sleep. I'm not strong like you, Dan."

. . . Billy Scott, in my opinion, might have been the bravest man among us. He lived with terror awake and asleep, but he continued to do his job.

The battalion surgeon, Doc Holley, took all his medics under his wing when they arrived incountry, but he had taken a special interest in Scott.

"Oh, Lord," he lamented. "Where are they getting these kids? He's such a sweet little kid, almost a mama's boy. Why isn't he back home teaching Sunday school?"

Scott was so frightened when he arrived in Dong Tam from Stateside that he hid out in the base chapel for two days. Doc Holley covered for him and went to the chapel and sat down with the kid in one of the pews where Billy had been praying.

"Billy, you have to come out. You can't stay here forever."

"Dr. Holley, I'm scared to death just *being* in Vietnam. I can't help it. I've prayed over it. I believe with all my heart that I will be killed if I go to the field."

Holley kept Scott in Dong Tam for as long as he could, then moved him out to a fire support base when his confidence improved. Soon battalion admin clerks shuffled a few papers and Scott found himself replacing platoon medic Ernest Osborne in Charlie Company. Osborne was big, macho, and a good combat aid man. . . . He found himself supplanted by a skinny wide-eyed conscientious objector who toted only an aid bag half his size. The platoon leader stared. Then he shook his head and walked away. . . .

Scott's first mission was a night ambush, as my first had been. Shivering from dread, battling against the jitters scratching around like a live animal inside his bowels, the new doc with a squad of Hardcore boonie rats set up their ambush patrol alongside a peaceful river.

It was a quiet moonless night. Billy worked to keep his mind occupied. He couldn't sleep when it was his half-squad's turn. He sat hunched on perimeter, peering through a starlight scope that collected available light and permitted its user to see in the dark.

Suddenly he caught his breath. Movement in the greenish light of the scope picture. He kept watching, thinking it might have been his imagination, hoping it had been.

He saw a Vietnamese man squatting in the undergrowth. Black clothing. Black sweat rag tied around his head. Short, stubby AK-47 with the characteristic swept-forward banana clip.

The VC crept toward the American position.

Billy reported what he had detected to his squad leader. The squad went on full 100 percent alert. Everyone scanned the terrain out front bush by bush, tree by tree.

Nothing. . . . The squad relaxed. Even Scott himself was beginning to think he hadn't seen a VC.

Shortly afterward the night erupted in gunfire and terror. Attacking VC caught the GIs by surprise and swarmed over the ambush position with the rapid-fire winking and blasting of their Chicom AKs. A Vietcong, the tree branches in his helmet silhouetted against the stars, charged at Scott, squeezing his weapon into full automatic.

Billy dropped to his knees and began praying. Flame blossomed point-blank. Lead slammed into the ground around the skinny medic.

He pitched forward, face down on the earth. Bullets kicked dirt into his eyes.

He lost all control over his muscles. Horror melted him into the ground. He lay unmoving, as in death. He thought he might not be breathing.

Terror turned to something beyond even that as he felt the enemy soldier squat and quickly rifle his pockets. The sour-fish stench of *nuoc mam* almost made him retch.

He managed to control the trembling in his limbs until the VC melted away. Then his trembling let him know he was still alive. He lay there, playing dead, until the firing ceased and the enemy left. Tears streaming down his boyish face, brave little Doc Billy mustered some inner strength fed by the springs of his religion and, instead of fleeing or hiding or breaking down entirely, found his aid bag and went to work. Dead and wounded GIs lay scattered everywhere in the jungle.

When rescuers arrived, they found the little medic covered with blood and gore, treating the survivors and offering spiritual comfort to the dying. His patients lay bandaged around him. Doc Billy knelt, gave thanks to God for his deliverance, and prayed for the souls of those whom God had seen fit not to deliver. . . .

KEY TERMS

A priori, 275 • Nosocomial, 266 • Solipsism, 266 • Thoracic, 271 • Uremic, 269

QUESTIONS TO CONSIDER

1. Following is a question often posed to bioethics students: Suppose you are on an ethics committee that must determine which patients should receive kidney dialysis. Only four openings exist, and you have nine applicants. Your applicants are male and female, from all age and ethnic groups, and from all walks of life. Denial of care is likely a death sentence. What criteria would you use to choose the lucky four patients? How would you justify your criteria? What would you say to the individuals not chosen?

2. Currently, we accept as a given that nobody should take part in medical experiments or drug trials unless they are fully informed about the procedures and risks, and that undue pressure must not be brought to bear. If this is the case, how do you think companies justify the use of men and women in prison—many of whom are functionally illiterate or minimally educated—who often participate in return for extra commissary privileges or reduced sentences? Does such use constitute undue pressure? Or is it informed consent? How can such research conform to the Nuremberg Code?

3. How do Dr. Spock's comments on the psychology of the adolescent compare with your upbringing? Did your parents raise you in accordance with Spock's child-care manual? How did their treatment and understanding of your issues compare with his advice?

4. What are your perceptions of the modern hospital? What do you believe are the five main problems with hospitals? Why do you choose these five over others? Are your selections based on experience? If so, what happened? What kind of changes do you think hospitals will undergo in the twenty-first century?

5. In one of the most important changes in medical history, modern consumers in developed countries have come to describe health as an inalienable human right—an entitlement—which is a new concept. Yet, most of the world's population does not have access to the most basic medical services. Why? What can be done to "even the playing field," to guarantee that every human being has access? Is such a goal realistic for the twenty-first century? Why?

RECOMMENDED READINGS

Adams, Mark B. *The Wellborn Science: Eugenics in Germany, France, Brazil, and Russia.* New York: Oxford University Press, 1990.

Berridge, Virginia, and Maurice Kirby, eds. *Health and Society in Britain Since 1939.* Cambridge: Cambridge University Press, 1999.

Colon, A. R. *Nurturing Children: A History of Pediatrics.* Westport, CT: Greenwood Press, 1999.

Drake, David F. *Reforming the Health Care Market: An Interpretive Economic History.* Washington, DC: Georgetown University Press, 1994.

Fessler, Diane B. *No Time for Fear: Voices of American Military Nurses in World War II.* East Lansing: Michigan State University Press, 1996.

Gallagher, Hugh G. *By Trust Betrayed: Patients, Physicians and the License to Kill in the Third Reich.* New York: Holt, 1990.

Gamble, Vanessa N. *Making a Place for Ourselves: The Black Hospital Movement, 1920–1945.* New York: Oxford University Press, 1995.

Goodman, Jordan, and Anthony McElligott. *Useful Bodies: Humans in the Service of Medical Science in the 20th Century.* Baltimore: Johns Hopkins University Press, 2003.

Hogan, Neal C. *Unhealed Wounds: Medical Malpractice in the 20th Century.* New York: LFB Scholarly Publications, 2003.

Howell, Joel D. *Technology in the Hospital: Transforming Patient Care in the Early 20th Century.* Baltimore: Johns Hopkins University Press, 1995.

Jacobs, Lawrence R. *The Health of Nations: Public Opinion and the Making of American and British Health Policy.* Ithaca, NY: Cornell University Press, 1993.

Leyton, Elliot, and Greg Locke. *Touched by Fire: Doctors Without Borders in a Third World Crisis.* Toronto, Ontario, Canada: McClelland & Stewart, 1998.

Marks, Harry M. *The Progress of Experiment: Science and Therapeutic Reform in the United States, 1900–1990.* Cambridge: Cambridge University Press, 2000.

Meade, Teresa A. *Science, Medicine and Cultural Imperialism.* New York: St. Martin's Press, 1991.

Rosen, Christine. *Preaching Eugenics: Religious Leaders and the American Eugenics Movement.* New York: Oxford University Press, 2004.

Rubin, Hank. *Spain's Cause Was Mine: A Memoir of an American Medic in the Spanish Civil War.* Carbondale: Southern Illinois University Press, 1997.

Sanger, Margaret. *The Selected Papers of Margaret Sanger.* Edited by Esther Katz, Cathy Moran Hajo, and Peter C. Engleman. Urbana: University of Illinois Press, 2002.

Scott, W. Richard. *Institutional Change and Healthcare Organizations: From Professional Dominance to Managed Care.* Chicago: University of Chicago Press, 2000.

Whorton, James C. *Nature Cures: The History of Alternative Medicine in America.* Oxford: Oxford University Press, 2002.

Chapter Thirteen

The Twentieth Century
New Enemies, Old Nemeses

INTRODUCTION

In addition to witnessing all the procedural and ethical challenges presented by modern medicine, the twentieth century endured some of the greatest epidemiological crises in history. Scientists and laboratory researchers discovered a host of vaccines for many diseases that had plagued humanity. They could examine the human body at the cellular, even the genetic, level without causing trauma to the patient, and reports were constantly made about discoveries of the causes of diseases such as cancer and Alzheimer's. Technology could support life almost indefinitely, and surgeons could even replace several types of failing major organs.

Yet, despite these enormous medical advances, infectious disease continued to destroy millions of lives every year. Some of these plagues were old foes, such as tuberculosis and malaria; others were new to the human race, such as polio and AIDS. Some were both old and new, such as influenza, which mutates so rapidly that it essentially reinvents itself every year. Most years, people get their flu shots and forget about the flu. However, the Spanish Flu of 1918 killed tens of millions of people, and although it vanished, scientists still do not assume that it has truly disappeared.

Some infectious enemies that had been thought vanquished reemerged. For instance, the incidence of tuberculosis decreased dramatically with the discovery of antibiotics, but the bacterium adapted to that threat, and tuberculosis reappeared in a dangerous multi-drug-resistant form. Likewise, with the development of the polio vaccine, cases of polio virtually vanished in the developed countries. Nevertheless, polio remained endemic in some areas of the world, although the World Health Organization (WHO) targeted 2005 as the year when polio would disappear from the planet—a goal that was not yet met at the time of this publication. In the meantime, people who had polio earlier in life were beginning to realize that the disease packed a secondary punch, seen in **postpolio sequelae.** The only disease considered eradicated from the world was smallpox, because not a single case had been seen from 1980 to the end of the century. Still, some of the virus was alive in U.S. and Russian laboratories, and it posed a terrible threat to the world through biowarfare.

AIDS was the single greatest danger to the human race at the end of the twentieth century. Emerging from the African rain forests into the sexual revolution of the 1970s, it claimed about fifteen million lives by 2000, and the numbers continued to increase. Scientists had developed a number of drugs to deal with the disease, extremely expensive and with miserable side effects, but no cure had been found. The AIDS virus is somewhat similar to influenza in that it changes so rapidly that medication can only treat symptoms, not cure the disease. AIDS robbed society of the most productive age group, the young adults, but also attacked the newborn, and cases began to skyrocket even among persons who were elderly. AIDS destroyed an entire generation in Africa, continued unabated, and thus created a unique generation of orphans.

Thus, the balance sheet for the twentieth century was a mixed bag. On the one hand were the incredible number of discoveries and improvements in medicine; on the other hand were all the questions of availability and use of these resources. In addition, the specter of infectious disease was more immediate than ever. Unquestionably, science and medicine would continue to improve responses to all these challenges, but the lesson of the twentieth century was that new problems would continue to emerge.

TIME LINE

1904	William Gorgas (U.S.) is put in charge of disease control on the Panama Canal project—wipes out malaria and yellow fever
1905–1908	Sixth cholera pandemic occurs
1907	Typhoid Mary (Mary Mallon; U.S.) is quarantined twenty-six years for being a typhoid carrier
1909	Bubonic plague finally ends in San Francisco—the last cases in a pandemic that began in 1897
1911	Last major outbreak of cholera in the United States is seen
1914–1918	World War I—many of the nearly eight million dead die from the Spanish influenza pandemic
1916	Polio epidemic occurs in New York City—twenty-three hundred children die
1917–1918	Famine strikes Ethiopia—again in 1927, 1956, 1972–1974, 1984, 1987, 2002
1918	Spanish Flu pandemic occurs—approximately 25 million are dead worldwide; in the United States, 675,000 people are dead
1932–1933	Russian famine results in about seven million dead (five million in Ukraine)
1932–1945	Biowarfare techniques are perfected through human experimentation at Japanese Unit 731 at Pin Fan, Manchuria; at least three thousand prisoners die

1938	March of Dimes is founded as the National Foundation for Infantile Paralysis
1941	Japanese attack Changteh with cholera; an estimated ten thousand civilians and seventeen hundred Japanese soldiers die
1942–1969	Life span of the U.S. offensive biological warfare program
1952	United States—polio epidemic results in 57,628 cases and 3,300 deaths
1956	Minamata disease—mercury poisoning caused by illegal dumping into fishing grounds—occurs in Japan
1957	Asian flu epidemic begins in Hong Kong
1958–1961	Chinese famine occurs, one of the worst in history—thirty to forty million are dead
1961–present	Seventh cholera pandemic occurs
1966	United States tests nonpathogenic anthrax in the New York City subway system; shows ease of spread
1967	New hemorrhagic virus appears in Marburg, Germany
1969	United States and United Kingdom officially end their offensive bioweapons programs
1971–1974	Famine strikes Bangladesh
1973	USSR begins Biopreparat bioweapons program
1976	First appearance of Legionnaires' disease, in Philadelphia: 221 are sick and 34 are dead; swine flu causes concern that it is the same as the Spanish Flu, which forces 50 million vaccinations in the United States in ten weeks; Ebola outbreak occurs in Sudan and Zaire—90 percent mortality rate
1977	Probably the first two cases of AIDS (which is not recognized by the Centers for Disease Control until 1981) occur; last case of smallpox outside the laboratory is seen
1977–1978	Ebola strikes Zaire; again in 1980, 1981, 1993
1978	Ricin is used in an assassination in London
1978–1980	Human anthrax epidemic occurs in Zimbabwe; infects six thousand and kills about one hundred people
1979	Anthrax epidemic at Sverdlovsk, USSR—caused by release from a nearby military facility—results in ninety-four cases and sixty-four deaths

1980	Toxic shock syndrome (TSS) is linked to tampon use; WHO declares smallpox is eradicated worldwide: Officially, stocks remain only in Atlanta and Moscow
1984	Bhopal Disaster occurs—causes approximately four thousand deaths, and some four hundred thousand individuals are still affected as a result of the chemical reaction and release; considered the worst industrial accident in history; salmonella outbreak in Oregon is traced to intentional contamination—first U.S. bioterrorism case
1984–1988	United States—women account for an increasing percentage of AIDS cases, rising from 6.4 percent to 10.4 percent
1985	Mad cow disease (bovine spongiform encephalopathy, or BSE) is first identified; Rotary International and WHO launch the PolioPlus program, aiming to eradicate polio from the world by 2005
1986	Chernobyl, USSR—reactor overheats and explodes, the worst nuclear accident in history, and the extent of the damage is still unknown; twenty-five thousand diagnosed AIDS patients exist in the United States
1988	One in six babies born in New York City is HIV positive
1989	Ebola virus infects monkeys in a research facility in Reston, Virginia
1990	United States and United Kingdom demand that the USSR end its biowarfare program; officially ended in 1992
1991	First diagnosis of Gulf War syndrome; in 1996, the U.S. Department of Defense announces no evidence for its existence
1993	Massive *Escherichia coli* outbreak is traced to fast-food burgers in four western states; hantavirus outbreak occurs in Four Corners country; Milwaukee—four hundred thousand people are sick from *Cryptosporidium*-contaminated water
1994	Pan American Health Organization declares the Americas free of polio; outbreaks of bubonic and pneumonic plague are seen in India
1995	Aum Shinrikyo cult looses sarin gas in a Tokyo subway; were also researching other bioweapons

1996	AIDS—U.S. death rate from this disease drops 26 percent, the first decrease, and a decrease or plateau occurs in Europe, Australia, and New Zealand; United Nations Special Commission on Iraq (UNSCOM) inspectors destroy Iraqi bioweapons
1997	WHO estimates 22.6 million people are HIV infected worldwide; 42 percent are women, and the percentage is still climbing
1999	WHO announces AIDS is now the world's leading infectious disease; West Nile virus appears in the U.S. northeast, including New York City

▲

Tuberculosis as a Disease of the Masses and How to Combat It

S. Adolphus Knopf

In the early twentieth century, of all infectious diseases tuberculosis was the greatest killer, accounting for approximately one in every seven deaths. It was generally recognized as extremely contagious and was assumed to have a hereditary component. For people who could afford treatment, the most common program was fresh air, rest, and wholesome food in an isolated sanitarium. Physicians devised a number of procedures to deal with the disease, including the use of chlorine gas and the surgical deflation of one lung. Because tuberculosis was extremely common among the poor and working class, however, most sufferers could not afford such treatments.

A real need existed for affordable public education about tuberculosis. In Germany, S. A. Knopf wrote an inexpensive paperback containing a wealth of information about the disease, how to avoid it, and how to treat it at home. The prize-winning book was subsequently translated and published in several editions in the United States. Instead of taking the popular, romanticized view of tuberculosis, he described it as a disease of the masses, a "social disease" linked to overcrowding, malnutrition, lack of sanitation, and alcoholism.

Books such as Knopf's were useful to the target audience of working poor, those most at risk of contracting the disease. Effective treatment continued to elude doctors and patients until after World War II, when antibiotics, particularly streptomycin, became widely available and extremely effective. Within twenty years, cases of tuberculosis were nearly a rarity.

Reprinted from S. Adolphus Knopf, *Tuberculosis as a Disease of the Masses and How to Combat It* (New York: Flori, 1908), 15–16, 25–27, 30–35, 40–42, 56, 61, 63–64.

However, near the end of the century, tuberculosis returned as a critical global health concern, and only partially because problems of poverty and malnutrition remained. The tuberculosis bacterium had evolved rapidly to the point at which many strains were resistant to nearly every antibiotic, and even a few strains could not be controlled by antibiotics. In addition, the AIDS pandemic had created a growing population of immunosuppressed individuals who were at extreme risk of getting tuberculosis. According to the WHO, in 1998, three million people died of tuberculosis and another seven million became ill, and going into the twenty-first century, an estimated one-third of the world's population was infected. Tuberculosis had become the leading infectious killer of youth and young adults, and the leading cause of death for women of childbearing age, causing three times the number of deaths resulting from HIV/AIDS. In a real sense, the medical field was back to square one, and much of the advice Knopf had offered remained relevant.

▲

What Is Consumption?

Pulmonary consumption, or tuberculosis of the lungs, is a chronic disease caused by the presence of the tubercle bacillus, or germ of consumption, in the lungs. The disease is locally characterized by countless tubercles, that is to say, small rounded bodies, visible to the naked eye. The bacilli can be found by the million in the affected organ. . . .

The important symptoms of pulmonary tuberculosis are cough, expectoration (spitting phlegm), fever (increased temperature of the body, especially in the evening hours), difficulty in breathing, pains in the chest, night-sweats, loss of appetite, hemorrhages (spitting of blood), and emaciation (loss of flesh). . . .

How May the Germ of Consumption (Bacillus Tuberculosis) Enter the Human System?

1. By being inhaled; that is, breathed into the lungs.
2. By being ingested; that is, eaten with tuberculous food.
3. By inoculation; that is, the penetration of tuberculous substance through a wound in the skin. . . .

How Can We Guard Against Germs of Tuberculosis in Our Food?

Whenever one is not reasonably certain that the meat he eats has been carefully inspected and declared free from disease germs, it should be very thoroughly cooked. By this means one is certain to kill all the dangerous micro-organisms. . . .

[Likewise], unless one can be reasonably sure that the cows from which the milk is derived are healthy and not tuberculous, the milk should be boiled or sterilized before use, more especially when it is intended as food for children. Milk obtained from stores and from milk peddlers should invariably be submitted to boiling or sterilization. . . .

In What Other Ways May the Bacilli or Germs of Consumption Enter the Intestinal Tract?

Since the tubercle bacillus may be found in the saliva of a tuberculous patient, it is best never to kiss such a person on the mouth. . . . Tuberculous patients should have their own drinking glasses, spoons, forks, etc. . . . Every consumptive patient should remember never to touch food before having washed his hands very thoroughly. Even with the greatest care, it is possible that he may have soiled his hands with tuberculous expectoration.

How May Tuberculosis Be Contracted Through Inoculation . . . ?

Inoculation of tuberculosis happens perhaps most frequently through injuries received while cleaning nicked or chipped glass or porcelain cuspidors which had been used by consumptives. . . .

What Protects the Healthy Individual from Contracting Tuberculosis?

After all that we have said of the contagiousness, or rather the communicability, of tuberculosis, and consumption in particular, one must not think that a breath in an atmosphere accidentally laden with bacilli would certainly render a healthy individual consumptive, or that by a swallow of tuberculous milk or a little injury from a broken cuspidor one must necessarily become tuberculous. The secretions of our nasal cavities, doubtlessly also the blood, and the secretions of the stomach of a healthy individual, have bactericidal properties; that is to say, they kill the dangerous germs before they have a chance to do harm. Therefore, the healthy man and woman should not have an exaggerated fear of tuberculosis, but they should, nevertheless, not recklessly expose themselves to the danger of infection.

How May One Successfully Overcome a Hereditary Disposition to Consumption?

The mother who fears for her future child a hereditary disposition to tuberculosis should lead a very healthful life. She should be as much in the open air as possible, breathe deeply and eat regularly of plain but nourishing food. Never should she wear garments which constrict any of her chest or abdominal organs. . . . The tightly laced corset should be banished forever from the dress of women. Not only is free and natural breathing interfered with by this article of dress, but indigestion and disturbances in the circulation follow excessively tight lacing. Anæmia, or poverty of the blood, so often observed in young girls, can very frequently be ascribed to this unnatural mode of dress, which does not permit either a free circulation or sufficient oxygenation of the blood. . . . It cannot be insisted upon too often that in an individual predisposed to tuberculosis nothing can be more injurious than an interference with proper digestion and assimilation. . . .

Whenever a mother has a tendency to tuberculous disease, the child should be given a healthy wet-nurse, or be fed artificially with modified cow's milk. . . .

. . . The careful, judicious, and regular application of cold water is perhaps one of the best preventive measures against taking cold. . . . Cold baths, especially bathing in a river or in the ocean, are, of course, to be recommended in warm weather. Weakly and elderly persons should not take cold baths, no matter at what season, unless permitted to do so by their physician.

To keep the skin clean and in good condition, cold baths, even when taken every day, are not always sufficient, and soap and warm water should be used at least once a week. The warm bath should always be followed by a rapid sponging off with cold water. . . .

The proper bringing up of children that have a tendency to become tuberculous is of the greatest importance. . . . The dislike to play outdoors, which is so characteristic of the little candidates for tuberculous diseases, can also only be overcome by discipline. To dress them too warmly and bundle them up all the time is as injurious as having them remain most of the time indoors. Such children should not work too hard during their school age. To spend too many hours sitting down, to do too much brain work, to spend too much time at the piano or in other musical studies, have [*sic*] a tendency often to weaken seriously the child predisposed to tuberculosis. . . .

When the time comes to choose a profession or trade for a young man who has a tendency to tuberculosis, one should bear in mind that gardening, farming, forestry, and all occupations which demand an outdoor life, are the most likely to make him a strong man and a useful member of society.

In connection with the precautions which should be taken to combat a tendency to tuberculosis, we must say a few words concerning the curability of consumption or pulmonary tuberculosis. The old idea—still, alas! very prevalent and deeply rooted in the minds of many people—that a tuberculous individual who has seemingly inherited his tendency to the disease, can have no hope of cure, is wrong. We desire to emphasize the fact that the chances for a cure of the consumptive individual does not at all depend upon whether he had a hereditary tendency, or has accidentally acquired the disease. There are hundreds of cases of healed tuberculosis in men and women who have lived to old age, and nevertheless their fathers or mothers had succumbed to consumption. . . .

How Can a Predisposition to Tuberculosis, Other than Hereditary, Be Created or Acquired?

1. By the intemperate use of alcoholic beverages, a dissipated life, excesses of all kinds, etc.
2. By certain diseases which weaken the constitution; for example, pneumonia, typhoid fever, smallpox, measles, whooping cough, syphilis, influenza, etc.
3. By certain occupations, trades, and professions, such as printing, hat-making, tailoring, weaving, and all occupations where the worker is much exposed to the inhalation of various kinds of dust, as bakers, millers, confectioners, cigar-makers, chimney-sweepers, and the workers in lead, wood, stone, metals, etc.

. . . For the intemperate man, the fast liver, or one inclined to excesses, there is no remedy except to change his mode of life. . . . The necessity of seeking medical advice holds good for all those who by intemperance or excesses of any kind have undermined their constitution, and thus diminished their natural resistance to the invasion of the tubercle bacilli. . . .

. . . We have already mentioned . . . that certain occupations, such as those of stonecutters, printers, and cigar-makers, render weak individuals particularly prone to consumption; therefore, any one inclined to this disease should, in his own interest, never pursue such an occupation.

Lastly, we must mention one more occupation in which tuberculous individuals should never engage, namely, that of keepers of animals in menageries. . . .

Can Tuberculosis, Especially in Its Pulmonary Form, or Consumption of the Lungs, Be Cured?

This question can be answered with a very decided Yes. . . . There are thousands of such cases where people, once declared consumptive by competent physicians, have ultimately recovered, and pursued their vocations in life with unimpaired vigor for many years afterward.

The statistics from sanatoria for consumptives, where patients in all stages of the disease are received, show that twenty-five per cent, leave as absolutely cured, and forty to fifty per cent, leave much improved, many of them being again capable of earning their living. . . . We do not think it an exaggeration to say that of all chronic diseases tuberculosis is the most curable, and of late years the most frequently cured. . . .

What Are the Modern Methods to Treat and Cure Consumption?

It is not cured by quacks, by patent medicines, nostrums, or other secret remedies, but solely and exclusively by scientific and judicious use of fresh air, sunshine, water, abundant and good food (milk, eggs, meat, vegetables, fruit), and the help of certain medicinal substances when the just-mentioned hygienic and dietetic means do not suffice in themselves to combat the disease. . . .

▲

America's Deadly Rendezvous with the "Spanish Lady"

JACK FINCHER

In the last months of World War I, influenza broke out in a U.S. military camp packed with soldiers awaiting shipment to the European front. What began as a flu outbreak rapidly spread from North America to Europe and on to the Middle East, Asia, and the rest of the world in a pandemic known as the Spanish Flu. *Completely misnamed (it had no connections with Spain), the Spanish Flu became the deadliest epidemic to that time, rivaled only by the Black Death as the greatest killer disease in human history. Exact figures are unknown, but at least six hundred thousand people died of the Spanish Flu in the United States, and worldwide estimates range from twenty million to one hundred million, with another one billion who caught the flu but recovered. What killed in such incredible numbers was not influenza per se, but the complications that accompanied it, particularly an extremely virulent and fast-acting pneumonia. Despite its impact, the Spanish Flu remains the "forgotten pandemic," as one author dubbed it.*

What is still particularly frightening about the Spanish Flu is that scientists do not know specifically how it evolved. Results of modern research suggest that the virus originated in birds, mutated, then jumped to human hosts. Further, it disappeared suddenly, for unknown reasons. No one knows whether the mutated form of the virus still exists. Because influenza can jump across species, as the Spanish Flu did, it may not have vanished forever. The avian flu outbreak of 2005 has shown a bird-to-human transmission similar to that of the Spanish Flu, although as of this writing it has not mutated to human-to-human transmission. World health authorities have maintained a vigilant watch for anything resembling the Spanish Flu, and so far the avian flu seems perilously close. Authorities admit that if the Spanish Flu were to reappear, the results would be far worse than in 1918. Some researchers even refuse to say "if" it reappears, but rather "when."

▲

Reprinted by permission of Claire M. Fincher, from Jack Fincher, "America's Deadly Rendezvous with the 'Spanish Lady,'" *Smithsonian Magazine* 19, no. 10 (1989): 130–45.

The brothers stood in the cooling dust of an East Texas autumn, hitting each other as hard as they could. Murlin, two years younger at 16, had struck first. Wright was their widowed father's favorite, and Murlin was sick of it. Yet with their little brother, Neal, looking on, it seemed somehow fitting that Wright should strike the last blow, battering Murlin, dazed and bloody, to the ground.

Wright, dreading what their stern sheriff father might do to punish him, did what many a young man has done to escape an unhappy household. He ran off and joined the Army. A few days later word reached home from the camp in Dallas: come at once, your son is gravely ill. His father found him lying unconscious on the cold stone floor of a makeshift military hospital, its exhausted staff too overworked by the influenza raging round them to notice. Wright died on October 18, 1918.

Murlin was so guilt-stricken at his brother's death that he never talked about it. I know. Murlin was my father. Only after he died did my cousin tell me the story. At that, it was but one small, sad design in the vast tapestry of a fatally infectious disease as common to the fabric of American family life then as it is rare today. Times were so different then. Grown-ups and children were so quickly subtracted from the world by so many diseases that we no longer have to fear. My grandmother, for instance, died before Wright. She sewed her tubercular sister's burial shroud and then died of the disease herself. Her youngest son was born tubercular. He died before his mother.

For millions of people fortunate enough to have escaped the horrors of World War I, the plague struck as the fighting neared its end and displaced war as the tragic centerpiece of everyday life. It was known as the Spanish flu and it spread worldwide. In just under a year, starting in the spring of 1918, it killed more than 22 million people, at least twice as many as died in the "war to end all wars." Some estimates, including people who died of complications, go as high as 30 million.

In America, with curiously little fanfare, the flu brought to death a half-million souls, five times as many Americans as died in combat in France. How we tried to cope with the flu and its side effects became what historian Alfred Crosby calls the "greatest failure of medical science" ever. . . .

The first mild wave of the epidemic began in March 1918 when a mess cook with chills and fever reported for sick call at Fort Riley, Kansas. Pvt. Albert Gitchell said his head and muscles ached and his throat felt sore. By week's end there were 522 such hospital admissions at the fort. Despite the quickening effect of fever, vital signs including heartbeat were slowed by a profound systemic depression. Doctors were puzzled. Disturbing, too, the illness seemed to hit hardest among robust people in their 20s and 30s, a period when resistance is normally high.

Yet nobody seemed terribly worried at first, not even when a dozen other overcrowded camps were struck. Military authorities and the government were still concentrating on how to get enough fresh troops to France, where Gen. John J. (Black Jack) Pershing was planning the first American offensive, one that everyone hoped would end the war. Besides, flu had been around since Hippocrates first noted a probable Athenian epidemic in 412 B.C. Centuries later, the Italians christened it *influenza di freddo,* "influence of the cold." Still later it came to be believed that some "vicious quality" or sudden shift in the atmosphere mysteriously communicated the disease to whole areas. Fort Riley was a famous cavalry post, and right before the outbreak, it had experienced just such an atmospheric change when gale-force winds shrouded the camp with a noxious pall of prairie dust and stifling smoke from burning horse manure.

But exactly what was communicated nobody knew. In fact, though flu shots are of some preventive help today, there is still no known cure for most of influenza's many forms. In 1892, Germany's Richard Pfeiffer thought he'd found the answer in throat cultures of flu patients in Berlin: a blood-nourished bacillus—a rod-shaped bacterium—

one-sixteenth the size of a red corpuscle. Other medical researchers weren't so sure. They suspected the existence of invisible microorganisms—viruses. But nobody had really pursued this early lead. Why should they have? Flu ranked a distant tenth among the world's causes of death and aroused little concern compared with dread diseases like diphtheria. By and large, too, its initial symptoms in 1918 produced a relatively mild and apparently temporary condition of the kind that used to inspire the old medical school quip, "Quite a godsend! Everybody ill, nobody dying."

People were used to death in 1918, not only at the distant fighting front but in crowded training camps. The 46 deaths that followed at Fort Riley were simply attributed to the complications of pneumonia, and the Army quickly went back to training two million men under crowded conditions and shipping them across the North Atlantic. Often they were packed into airless freighter hulls, floating test tubes for breeding virulent, improved mutations of an infection whose only constant, epidemiologists would learn to their dismay, was change. By the summer of 1918, when the latest batch of U.S. troops landed in France, plenty of flu got off with them.

By fall, vomiting, dizziness, labored breathing and profuse sweating were added to the previously mild symptoms. Sometimes purple blisters appeared on oxygen-starved skin. Projectile nosebleeds from pulmonary hemorrhages occurred, too. Victims often went into paroxysms of coughing. . . . Flu victims began dying in larger and larger numbers, some violently within a few days. . . .

From France this second wave of flu spread west to England and south to Spain where it killed eight million Spaniards, which is how it came to be known as Spanish flu, and even, ungallantly, "Spanish Lady." It was called *Blitz Katarrh* when it struck eastward into the ragged ranks of the Kaiser's army in Germany. . . . On it swept, to Russia, China and Japan; down to South Africa and across to India (where 12 million people died of it) and soon to South America. The Spanish Lady's speed beggared belief. . . .

Among Americans the disease was primarily confined to the Army for several months. On September 3, 1918, a civilian case was documented in Boston. A week later, as Babe Ruth and the Red Sox beat Chicago in the World Series, three men dropped dead on the sidewalks of nearby Quincy. From Maine to the Gulf, from Florida to Puget Sound, fed by the mass movements of uniformed men and by their contact with civilians, cases began popping up first by hundreds, then by thousands. Statistics pyramided to roughly 10,000 domestic deaths in September. Up to 90 recruits a day were now dying at Camp Devens, Massachusetts, and Dr. William Henry Welch, the nation's most renowned pathologist, was called in to perform autopsies on bodies "blue as huckleberries." Afterward, shaken, he admitted a truth that the medical establishment hates to share with the public: "This must be some new kind of infection."

For the government and American medical authorities, it was crucial not only to find a cure and a preventative but to insure against possible public panic. Then, as it would now, the main official responsibility lay with the Surgeon General of the United States, Rupert Blue, a quietly competent 26-year career veteran, who had fought bubonic plague in San Francisco and yellow fever in New Orleans.

. . . In 1918 Blue had only a relative handful of doctors and researchers to help him, and a yearly budget—even then regarded as a pittance—of less than $3 million.

Flu was not then a reportable disease anywhere in the United States, and many states did not even bother to file death statistics with the federal government—or to keep them at all. Because it was viewed as a common and usually mild disease, it was unlikely that Blue would have had the authority to impose a quarantine or to prevent ships carrying influenza cases from docking. The federal government was far less powerful and pervasive than it is today. Blue's office lacked not only funds but the necessary medical data to do much. He finally decided that it would be impractical to attempt a massive quarantine, a decision that, in retrospect, was probably wise. . . .

Alas, other dangerous infections were in the air—fatuity, folly, finger pointing and wishful thinking. Cities as diverse as Santa Fe, San Francisco, Philadelphia and Seattle bragged that they need not worry—the flu would be kept at bay by their ideal climates. People were presented with a welter of official commentary and patronizing reassurance, much of it nonsense. A community doctor in Arizona, perhaps trying to keep the lid on panic, reported 50 fresh cases as follows: "all mild, four deaths." Mild? An *8 percent* death rate?

The New York City Health Commissioner, Royal Copeland, seemed hell-bent on single-handedly jawboning the epidemic into remission by blaming it on unsanitary Europeans. "You haven't heard of our doughboys getting it, have you?" he asked in airy disregard both of the evidence and the fact that existing rules of censorship forbade any such news from being published. "You bet you haven't, and you won't. No need for our people to worry." Copeland was not the only one who opposed Blue's flu alarms. In Missouri, one official even dismissed the flu as "Hun propaganda." Partly to avoid panic, mainly because it was overshadowed by the war, some newspapers tended to downplay the epidemic, just as the country would at first downplay the spread of AIDS.

In general, Blue's plea for enforced limitations on public gatherings to prevent spread of the disease fell upon ears deafened by the din of martial music. Thirteen million young men—ideal fodder for infection—were still jamming public buildings to register for the draft. In late September, a national subscription to finance the war effort got under way from coast to coast with mammoth rallies, parades and canvasses. In Philadelphia 200,000 marched; in San Francisco, 150,000. . . . Evangelist Billy Sunday joined the patriotic rush and dismissed the whole affair as a German ploy: "There's nothing short of hell they haven't stooped to do since the war began. Darn their hides!"

It wasn't long before the nation's thin, blue line of surrogate health officers started fining public spitters as well as handkerchiefless sneezers and coughers, and issuing calls for mandatory face masks. Sales and production of masks exploded. Workers wore them in offices and in factories, and in some cities you couldn't climb on a bus or a trolley without one. But there was plenty of heated argument and plenty of backsliding from people who didn't believe masks helped; or didn't like being told what to do.

And, as so often happened with the flu, tragedy was marked by comic oddities. A pair of newlyweds in San Francisco left an indelible impression on a young doctor friend by telling him they'd worn therapeutic masks—and nothing else—when they made love. In Tucson, Judge L. C. Cowan fined a window washer for removing his mask to blow the panes dry. Widely worn, masks probably were marginally helpful in the general way of hygiene and as a discouragement to intimacy.

As flu hopscotched around the country, the death toll mounted; from 2,899 in August to 10,481 in September to 195,876 in October; in the last four months of 1918, well over 300,000 died. Both sexes and all races were hit. Surprisingly, a general exodus failed to occur; the poor couldn't afford to run, and because the disease seemed so quixotic, the rich never knew where to go to avoid it.

Historians still ask themselves how more than a half-million Americans could die in hardly more than ten months, in the most lethal internal convulsion since the Civil War . . . , without laying a comparable mark on the country's psyche. But the astonishing truth is that during the epidemic few people were in a position to see the big picture, and not one of the few was actively in charge overall. . . . Moreover, only one man, President Woodow Wilson, possessed the means to mobilize national consciousness. But except when the flu threatened to disrupt troop movements or hamper vital arms production, Wilson was far too busy prosecuting the "war to end all wars" to bother with a silent foe that ebbed and surged like wildfire, burning itself out here, moving on there. And where it concerned soldiers, this foe was often protected by the cloak of official censorship.

Not that any of that would have mattered in the end. For nothing helped, really. . . . Phone booths were padlocked and streets sprinkled; cashiers were equipped with finger bowls of disinfectant. Public places from dance halls, pool rooms and movie houses to libraries, schools and ice cream parlors, even red-light districts, were buttoned up. Churches and saloons were shut tight, too, though not without spirited resistance.

But controlling possible contagion on such a scale was virtually impossible. One sanitation officer counted 199 individual chances for exposure in any citizen's average day. . . .

At a West Coast Navy base, guards were ordered to shoot to kill anyone attempting to enter or leave without official permission. Drinking fountains were sanitized hourly by blowtorch, telephones drenched in alcohol. Draftees were given "close order drill," keeping a 20-foot interval. Yet such Herculean efforts were mocked by inexplicable immunities. Waterbury, Connecticut, suffered 753 deaths in one month alone. Milford, 20 miles away, escaped completely. In Montana, people were baffled by the relative lack of flu among butchers, Methodists and underground miners.

. . . Across the land, doctors rushed to create prophylactic solutions. Certain he had located the best, the mayor of Boston ordered his secretary to carry a batch to San Francisco via the 20th Century Limited, a crack express train. Seventeen thousand Bay Area hopefuls lined up for doses despite widespread assertions that such "soups" offered nothing more than a sore arm. . . .

. . . Naturally, good old American home medicine bulged with all sorts of cures, from tiny doses of strychnine and kerosene to red-pepper sandwiches and something called Bulgarian blood tea. Nostrums ranged from the bizarre to the superstitious. As a preventative, people variously sprinkled sulfur in their shoes, wore vinegar packs on their stomachs, tied slices of cucumber to their ankles or carried a potato in each pocket. Ac-

cording to one belief, if you placed a shotgun under the bed the fine steel in it would draw out fever. In New Orleans, people bought voodoo charms and chanted, "Sour, sour, vinegar V, keep the sickness off of me." One Volunteer Medical Corps general championed "breathing through the nose, chewing food well, and avoiding tight clothes, shoes and gloves." One mother in Portland, Oregon, buried her 4-year-old girl from head to toe in raw, sliced onions. An appalled Chicago physician summed it all up as "poly-pharmacy run riot." . . .

The tragic stories accumulated. Years later in San Francisco, Henrietta Burt, a secretary, would recall a fateful bridge game: "We played until long after midnight. When we left we were all apparently well. By 8 o'clock in the morning I was too ill to get out of bed, and the friend at whose house we played was dead." A stricken Congressman and his bride, clinically gowned and masked, were married at his hospital bedside; seven hours later he succumbed.

"Hunt up your woodworkers and cabinetmakers and set them making coffins," one health department was morbidly advised. "Then take your street laborers and set them to digging graves." Devastated Pennsylvania had learned the wisdom of that counsel through grim experience. In one week a total of 5,000 people died in Pittsburgh and Philadelphia. So overwhelmed was the latter city that 528 bodies piled up in a single day awaiting burial. More lay beside the gutters or in rooming houses.

As fear spread, laws and law enforcement in some cities grew savage. In Chicago, charges of murder were demanded against landlords whose sick tenants died after their heat was turned off for nonpayment of rent. In New York City, 500 people were arrested for violating "Spitless Sunday"; doctors were fined for failing to report new flu cases.

Violence and vigilantism flourished. Strangers from notoriously infected states who got off the train in some New Mexico towns were told to move on. A Montana rancher intercepted a doctor on the road and forced him at gunpoint to treat his family. . . . San Francisco's authoritarian, chief public health officer, who was a stickler for masks, was sent a bomb containing black gunpowder, buckshot and broken glass. Frontier justice may have reached some sort of zenith when Prescott, Arizona, made it a jailable offense to shake hands. . . .

By mid-autumn, public services were crippled everywhere. . . . In Pennsylvania and Kentucky, officials demanded that the Army send medical help to coal-mining towns to sustain the vital war effort.

For every 1 who died in the United States, an estimated 50 had the disease. Some took advantage of the pandemonium to steal or to seek oblivion in drink for weeks on end. . . .

All that could really be done, it turned out, was to keep the patient quiet, warm, fed and medicated against other life-threatening complications, but even that put a terrible burden on the people who were well, or though sick, still able to get about. Everywhere the call went out for anyone with two hands and a willingness to work. Helping their prostrate relatives, small children cooked, kept house, cared for and cleaned up after the sick. Some, like those of their elders unable to face the plague, wandered the streets in a daze. Minneapolis police set up a special search for parents of a hundred homeless youngsters found alone and hiding. In Chicago, a laborer crazed by the illness of his wife and four children screamed, "I'll cure them my own way!" and cut their throats. Families called the authorities to report the terminally ill, then quickly fled their homes in terror.

With churches closed, people prayed elsewhere, sometimes using rude outdoor altars as they did in Maine where a priest set up a table and a cross in a garage doorway, and worshipers knelt in the snow. Some deeply believed that the plague had been visited on the world as Divine punishment for human sinfulness. Acting Army Surgeon General Vaughan gave voice to a different, but statistically chilling, thought: "If the epidemic continues its mathematical rate of acceleration," he announced, "civilization could easily [disappear] from the face of the Earth."

Stretched to the breaking point and worked to exhaustion, doctors and nurses labored on. They pumped railroad handcars to reach isolated cases, made their rounds by horse and newfangled airplane. Not only did they treat whole families, they assembled and handed out food and blankets; they milked cows, cooked, built fires, heated water, and bathed and dressed the helpless. They grabbed meals from the family stew pot and fell asleep on the nearest couch. Or dozed upright in their buggies, warmed by heated bricks wrapped in newspapers as their horses were given free rein.

And gradually a kind of dogged selflessness, sometimes amounting to heroism, became commonplace. Businesses, hotels, fraternity houses, private clubs, even the exclusive Vanderbilt farm in Rhode Island donated their premises for emergency hospitals. Private automobiles and taxicabs, as well as the limousines of society matrons, chauffeured medics and served as ambulances. Off-duty police and firemen drove ambulances and carried stretchers. Department stores distributed relief supplies and opened phone banks so people could make emergency calls. Volunteers canvassed house-to-house searching for those too weak to cry out for help.

Fitfully, the long day's night began to fade. People who had the disease and survived, either by chance or because of care that prevented pneumonia, the most common and most deadly complication, seemed to be immune from further episodes. Like a storm, the Spanish flu eventually blew itself out. On November 7, a false Armistice sent a million people streaming into the streets of Philadelphia to kiss and hug and dance in defiance of every public health tenet. When the real Armistice was signed four days later there was no holding back a war-weary nation. Factory whistles blew, church bells and fire bells rang, and in Chicago 16,000 police could not keep the joyous crowds from jamming together. A third wave of flu—harsher than the first yet milder than the second—was still to come by year's end. But as far as the people were concerned, the real crisis had passed. Psychologically, at least, the end of the war had upstaged it. . . .

More than 25 million Americans were infected; perhaps a billion beings worldwide. Direct U.S.

economic losses have been put at $3 billion, but an insurance industry expert calculated the influenza epidemic as an "actuarial nightmare," which would ultimately cost the United States alone *ten million years* in productive lives cut off in their prime. . . .

As for the mysterious Spanish flu virus, it seemed to vanish from the planet as if it had never been. Since then there have been plenty of milder flus, of course. Today we know that influenza viruses have a genius for assuming new forms when an old one has run its course. The World Health Organization isolates each new flu strain, analyzes it and, if antibodies prove low in global population samples, annually modifies the effective, existing vaccine to combat what might otherwise become another universal contagion. It is tedious work, and even now there are no guarantees for the future. The existence of antibiotics, however, would probably minimize the number of deaths from complications such as pneumonia, which killed many of the victims in 1918.

As evolutionary biologist Stephen Jay Gould recently told an AIDS-lecture audience: "We've had a couple of generations of great fortune: since the . . . flu epidemic of 1918, there has not been a [lethal] pandemic disease that struck the human population. If you look through human history, a pandemic is everyday biology. With our usual hubris we felt that we'd learned through technological advances to be free of it forever. But we're not." . . .

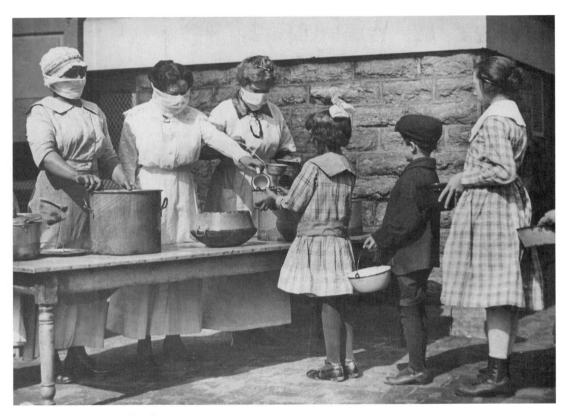

FIGURE 13–1   Spanish Influenza
At the height of the 1918 Spanish influenza pandemic, public services were overwhelmed at the same time that thousands of families were in desperate need of assistance. Volunteerism provided vitally needed help for such families, as in this soup kitchen in Cincinnati that fed children from influenza-stricken households.

▲

In the Shadow of Polio

A Personal and Social History

KATHRYN BLACK

Poliomyelitis, more commonly known as polio, *was one of the most feared infectious diseases during the first half of the twentieth century. It was a mysterious disease that appeared during the summer, and for many years its mode of transmission was unknown. Research subsequently indicated that the virus is spread by the oral-fecal route and that exposure is often correlated with lack of proper sewage treatment. Although it was popularly perceived as primarily attacking young children, polio was in fact more common among young adults. Most people who contracted the disease had only minor respiratory and gastrointestinal symptoms with fever and headache, and they recovered in a few days. However, what made polio so terrifying was the cases of paralysis that it caused. Most often paralyzing the legs, polio also could paralyze normal breathing. In such instances, patient survival depended on mechanical ventilation in the devices called* iron lungs.*

The first major polio epidemic in the United States came in 1894, and a larger outbreak in 1916 affected some nine thousand people in New York City alone. In 1921, it claimed its most famous patient, Franklin D. Roosevelt, who put a great deal of time, effort, and his family fortune into treatment and research for a cure. The famous March of Dimes Birth Defects Foundation was one of his contributions. Research continued until World War II, but little progress was made. Another outbreak hit Los Angeles in 1934, with about 2,500 cases. Polio claimed a number of victims among the troops, but the worst epidemics occurred in the postwar years. From 1945 to 1949, there was an average of 20,000 cases a year. The worst outbreak occurred in 1952, with 58,000 cases in the United States, and the following year saw an additional 35,000 cases. The public was terrified as parents tried desperately to protect their children. Finally, in 1954, the Salk vaccine was tested and found to be extremely effective. After a massive immunization campaign by the March of Dimes in 1957, the incidence of new cases dropped to 5,600 nationwide. In 1962, an improved vaccine developed by Albert Sabin replaced the Salk vaccine, and in 1964, only 121 cases were reported. Polio appeared to have lost its hold.

The story did not end there, however. Even though polio virtually disappeared from Europe and the United States, it remained a major threat, attacking 350,000 people worldwide in 1988. That year, the WHO, together with Rotary International, resolved to eradicate polio by 2000. The deadline was not met, but was extended to 2005. In 2001, 575 million children were vaccinated. As of publication of this book, total eradication of this disease still had not been realized.

The other postscript to the story was the appearance, starting in the 1970s, of what was named postpolio syndrome. *Former polio victims experienced new symptoms, some debilitating, which brought polio back into the news.*

The events in the following excerpt took place in the 1950s when the author's mother was stricken. The impact, not only on the patient, but also on the whole family, was devastating, as her mother fought the severe symptoms before dying just two years after the onset of her disease.

▲

Backache

. . . When my grandmother received the letter saying our family now most certainly was returning to Colorado, she splurged on a long-distance call. She and Mother chatted and made plans for their reunion. Mother's exuberance over the move, and the pool party Dad's office mates were throwing for him, however, was dampened by a backache that had worsened over the past couple of days. She wasn't feeling well and hoped that whatever was ailing her would pass quickly. Mother would have to drive our Chevy sedan to Colorado while Dad drove the pickup. That long trip, she said to her mother, would be no fun with a bad back.

As my father remembers the story, the backache soon took a bad turn. He tried rubbing her muscles, and when that didn't help, he drove to a distant drugstore—the only one open on a Sunday evening—for aspirin and liniment, confident they would ease her discomfort. Groping for a simple, ordinary explanation for this intrusion, they told each other the packing must have strained her muscles. . . .

Despite the drugstore aids, Mother passed the evening in increasing pain. Lifting her arms to put her hair in pincurls reminded her how stiff and achy her neck and shoulders were. Straightening up after bending over to pull off her shoes was difficult. Deep, cramping spasms ran up and down her legs and twitched in her back. As the night lengthened, the symptoms accumulated: pounding head pain, aching joints, shortness of breath, a strange sour taste, thirst. Her mind drifted and blanked, refusing her efforts to focus. She paced uncomfortably. After she finally dropped into bed, she noticed that she had trouble moving her legs when she rolled to her side. In the morning, Dad took her to a doctor. It was June 21. . . .

The doctor examined mother in his office and quickly made a diagnosis that startled my parents: polio. It had never occurred to them that *polio* could be the cause of her misery. Their experience with the disease was limited. They had had a high school classmate who, after graduation, had been paralyzed with polio, and our family had a five-thousand-dollar polio insurance policy through Dad's office, which they certainly hadn't expected to need. Almost daily the disease made the news, but never had they dreamed that polio would find our family.

The doctor was matter-of-fact and unalarmed as he ordered a spinal test for confirmation. Also called a lumbar puncture, the procedure required patients to curl into a fetal position to expose the spine to a needle through which fluid was drawn for analysis. If the patient had polio, the fluid showed cellular and chemical changes consistent enough for physicians to diagnose the disease. During epidemics, hospital emergency rooms were set up to do the taps to anyone coming in with fever or lassitude. The procedure was so common in one hospital that a jaded technician kept a book propped up to entertain himself while a patient's liquid dripped. For those whose spines were penetrated, however, the procedure was singular and not easily forgotten. Mother's puncture went smoothly, though not without discomfort.

Although the symptoms of headache, fever, **malaise,** upset stomach, and muscle pain were common to many viral infections, Mother's doctor probably suspected polio simply because the warm-weather polio season had begun. Arizona was not, however, having an epidemic, and 1954 was not expected to be a bad polio year for the state. When Mother fell ill, there were only twenty-eight other cases reported, compared to thirty-nine by the same date the year before. Many of those patients had been or were being cared for at Phoenix Memorial Hospital, one of the few hospitals in a wide area of the Southwest equipped to care for polio patients.

"Try not to worry," the doctor said, assuring Mother and Dad that she appeared to have a light case of nonparalytic polio, which, like most viruses, would run its course in a few days. "Expect full recovery," he told them. Yet despite his casual reassurance, the doctor immediately ordered Mother to Phoenix Memorial. No one knew how polio passed from person to person, but as it was clearly a contagious disease, health officials considered isolation of patients in the acute stages only prudent. Dad took Mother to the hospital, where a nurse led her to the polio ward. . . .

The hospital had begun as St. Monica's Mission, founded in 1934 by a Franciscan priest as a clinic for the poor. . . . The nonprofit, private St. Monica's had been sold to the federal government in 1947, and in 1949 it had been renamed Memorial Hospital to honor the war dead. In 1951, because of the growing legions of polio victims, a wing once set aside solely for pediatrics had been converted to a polio ward for both children and adults. What the hospital lacked in physical amenities, it made up for in services. By 1954, when Mother lay in the polio ward, the hospital staff had had ample experience caring for polio victims. At times, up to seventy iron lungs packed patient rooms, a **solarium,** and the hallway. On staff were nurses and doctors with special training in the care of polio patients. Their wing was equipped with a rocking-bed ward, an iron-lung ward, and a physical therapy room. The day Mother arrived, nurses applied moist hot packs to her back and legs, bringing relief from the pain and spasms. A board placed under the mattress gave additional comfort to her back.

Dad finally waved goodbye to her from the window and went home to call her parents, Maurine and Hayes Royce, with the news. Even though he tried to reassure them, repeating what the doctor had said about it being a mild case, they were horrified by the possibilities that hung on the word *polio.* In 1954, few people could hear the diagnosis and not be dismayed. A decade of polio summers, the high-profile March of Dimes fund-raising, and word of a vaccine's development had kept the disease in the news. Almost everyone knew someone who had been touched by polio—a friend, a neighbor, a colleague. Still, most people, like my grandparents and parents, knew only that the disease could cripple. What this diagnosis of polio meant, what Mother's outlook might be, and how long it would be before anyone could say for sure were all mysteries to my family. . . .

When she heard the news over the telephone that Virginia was in the hospital with a case of polio, my grandmother could not be reassured. Nor would she sit home waiting for further word; she and Hayes packed the car and started the eight-hundred-mile drive to Phoenix the next day. They were already on the road when early the following morning Dad answered a knock at the door and was startled to see a police officer standing on our step. "Mr. Black?" he said. "You're needed at the hospital."

Mother was worse. Much worse. Her case was *not* mild. She had bulbospinal polio, a combination of two types of paralytic polio, spinal and **bulbar.** This was the most dire of diagnoses.

My grandparents arrived the next day and learned the bad news: Mother was gravely ill. They went straight to the hospital. Maurine still balks at talking of that day, and I can only imagine the fear she and Hayes must have suffered when they were told to put on white sterile gowns and masks and were led down a corridor smelling of disinfectant and littered with metal medicine carts and wheelchairs. A nurse guided them past rooms of polio patients to an iron lung. Wards of tank respirators looked something like the boiler rooms of giant ships, with the blur of gauges, tubes, latches, and dials. The six-foot metal cylinders that breathed for patients lay like coffins on stands that raised them to table height. Intravenous bottles hung from aluminum poles next to respirators, and at one end of each lay a head. Rectangular windows, through which parts of bodies could be glimpsed, and a row of three or four portholes, used by nurses to tend to the bodies inside, lined the sides of the iron lungs.

A respirator's rhythmic *ka-thum-pa* sounds and the cacophony of mechanized, wheezing breath led them to Mother. The iron lung encased Virginia in a vacuum. Pumps working at regular intervals applied first positive, then negative pressure, pushing on her lungs to expel air, then pulling on them to draw more in—an awkwardly consistent cadence. In this acute, dangerous stage of the disease, Mother likely lay semiconscious, unable to speak. One tube entered her nose, and another penetrated her neck.

At the sight of her daughter's gaunt face protruding from the massive iron cylinder, my grandmother gasped, then paled as she reeled with dizziness. A nurse took her arm and led her to a chair, commanding her to lower her head. The hospital allowed only short visits to patients still in the acute stages of polio, and time was almost up when my grandmother felt steady enough to cross the room to Mother.

My grandmother had brought along a gift for that first hospital visit: a white quilted bathrobe with white velvet ribbons. When she told me that detail, I wept, imagining my grandmother selecting that pristine and utterly inappropriate gift for the daughter who, any day up to that one, would have loved its elegance and beauty. The robe would have been jarringly out of place amid the metal and glass and rubber tubing, where the space between life and death pressed to a thin line. How little my grandmother knew—how little most people knew—of the grim particulars of this disease. The last time she'd seen her, Mother had been a healthy, active woman, concerned that she didn't have a new bathing suit for the upcoming office pool party and pleased that her son had joined the best readers in his class.

Polio had not left Mother lying prettily against fluffed white pillows but **palsied,** in a **torpor.** A rubber collar separated her head from her body, her brown hair was matted from perspiration and fell back from her face, and her long, slender neck was marred by a raw, sunken hole and a metal fixture holding a rubber tube. During her first night in the hospital, when the virus had raged through her body, deadening muscle after muscle but leaving her on fire with pain, doctors had performed an emergency tracheotomy to keep her from suffocating. The incision, a slice in the throat just below the Adam's apple, made a hole in the windpipe where an oxygen tube could be inserted and from which phlegm could be drawn, saving her from drowning on the mucus that obstructed her upper respiratory passages. Her throat muscles useless, she was unable to breathe, cough, or swallow on her own. The tracheotomy signaled to all at the hospital that Mother was among the sickest, highest-risk polio patients. . . .

In spinal polio, any combination of anterior horn cells can be affected, but legs are more often involved than arms, and the large muscle groups of the hands more often than the small ones. Any combination of limbs might be paralyzed, though most commonly it is one leg, followed by one arm, or both legs and both arms. Paralysis sometimes occurs within a few hours, but it often spreads over two or three days and ends with the breaking of the fever. During the first night Mother was in the hospital, the virus had swept through her body, disengaging muscle after muscle, including her **intercostals** and diaphragm.

All that would have been bad enough, but the virus worked at the bulbar cells of her central nervous system also, causing severe respiratory difficulties by another route. When the poliovirus heads for the brain, it can attack cranial nerves that control eye and facial muscles and interfere with chewing, which causes victims considerable difficulty but is not life-threatening. More commonly, however, bulbar polio attacks cranial nerves that operate the pharynx, the soft palate, and the larynx, making swallowing, breathing, and speaking difficult or impossible, and endangering the life of victims.

At the initial onslaught, Mother struggled to maintain even slow, irregular, shallow breaths. The doctors and nurses at Phoenix Memorial stood by, knowing that at any moment she could die. No case of polio was considered routine, but respiratory cases caused considerable turmoil. As paralysis overtook Mother, aides lifted her onto the bed of an iron lung, on hand for just such an emergency. They carefully straightened her body and rolled the cotlike slab into its cylindrical tank, clamping it shut tightly. The rubber collar around her neck prevented air from escaping, and cotton padding reduced chaffing as the rubber slid up and down her neck with each breath. Her shoulders wedged against one end of the tank, her feet set firmly against a foot board at the other, she lay entombed, but alive.

How to help victims suffering bulbospinal polio sometimes posed dilemmas for physicians, because treatments for the two kinds of paralysis conflicted. . . .

Iron lungs also posed risks for bulbar patients, who sometimes died in the tanks as they lay flat on their backs and aspirated their own secretions. Others died of exhaustion, fighting the machine that did not synchronize with the efforts of their unaffected breathing muscles.

In my mother's case, however, the virus so ravaged her body with both spinal and bulbar paralysis that her physicians had no qualms about placing her in an iron lung and doing a tracheotomy. Her rapid pulse, high blood pressure, irregular breathing, and bluish discoloration of the skin all called for life-saving measures. The tracheotomy and the tank respirator saved her that first night, but no one caring for her had confidence she would survive, nor could they predict what her condition would be if she did.

Mother hovered near death for days, her temperature and blood pressure dangerously high. She received around-the-clock care, but no medication could check the progress of the poliovirus, and no doctor dared give a barely breathing patient a sedative or painkiller. All her attendants could do was suction her fluids, monitor her breathing, and wait for the crisis to pass. The overall mortality rate for polio victims was less than one in ten, but 60 percent of those stricken with

bulbospinal died. Twenty-five percent of polio deaths came in the first twenty-four hours, and Mother had passed that marker. But another lay ahead: 85 percent of deaths occurred during a victim's first twenty days in the hospital. Mother lay through those three weeks, in her tank, eyes closed, saliva from her parted lips carving a pink, raw line across her face, inhaling, exhaling, inhaling, exhaling.

She survived night after night. And the fever retreated. With the initial crisis past, she regained consciousness, but given her circumstance, which took her far from all familiar landmarks in her life, her awareness was limited. She couldn't move a muscle below her neck. Watery noises escaped through her tracheotomy tube; her tank pumped and whooshed. My grandparents and father continued their vigil through long, uneventful days. "The nightmare commenced," Dad recalled. "We watched her go from a healthy girl to a skeleton who couldn't breathe, strangling on her own saliva."

Time lost its familiar context, and uncertainty and foreboding colored those who kept vigil. Doctors had no news. My grandparents and father entreated the doctors to tell them how she fared. How long would she be in the hospital? What would happen to her?

"She's doing as well as can be expected," came the answer. "Only time will tell."

The unspoken and unquestioned implication was that "time" meant "a long time." . . .

▲

Famine and Totalitarian Dictatorships in the Twentieth Century

Andrew S. Natsios

Not all the great killers of the twentieth century were infectious diseases. Even in a world that had space travel, computers, mechanized agriculture, and nuclear energy, one of the oldest enemies of humankind still visited the planet: famine. In virtually every decade, famine could be found somewhere in the world, most often in Africa. Ethiopia probably experienced more famine years than did any other country in the twentieth century, the result of war, overpopulation, and the southward march of the Sahara Desert.

The worst famines occurred in countries ruled by totalitarian governments. In Stalin's Russia, seven million people died in the 1932–1933 famine that accompanied his ruthless collectivization of agriculture. Probably the worst famine of modern history took place in 1958–1961 in China under Mao Zedong during the Great Leap Forward: An estimated thirty to forty million people died. Nearly three million starved in India in 1943. Ethiopia lost a million people in 1984–1985. The last great famine of the century occurred in North Korea; it began in 1994 and continued into the twenty-first century. Figures were nearly impossible to attain, but estimates claimed close to one million famine deaths per year, and North Korea had not emerged from the incident at the turn of the century. Famine would continue to stalk people in the twenty-first century as world populations expanded beyond the carrying capacity of the land, food supplies could not meet the needs of local populations, and wars continued to displace people.

Historical Precedents: Totalitarian Famines of the Twentieth Century

Had this been the first successful attempt by a totalitarian regime in the twentieth century to disguise a famine of this magnitude from the outside world, one might wonder how the North Korean government had succeeded in such an implausible task where others had failed. But in all four of the century's previous totalitarian famines—in Soviet Ukraine (1930–33), the People's Republic of China (1958–62), Ethiopia (1984–85), and Cambodia (1975)—exactly the same pattern of government behavior was apparent.

Dekulakization and the Ukrainian Famine

Robert Conquest, the great scholar of the dekulakization and forced collectivization in the Soviet Union that killed 14.5 million people nationwide between 1929 and 1933, described in painstaking detail the lengths to which Joseph Stalin went to disguise the consequences of his policies in Ukraine. Between August and Sep-

tember 1933, the French Socialist leader Edouard Herriot, who twice served as his country's prime minister, visited the Soviet Union; he spent five days of the trip in Ukraine. Conquest wrote of the trip:

> A visitor to Kiev describes the preparations for Herriot. The day before his arrival the population was required to work from 2 a.m. cleaning the streets and decorating the houses. Food-distribution centers were closed. Queues were prohibited. Homeless children, beggars, and starving people disappeared. A local inhabitant adds that shop windows were filled with food, but the police dispersed or arrested even local citizens who pressed too close (and the purchase of food was forbidden). The streets were washed. . . . At Kharkov he was taken to a model children's settlement. . . . Certain villages were set aside to show to foreigners. These were model collectives . . . where all peasants were picked Communists and *Komsomols*. These were well housed and well fed. The cattle were in good condition.

Herriot announced that no famine existed and "blamed reports of such on elements pursuing anti-Soviet policy." *Pravda* announced that

Herriot "categorically denied the lies of the bourgeois press about a famine in the Soviet Union." Conquest provides other examples:

> On another occasion a delegation of Americans, English and Germans came to Kharkov. A major round up of peasant beggars preceded it. They were taken off in lorries and simply dumped in a barren field some way out of town. A Turkish mission, on its way home, was scheduled to eat at the junction of Lozova. In anticipation of their stay, the dead and dying were loaded in trucks, and removed to an unknown fate. The others were marched eighteen miles away and forbidden to return. The station was cleaned up, and smart "waitresses" and "public" were brought in.

The Great Leap Forward and the Chinese Famine

Mao Zedong launched the Great Leap Forward in 1958 after having begun forced collectivization of agriculture in 1956. Mao designed the Great Leap Forward to accelerate China's achievement of the marxist utopian paradise through, alongside other initiatives in the industrial sector, "innovative" agricultural practices. Mao borrowed these practices from Stalin's notorious minister of agriculture, Trofim Denisovitch Lysenko, and other pseudo-agronomists. To pander to Mao's ego, the sycophants in the party structure kept information on the famine's devastation from Mao. Indeed, they insisted that his policies were responsible for such a massive increase in production that food, forcibly requisitioned from the starving peasantry, was exported.

During this period, refugees escaping into Hong Kong with stories of famine were dismissed as "biased, rarely accurate, usually interested in painting an adverse picture," according to *The Times* of London. Jasper Becker devoted an entire chapter in his book on the Chinese famine to the story of leftist Western political leaders who admired the radical egalitarianism of Mao's China.

China scholars also dismissed reports of the famine as baseless, anticommunist propaganda. While a few journalists such as Joseph Alsop and newspapers such as the *New York Times* accurately reported the Chinese catastrophe, most chose to ignore the evidence. This dismissal of compelling evidence reflected the nearly absolute control the Chinese government—like the Soviet government before it—exercised over any outside visits; foreigners saw only what the security apparatus wanted them to see. And, as previously stated, the authorities' success at disguising the famine in China was not limited to foreigners, but extended to Mao himself. When he visited rural areas, party bureaucrats hid evidence of the famine and provided him with fictitious reports of increased grain production, when production was actually dropping precipitously. Only in 1960 did Mao hear from senior officials like Marshal Peng Dehuai how devastating the famine had become. Even so, it was not until 1962 that he abandoned his schemes, changed policies, and allowed agricultural production to increase. Thirty million people lay dead in the wake of his ideological catastrophe.

Ethiopian Resettlement and Famine Under Mengistu

Another hidden famine killed several hundred thousand people in Ethiopia in 1972–73, precipitating a coup by military officers in 1974 that unseated Emperor Haile Selassie. The subsequent famine of 1984–85, which killed one million people, was reportedly a consequence of drought-induced crop failure. But as Robert Kaplan reported in his book on the famine, the forced resettlement schemes of the central government were a major factor contributing to the disaster. Colonel Mengistu Haile Mariam's marxist regime attempted to resettle hundreds of thousands of people from the Amharic and Tigrayan highlands—people who coincidentally supported the rebel movement seeking to overthrow the regime—to more fertile lowlands. The regime also tried to move family compounds in the highlands into planned villages, ostensibly to improve the "efficiency" of the farms, but in fact the scheme had precisely the opposite effect. The marxist agricultural system prohibited the trading of food across provincial lines, so surpluses from one region could not be moved to another suffering a deficit.

The central government's responsibility for the 1985 famine was never made clear in journalistic reporting. Cultural Survival, a Cambridge, Massachusetts–based organization formed by Harvard University academics to conduct research and publicize reports on endangered ethnic groups in the developing world, interviewed thousands of refugees streaming across the Ethiopian border into Sudan to escape the brutal resettlement program. Perhaps as many as one hundred thousand people had died by July 1985 because of this campaign, according to the Cultural Survival report:

> Some of the resettled people were undoubtedly malnourished as a result of declining agricultural production in their homelands, but many had not experienced famine until they were captured for resettlement. . . . Perhaps it is more important to note that the settlers received minuscule amounts of food for as long as a month before they arrived in the resettlement camps and then were expected to work 11 hours each day for six and a half days each week.

Yet, international relief agencies summarily dismissed the testimonies of the Ethiopian refugees reporting these conditions, because they contradicted the information provided by the central government NGOs [nongovernmental organizations], dependent on central government approval to conduct their relief work in the country, claimed they had seen no evidence of these policies being carried out or no evidence of the high death rates.

The Cambodian Famine and the Killing Fields of the Khmer Rouge

The Cambodian "killing fields" was the fourth great totalitarian famine of the twentieth century—

or the fifth, if one includes V. I. Lenin's abortive attempt to collectivize agriculture in the early 1920s, which killed millions. Although the 1976–79 killing fields period in Cambodia was not a famine in the traditional sense, the Khmer Rouge did use starvation as one of several means of execution of the urban elites they were attempting to liquidate. Sichan Siv was a Cambodian national who assisted American foreign service officer Charles Twining in interviewing Cambodian refugees escaping the Khmer Rouge atrocities. He said that perhaps as many as a third of the victims of the atrocities actually died of deliberately planned starvation. The Khmer Rouge worked the victims to death in the countryside and provided such meager rations as to ensure their ultimate death. To increase the death rates further, the communist cadres prohibited these victims from scavenging for food from the countryside, which was rich in wild foods that could have sustained them through the terror.

What is most relevant for the purposes of this study is the international reaction to the refugee reports that leaked out of Cambodia beginning in 1977. In *The Quality of Mercy*, a classic book on the humanitarian relief effort following the Vietnamese invasion that ended the Khmer Rouge nightmare, William Shawcross records this reaction in some detail. Some of the critics refused to believe the apocalyptic refugee reports because they described events that could only be called demonic; even tyrants do not do the kinds of things the Khmer Rouge were being accused of doing. Other critics, such as the left-wing professor Noam Chomsky, dismissed the reports for ideological reasons. Chomsky declared that "from the moment of the Khmer Rouge victory in 1975 the Western press colluded with Western and anti-Communist Asian governments, notably Thailand, to produce a 'vast and unprecedented' campaign of propaganda against the Khmer Rouge." Other academics and journalists on the left took the same view, associating the attacks on the communists with the Vietnam War. . . .

⋏

Giving Care to People with Symptoms of AIDS in Rural Sub-Saharan Africa

A. F. Chimwaza and S. C. Watkins

Certainly the most famous epidemic of the twentieth century was acquired immunodeficiency syndrome, or AIDS. Not only was it a pandemic of historical proportions, but AIDS reached, in some way or another, into nearly every household in the world. Everyone knew people who were HIV positive, who had AIDS, or who had died of AIDS. The public received constant education about using universal precautions and practicing "safe sex." Pictures of the AIDS Memorial Quilt and books or movies about victims of AIDS were abundant. On the evening news, announcers described the research of scientists who were constantly trying to find a cure, conferences held to disseminate new scientific knowledge, or new horrifying statistics on the number of cases worldwide. No corner of the globe had escaped this disease. It was all around everyone. At best, society learned to live with it in a world newly redefined by one of the greatest plagues in human history.

Although the first cases of what became known as AIDS occurred in the United States and Europe in the 1970s, the greatest impact was not felt in the developed countries, but rather in Asia, Africa, and Latin America. The statistics for Africa were particularly frightening: Sub-Saharan Africa had 10 percent of the world's population and nearly 70 percent of the world's HIV-positive people. More than 80 percent of all AIDS deaths occurred there. AIDS reached Asia in the 1980s, and approximately 20 percent of all new cases occurred in that region. For an area holding nearly 60 percent of the world's population, the potential for a catastrophic die-off was real.

Yet, numbers alone are not adequate to clarify how AIDS was devastating the African people. There, where the virus originated, and where an entire generation was disappearing, little could be done for victims of AIDS. The medications that could help limit the symptoms and delay inevitable death were far too expensive for the average African family to buy, costing nearly twenty thousand dollars per person per year, even if they were available in sufficient quantities. Instead, as the people interviewed in this selection so poignantly describe, families could only try to care for their members with the most minimal resources, and the faces of the AIDS epidemic continued to be seen in the twenty-first century.

⋏

Introduction

In most of the countries of sub-Saharan Africa there is little alternative to caregiving by family members due to the lack of well-developed health services. Little has been published on home-based care in the countries in this region that have been most affected by the AIDS epidemic, although it is reasonable to assume that the social safety net has been stretched to its limit by the burdens of

Reprinted by permission of Taylor & Francis Ltd., Susan Cott Watkins, and Angela Chimwaza, from A. F. Chimwaza and S. C. Watkins, "Giving Care to People with Symptoms of AIDS in Rural Sub-Saharan Africa," *AIDS Care* 16, no. 7 (2004): 795, 801–805. Available from http://www.tandf.co.uk/journals

caring for the dying and for orphans. . . . In this study of home-based care for people with AIDS in rural Malawi, we find that the social safety net is still functioning. The 15 caregivers, all close female relatives of the patient, gave basic and compassionate care for the few months before death that the patients required their care. Other kin and members of the community provided social and moral support for patient and caregiver, as well as modest financial and physical assistance. Most caregivers said that they did not consider caregiving to be a problem, although it was clear that they suffered, from the physical strain, from the emotional consequences of their inability to provide for their patient as they wished, and from their patient's failure to improve.

. . . The physical care provided by the caregivers was similar across all of the caregivers, and was extremely basic. It consisted almost exclusively of preparing food and traditional medicines for the patient, feeding the patient meals and medicine (both Western and traditional), heating water and bathing the patient, cleaning sores, massaging and exercising his or her limbs, carrying patients who were immobile to the pit latrine or to sit in the sun, and washing soiled linen in a stream or in a bucket of water (none of the houses had running water). Even more time-consuming than these activities was simply being available to patients, as most of the patients were considered to be too sick to be left alone. The majority of the caregivers (8/15) complained of the physical strain—"taking the patient in and out of the house"—painful hips from sitting in one place watching the patient, and washing soiled sheets.

Despite some complaints, the care seems to have been provided empathetically and lovingly. When Charity, who has described the primary symptom of her daughter as sores, is asked her major problems in caregiving, she answers: "The only problem that I see is that when the sore bursts, you will see another one swelling on the same part and it bursts even at night and the patient always cries in agony". Doreen, when asked "What do you do in day to day life as a caregiver", answers:

OK, let's say she has vomited, then I make sure that I remove the things that she vomited and [with] warm water then I bathe her. In the course of bathing her, I bend and stretch her limbs. After that, I also warm the herbs and give them to her to drink. I then make her bed and leave her to sleep. That's what I am doing daily.

In addition, the caregivers provided emotional and moral support to their patients. They worried about their aches and pains, and regretted that they could not fulfil some of their patients' demands, such as the desire for a tasty meal or soda. . . . Even Falesi, who believed her aunt had brought AIDS on herself through promiscuity, nonetheless joked with her patient to keep her from worrying.

When asked who else provided physical care, most of the caregivers initially answered that they alone provided the care. After probing, however, only five lacked support with physical care. Manesi, who cared for her son, was asked whether relatives assisted her with caregiving:

MANESI: The relatives just come and say good morning and leave, but they don't take part in caring for the patient like cooking him porridge. I do all these myself and there is no one else. . . .

INTERVIEWER: You have said your husband assists you in bathing him?

MANESI: Yes.

INTERVIEWER: Is there any other thing that your husband does apart from bathing him?

MANESI: No, he only assists with bathing the patient.

INTERVIEWER: Are there any friends of yours or of the patient that give you support with caregiving?

MANESI: His friends gave him Coca-Cola, K5 for buying medicine, these friends do assist him when they have something. . . .

Manesi's answer is typical in following an initial claim to be the sole caregiver with a variety of others who provided support, and suggests the importance of ethnographic interviewing techniques that permit flexibility in questioning and extensive responses, rather than structured, short-answer surveys. Since Balaka District is primarily matrilocal, caregivers often had other female relatives living in the same house or nearby. These female relatives sometimes bought food or prepared it, helped with bathing the patient, or sat with the patient in order to free the caregiver to leave the house temporarily. In addition, and consistent with the expectation that it is men who provide the financial support for a household, male relatives sometimes provided small amounts of money for transport to the hospital, for buying foods for the patient, or to locate and buy medicines, as well as occasionally sitting with the patient when the caregiver was out.

This division of labour—the female relatives responsible for domestic work, the males for providing money—is typical of eastern and southern Africa. Husbands of the caregivers provided support, but husbands of the patients were notably absent. Some were divorced or widowed earlier, but three of the female patients had been abandoned by their husbands when they became seriously ill. This is consistent with findings of a study in Rakai, Uganda, that showed divorce to be significantly higher in serodiscordant couples where the man was HIV+ but the woman was not than in serodiscordant couples where it was the woman who was infected. In addition, caregivers told of other relatives who were expected to provide support but did not. For the five caregivers who had no support with physical care, some relatives were said to be afraid of contagion, although it was not clear whether they feared AIDS specifically or whether they had absorbed public health instruction over the decades to avoid contagion from any illness.

In addition to the physical and financial support provided by relatives, neighbours, friends, and visitors provided emotional support for the patient and caregiver:

INTERVIEWER:	So, do friends come to see her here or are there others who don't come lest they catch the disease?
MARY:	No, they do come here. They do enter into the hut, chat with her, and off they go.

Another caregiver, Eda, talked about the emotional support that others provided her:

INTERVIEWER:	What do other people say about the patient?
EDA:	Other people just feel sorry.
INTERVIEWER:	What do they actually say with their "sorries"?
EDA:	They feel sorry, saying that [it is a shame that] my responsibilities were so great.

Most of the caregivers had this type of support. Rather surprisingly, no caregiver identified visitors as members of their or their patient's religious group.

. . . When the interviewer asked what problems the caregiver experienced, some answered with the patient's illness—"the patient is not getting better"—but most (9) answered that there were no problems. They simply explained: "Even if I meet with problems, this is my daughter, therefore these problems are not problems any more". It may be that this is a form of 'courtesy bias': to complain about washing clothes for one's close relative would, in this cultural context, be interpreted as a sign of insufficient love or not wishing the patient well.

Nonetheless, with probing and on occasion without, the burdens of caregiving usually became evident. Perhaps the greatest burden was poverty, and in particular the inability of the caregiver to provide the patient, who had often lost his or her appetite, with foods that they would eat. Although some of the references to poverty may have been provoked by their perception of the interviewers as representing those with money sufficient to do such a study, when the caregivers talked about their inability to provide foods for their patients, the combination of financial and emotional burdens appeared genuine and moving. Most said their patients had little appetite for the ordinary diet; they wanted special foods—fish, meat, sodas. It was clear that caregivers believed that proper nutrition would prolong the life of their patient. But all of these tempting foods had to be bought, and it pained the caregiver not to be able to provide them: "Sometimes when my son tells me 'I want such and such a thing', I cry after I fail to think how I can find the things that he wants."

The caregivers who seemed to suffer the most from the combination of financial and emotional burdens were Lois and Jessie:

LOIS: Since I am alone, I do lack someone to help me . . . my daughter sometimes asks for something to eat and yet I don't have money to buy the food. . . . Right now, I am at a loss, I don't know what to do because I don't have anything to assist her with. Even when I make porridge for her, I just apply salt, instead of sugar because I do not have money to buy sugar. Money is a problem. With a patient like that one, you need to have money so that you can be able to buy the types of food to make her body function well. . . . Sometimes she wants to eat meat, or drink Fanta, or eat chicken or catfish. You see, since I am alone here it's a bit tough for me. . . . I just wash without soap. It is really hard to get soap and when I am bathing her, it's the same thing, I just bath her without soap. . . . Whenever the patient asks for something, you just feel pain in your heart since you don't have the means to get it. Milk is important for her and other foods but how can I get them?

JESSIE: The problems are many, due to poverty. As you know, I'm a single woman. I really struggle to get money. It is either borrowing from someone or selling something so that I can get money. I had a radio but I sold it. I also had some sheep but I sold them too to get money.

And right now I no longer have something to sell. The maize that I had is finished . . . and I have four orphans whom I am also caring for. Yet the maize is finished. I really don't know what to do.

At the other extreme was Kitty, who mentions God more than any of the other caregivers. Although Kitty's patient has diarrhoea and vomiting, and is not improving, and although her patient had been providing financial assistance before she became ill, when she is first asked about her problems with caregiving, she says:

KITTY: Ah, to me, I don't see any problem, my only request to God is that he should help me with my patient. I only request God day and night.

INTERVIEWER: Oh, there is nothing that you see as a problem?

KITTY: Not at all.

Even as the interviewer continues to probe, Kitty repeatedly says that she is not facing problems: she feeds the patient with *nsima,* adding other foods if they are available; she does not complain of the lack of soap or gloves; she says she has enough help with caregiving—all she wants for her daughter "is help from God so that she should be OK".

The economic burdens of caregiving—expressed in expenditures and loss of income—appear relatively small compared to those in more developed settings, including urban Malawi, because incomes were so low and so little was spent. Transport is much more expensive than soap or sodas (the cost of a round trip to a local hospital was about K100, twice that for both patient and caregiver). No caretaker had a formal job, only two had previously received remittances from the patient, and only two had small businesses (one was able to continue working, the other was not). The interviews were conducted during the months of active cultivation, and some caretakers complained that they were unable to cultivate their gardens fully. Again, however, others helped—'well-wishers' who cultivated for the caretaker or members of the household who sat with the patient while the care-taker herself worked on her land.

Despite what may appear to be the modest costs of caregiving, these burdens loomed large from the perspective of caregivers who were unable to buy a soda for the patient or soap for washing. The wants of the patients and the caregivers were limited: the patients wanted special food, the caregivers wanted to provide these foods, and some wanted money for transport to the hospital (although most of the patients had been to a hospital and had been sent home uncured). Even with these simple wants, however, without more

income they simply did not have the money to spend, and they had little to sell.

Almost as burdensome as the economic and emotional costs of caregiving was the disruption of ordinary social life that caregiving imposed. When asked about problems with caregiving, one began:

> The problems are there since I have no time to sleep at night. And during the day you don't have time to do your job and even if you would like to see your friends you don't have time to go there. When you hear that there is a funeral at your friend's home, still you cannot go.

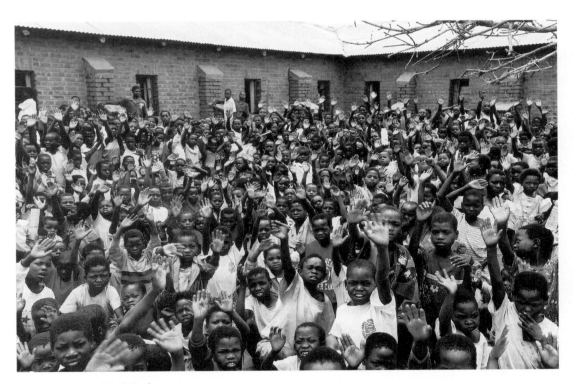

FIGURE 13–2   AIDS Orphans
Although the AIDS epidemic gets considerable publicity in the developed world, its impact is being felt the most severely in the less-developed countries. One of the most long-lasting effects of this pandemic is the staggering number of orphans it has created. According to WHO and UNAIDS (Joint United Nations Programme on HIV/AIDS) statistics (2002), some sub-Saharan countries have nearly a half million orphans, as in Malawi and South Africa, whereas a few countries such as Kenya and Zimbabwe have more than a half million each. The demographic and economic impact of these orphans can overwhelm both government finances and attempts to limit the spread of AIDS, which will extend the effect of the pandemic for generations to come.

Another said:

> Problems are there, because on Sundays I do fail to go for prayers, [I am] just seated looking after the patient, and my hips do hurt, and I fail to make journeys because she is ill, such are problems too.

The interviewer asks what kind of journeys, and the respondent answers: "Journeys like going to the market or visiting friends and chatting, such journeys".

Despite their initial disclaimers that caregiving was not a burden, all respondents eventually identified problems. It is noteworthy, however, that for many caregivers the duration of caregiving was typically short. Although the caregivers were often not precise about the history of their patient's illness, most of the patients had been ill off and on for some time, but with the caregiver for less than four months. Once they required continual care, the progression to death appeared rapid. Although we were not able to follow all of the patients, by the end of the five months of data collection, at least 10 had died. . . .

KEY TERMS

Bulbar, 303 • Intercostals, 304 • Malaise, 302 • Palsied, 304 • Postpolio sequelae, 286 • Solarium, 303 • Torpor, 304

QUESTIONS TO CONSIDER

1. Throughout this reader, we have learned about epidemics that have suddenly attacked virgin populations with little warning. What similarities and differences do you see among the stories of the Black Death in Europe, smallpox in the Americas, and AIDS today? How have interpretations of these events and responses to them changed? Had you somehow been alive through these three events, how would you have reacted? Would your reactions have been different during different episodes? Why or why not?

2. About thirty years ago, scientists confidently boasted that the absolute conquest of infectious disease was imminent. With hindsight, that prediction appears to be pure hubris and completely untrue. Why? Why are we today no closer to eliminating infectious disease than we were fifty or even a hundred years ago? What has changed? Do you think that such a feat is still possible in the future? Why or why not?

3. Most major modern-day infectious diseases are spread by person-to-person contact or human contact with an animal host. An enormous amount of advice is available on how to reduce such exposure—cover your mattress with plastic, do not wash towels and underwear together, wipe off your shopping cart handle before touching it, and, above all, wash your hands. Are we becoming a nation of paranoid people nearly immobilized by fear of the microbe? Or, conversely, have we become so inured to such advice that we are bored and simply ignore it? Is such vigilance necessarily a good thing—should we try to achieve a sterile environment? What might be disadvantages to this approach?

4. The Internet has been an essential tool in the age of instant information, particularly in the area of health. We can instantaneously find out more than we ever wanted to know about the rarest of diseases. Run a search on rare diseases, choose any four of them, and research them on the Internet. What have you learned? How do you evaluate the sources and information? What are your reactions to all this new information?

5. Look carefully at the photo of AIDS orphans taken somewhere in sub-Saharan Africa (Figure 13–2). How many nonextant families do you think this single photo represents? What do you think lies ahead for each of these children (remember, these youths are the lucky ones who are living in an orphanage)? How does this photo put a clearer face on the AIDS epidemic?

6. Note the gauze masks worn by the volunteers in Figure 13–1, and the children, who are not wearing masks. How do you explain the difference? What other counterinfection methods would probably be used today in a similar situation? Why do you think they were not used in 1918?

RECOMMENDED READINGS

Brower, Jennifer, and Peter Chalk. *The Global Threat of New and Reemerging Infectious Diseases: Reconciling US National Security and Public Health Policy.* Santa Monica, CA: RAND, 2003.

Crosby, Alfred. *America's Forgotten Pandemic: The Influenza of 1918.* Cambridge: Cambridge University Press, 1989.

Garrett, Laurie. *The Coming Plague: Newly Emerging Diseases in a World Out of Balance.* New York: Penguin Books, 1995.

————. *Betrayal of Trust: The Collapse of Global Public Health.* New York: Hyperion Books, 2001.

Greenblatt, Charles L. *Emerging Pathogens: The Archaeology, Ecology, and Evolution of Infectious Disease.* Oxford: Oxford University Press, 2003.

Guillemin, Jeanne. *Anthrax: The Investigation of a Deadly Outbreak.* Berkeley: University of California Press, 1999.

Kolata, Gina. *Flu: The Story of the Great Influenza Pandemic of 1918 and the Search for the Virus That Caused It.* New York: Touchstone, 1999.

Levy, Elinor, and Mark Fischetti. *The New Killer Diseases: How the Alarming Evolution of Mutant Germs Threatens Us All.* New York: Crown, 2003.

Morse, Stephen. *Emerging Viruses.* Oxford: Oxford University Press, 1996.

Preston, Richard. *The Demon in the Freezer.* New York: Ballantine Books, 2002.

Rogers, Naomi. *Dirt and Disease: Polio Before FDR.* New Brunswick, NJ: Rutgers University Press, 1992.

Ryan, Frank. *Virus X: Tracking the New Killer Plagues Out of the Present and into the Future.* Boston: Little Brown, 1997.

Sass, Edmund J. *Polio's Legacy: An Oral History.* Lanham, MD: University Press of America, 1996.

Shepard, Benjamin H. *White Nights and Ascending Shadows: A History of the San Francisco AIDS Epidemic.* London: Cassell Books, 1997.

Shilts, Randy. *And the Band Played On.* New York: Penguin Books, 1987.

Thomas, Gordon, and Max Morgan-Witts. *Anatomy of an Epidemic: The True Story of a Town, a Hotel, a Silent Killer, and a Medical Detection Team.* Garden City, NY: Doubleday, 1982.

Walters, Mark J. *Six Modern Plagues and How We Are Causing Them.* Washington, DC: Shearwater Books, 2003.

Yam, Philip. *The Pathological Protein: Mad Cow, Chronic Wasting, and Other Deadly Prion Diseases.* New York: Copernicus Books, 2003.

Other References on Historic Epidemics

Bollet, Alfred J. *Plagues and Poxes: The Impact of Human History on Epidemic Disease.* New York: Demos, 2004.

Diamond, Jared. *Guns, Germs and Steel: The Fates of Human Societies.* New York: Norton, 1997.

Karlen, Arno. *Man and Microbes.* New York: Touchstone Books, 1995.

Kohn, George C. *Encyclopedia of Plague and Pestilence.* Hertfordshire, UK: Wordworth Editions, 1998.

Kiple, Kenneth F. *The Cambridge World History of Human Disease.* 2 vols. Cambridge: Cambridge University Press, 1993.

———. *Plague, Pox, and Pestilence: Disease in History.* London: Phoenix Books, 1997.

MacNeill, William. *Plagues and Peoples.* New York: Anchor Books, 1998.

Scott, Susan, and Christopher J. Duncan. *Biology of Plagues: Evidence from Historical Populations.* Cambridge: Cambridge University Press, 2001.

Chapter Fourteen

A Brave New Century
Dilemmas in Twenty-first-Century Medicine

INTRODUCTION

As we have seen, progress in medicine in the twentieth century came at the cost of new and difficult problems, and we have no reason to assume that such a pattern will change in the twenty-first century. The invention of every new device and procedure carries with it ethical questions about how, where, and when it will be used. New definitions and parameters have to be written. For example, a person can now be kept alive on life support indefinitely, but the "quality-of-life" issue, and the ethical issues surrounding an individual's desire to be kept alive by artificial means, must be addressed. Definitions of what constitutes death have to be rewritten, and a decision about whether a person has a "right to die" must be made. Likewise, the conditions under which euthanasia or physician-assisted suicide might be a viable alternative to artificial life support must be determined. These topics are only a few of the many ethical issues of the twenty-first century.

Numerous other concerns exist. One major danger is the use of disease as a weapon of mass destruction. Biological warfare and bioterrorism are real threats posed by individuals and small groups as well as nations, as evidenced by the 1995 **sarin** gas attack by the Aum Shinrikyo. Pollution and contamination of the food supply poses another potential danger, as seen in the *Escherichia coli* 0157 outbreaks. Diseases such as anthrax and BSE (bovine spongiform encephalopathy, or mad cow disease) pose further threats to the food supply.

New diseases continue to appear. We are already familiar with the viral hemorrhagic fevers such as Ebola, and the drastic increase in dengue hemorrhagic fever. Undoubtedly, other microbes exist in the world that have not yet touched humans. Crowded cities and the ease of modern transportation make the spread of new pathogens easier than ever, so that an attack of SARS (severe acute respiratory syndrome) in China or new victims of avian influenza in southeast Asia become an immediate threat to England or Brazil.

Another problem, the availability and distribution of food, promises to be one of the most critical problems facing the twenty-first-century world. For a variety of natural and man-made reasons, famine is becoming increasingly common outside the industrialized countries. Conversely, because of changes in lifestyle and working conditions, obesity has become a major concern in the developed countries, particularly in the United States. Both situations pose profound medical problems.

Finally, there is the issue of health-care costs. Even in developed countries such as the United States, a significant portion of the population cannot afford basic health care and medications. Pharmaceutical prices are skyrocketing, and drug research focuses on profitability rather than on supplying the antiviral agents so badly needed in Africa to combat AIDS or on developing new antibiotics to combat the many drug-resistant diseases. The list of problems is nearly endless. Medicine will continue to modernize in the twenty-first century, and new challenges will continue to accompany this modernization. Medically speaking, this century is in fact a brave new world.

TIME LINE

2000–2001	Ebola outbreak occurs in Uganda
2000	World Health Organization (WHO) announces that polio has been eradicated from the western Pacific region, home to one-third of the world's population; United Kingdom—farm animals are mass slaughtered to prevent a further BSE (mad cow disease) outbreak
2001	United States—letters containing anthrax spores are sent to members of Congress; the Netherlands becomes the first country to legalize euthanasia; a California jury awards three billion dollars to a smoker with lung cancer; after 9/11, the U.S. government receives increasing power to quarantine in the event of a lethal bioterrorist attack
2002	United States—smallpox vaccination is ordered for military and health workers; the WHO reports that nearly 11 percent of all childhood deaths in developing countries are due to malaria, the fourth greatest killer
2003	SARS outbreak occurs; first case of mad cow disease in the United States is seen; Dolly the sheep—the first cloned mammal—dies prematurely
2004	Human Genome Project is finished

2005	Asian avian influenza A, which first appeared in 2003, spreads to non-Asian countries—attracts worldwide attention and causes fear of a flu pandemic on the scale of the Spanish Flu of 1918

⋏

Cloning: Ethics and Public Policy

R. Alta Charo

One of the most heated debates in modern medicine is over cloning. Both professionals and laypeople have definite opinions on cloning, particularly the cloning of human embryos. The basic ethical issue is whether cloning is morally right or wrong, an issue taken under consideration by the National Bioethics Advisory Commission. This selection, written by a member of that board, presents a balanced analysis of three arguments against cloning. Ultimately, the larger question remains: Should government have the power to limit or direct scientific advances, or are scientists capable of governing their own activities? Although this question is currently applied to the issue of cloning, it has far wider implications for future medical research.

⋏

Much of the discussion about cloning focuses on whether the act of cloning is right or wrong, according to some theory of morality. This is a worthy debate, and one that should help people to decide for themselves whether to take advantage of this technology, should it become available to them. But at the level of public policy, there is a different debate, for example, whether cloning should be forbidden or permitted. It is insufficient to argue that cloning is wrong and therefore should be forbidden. Many things are wrong but nonetheless are permitted, including bad manners, lying (except, for example, when under oath), and having a child when one is too young or impoverished to care for it as one should. The reasons for avoiding a governmental prohibition of such bad acts are many; governmental action might, for example, be ineffective, overly intrusive, oppressive, or harmful to third parties. In

other words, at times, governmental prohibitions represent a cure that is worse than the disease.

In the public testimony and submissions to the National Bioethics Advisory Commission ("NBAC"), three kinds of arguments were heard. Each represented a different kind of analysis that led to a conclusion that cloning is wrong. And each was linked to a particular set of policy concerns. In the end, the NBAC found that all but one of the arguments for the wrongness of cloning failed to overcome the obstacles to enshrining that moral conclusion in law.

The first set of arguments focused on the motivations of those who might want to use cloning, a so-called "relational" argument. By this analysis, cloning is neither intrinsically good nor intrinsically bad. Rather, when done for good reasons, it is ethically acceptable. When the motivations are bad, the act itself is bad as well.

From R. Alta Charo, *Cloning: Ethics and Public Policy,* 27 Hofstra L. Rev. 503 (1999). Reprinted with the permission of the *Hofstra Law Review Association* and R. Alta Charo.

By way of example, some people argued that if cloning were used to circumvent infertility, it is being pursued for a worthy reason, and is not a bad act. Others suggested that having a child who is a genetic twin of a sibling in need of a bone marrow transplant is arguably good, as it can save the life of one person without undue pain or suffering to the other. Here, too, the suggestion was made that in such cases, cloning is not a bad act and need not be forbidden. On the other hand, these people argued, when cloning is used to satisfy one's ego, or when it is used in conjunction with commercialized eugenics (as, for example, by selling embryos cloned from "desirable" people at a price higher than that of "undesirable" people), then it is evil and should be outlawed.

In many ways, this approach accords better with moral intuition than many of the analytical arguments that follow. As a matter of public policy, however, it is just not feasible to implement. There is a history of miserable experiences when trying to create rules in which the government defined which acts are permitted and prohibited based on the motivations of the actors. For example, many people who support legal abortion are appalled at the notion that it could be used by someone who simply wants to select the sex of a child. They find this inherently sexist, or, at least, unacceptably gratuitous as a justification for abortion. Therefore, these people often want to prohibit abortion for this one particular reason while preserving all other reasons for allowing abortion.

But the states have found the implementation of this public policy unworkable. It requires an inquiry into the hidden psyches of people who propose to have an abortion—an inquiry that is inherently intrusive and subject to fraud and manipulation. Indeed, it hearkens back to the pre-*Roe* era, in which the "liberal" states permitted abortion if a woman could persuade a panel of physicians that her reasons were adequate, a process that invited women to dissemble in order to obtain permission. In the end, the procedure was demeaning to the women and failed to achieve its purposes. One could predict a similar phenomenon should a relational ethic undergird a

public policy that premises permission to use cloning on a sufficiently persuasive case being made to some appointed body of judges.

The second type of argument heard by the NBAC was **deontological,** the so-called "thou shalt not" school of reasoning. Simply put, according to this analysis, cloning is wrong because it violates certain fundamental rules about the appropriate relationship between humans and nature, or humans and God; because cloning takes away the necessity of sexual intercourse; and because it confuses our common understandings of kinship and the separation of generations. These assertions were well illustrated by the moral repugnance arguments of Leon Kass. He, and others like him, argued persuasively that we should take moral intuition seriously, as it bespeaks a deep attachment to certain fundamental values that, however poorly articulated, nonetheless bind us together as a culture.

But whether these intuitions can be a sufficient basis for public policy is a separate question. To the extent that they are premised on explicitly religious convictions, they are insufficient because no one religious view can be imposed on others. The First Amendment to the Constitution guarantees that. Of course, if religious views can be supported by arguments that even nonbelievers can understand and accept, then they can become a basis of public policy; all that is needed is a widespread consensus.

But a consensus, backed up by a popular vote, can become something more than popular democracy at work—it can become oppressive if it stifles the preferences of a dissenting minority. This is tolerated for most situations, where a simply process of "majority rules" is accepted. It is not tolerated, however, when the interests being stifled are considered fundamental to our notions of liberty.

These so-called "fundamental" interests have been identified, albeit imperfectly, by the Supreme Court. They include those things specifically mentioned in the Bill of Rights, such as freedom of speech, assembly, worship, and association. They also include those things so basic that no one would think they need to be listed in the Constitution, such as the right to marry and form a family. And they include those things that are implicit in the decisions of the Supreme Court, by virtue of their close relationship to these aforementioned rights; the fundamental right to privacy falls into this category.

Thus, before one can accept a public policy based upon a consensus that cloning is wrong and a popular vote to prohibit its use, one must ask whether such a prohibition will impinge upon a fundamental right. Here, the waters become murky. Cloning is, arguably, just another form of reproduction. The Supreme Court decisions since the mid-twentieth century have carved out a large area of family life and reproductive decision-making as beyond the appropriate scope of governmental authority, on the basis that these implicate fundamental rights. But there has never been a clear statement that there is a fundamental right to procreate, especially to procreate by means that require third party assistance.

Further complicating matters is the question of whether cloning is a form of procreation, in either the biological or social sense. While it surely is a form of making a new person, it is divorced from the sexual interaction that forms the emotional and social underpinnings of the experience that has led courts to claim a zone of "privacy" for American citizens. Thus, it is worth questioning whether the Supreme Court, were it to revisit those earlier cases in light of this new development, would premise its decisions on a right to make a new person or on some other kind of right, such as the right to form intimate associations with others that may entail family formation.

If it is true, though, that cloning is, at least arguably, a form of exercising a fundamental right, then reasons for its prohibition must go beyond moral repugnance. They must be consequentialist, the third category of argumentation heard by the NBAC. In other words, to abridge a fundamental right, one must show that there is a compelling state purpose to be achieved—such as the prevention of a probable and serious harm—and that the only way to achieve this purpose is to abridge the right.

Thus, many people argued that cloning would harm children and society. Children, they argued, would be harmed by the excessive expectations brought to their births by the adults who believed that genetic duplication guarantees duplication of all physical and even psychological traits. Even though this is untrue, it would be the expectations of the parents that would cause the harm. In addition, they argued, the child itself might have false expectations based on the circumstances of its birth, and thus lose the unexpected quality of an open future that is the norm for children. Others argued, too, that a child conceived through cloning would suffer a form of genealogical bewilderment, as it might well have a rearing parent who was a biological sibling. People argued, too, that cloning would be harmful to society, as it would encourage a kind of commercialization, or, at least, commodification, of children. Images of mass marketing in cloned embryos are featured heavily in testimony and newspaper letters to the editor. And the merging of images of cloning and images of soulless drones gave rise to widespread fears of whole populations being created for slave labor.

Should all these things come to pass, they might well be harmful, and some might even meet the test for a compelling purpose. But these harms were both vague and uncertain, hardly enough to overcome the obstacles to abridging what might be a fundamental right. In the end, the NBAC identified only one kind of harm that met this test, and this was the possibility of physical side-effects from the cloning procedure that could result in injury to the children. In the near total absence of animal data, and in the presence of suggestive hints of physical problems that might be associated with cloning (ranging from atypically high mutation rates to shortened life span), it seemed appropriate to limit use of the technologies. In keeping with a policy of limiting rights as little as possible, however, the NBAC recommended that the prohibition be of five years duration only, while animal data accumulated. Then a reassessment could take place. The NBAC did consider other ways to protect children from harms associated with premature use of cloning in humans. For example, it considered whether the threat of medical malpractice suits would be sufficient to dissuade careless use of the technology. If a person acted in a way that was unreasonably careless, then that person could be punished in the form of monetary damages. This result would send a signal to the rest of the community and serve as a deterrent for similar behavior. By retrospective punishment of an individual, society deters similar acts in the future and changes the standard of care. Unfortunately, this is not a particularly satisfying solution. Judging somebody to be unreasonably careless is a difficult task. It is easy to imagine that driving significantly above the speed limit is unreasonable behavior. In a rapidly evolving field, however, there is no professional speed limit, no point of reference established for comparison. For this reason, among others, **tort** and malpractice law were unlikely candidates for effective regulation of human cloning.

Alternatively, the NBAC considered a voluntary moratorium, in which physicians and researchers in the United States would agree not to attempt human cloning until a certain period of time had elapsed to allow sufficient data of animal cloning to accumulate. The NBAC commissioned a study on the history of voluntary moratoria in the area of genetic engineering. With a few exceptions, this method worked extremely well in terms of achieving self-restraint in the biological community. However, the NBAC could not ignore the lack of federal oversight in the field of in vitro fertilization, which was an artifact of attempts by the federal government to divorce itself from abortion politics. An absence of federal funding has meant an absence of federal oversight. Reproductive technologies are characterized by a confusion between research and therapy, experimental and

standard care, all of which means that patients are poorly protected from overly zealous practitioners and from the exigencies of the marketplace. The NBAC was unable to get a statement from any relevant professional society in that field to try to achieve a voluntary moratorium on the part of their members. The absence of such a statement from one of the societies representing the very professionals who might be interested in offering the technology meant that a voluntary moratorium was not a realistic means for curbing premature and possibly unsafe experimentation.

At the end of the day, many people complained that the NBAC had failed in its duty. By never issuing a stinging condemnation of cloning, by never endorsing any one of the many arguments claiming its inherent wrongness, the NBAC had failed to grapple with the issues, they claimed. But that is not the case. The NBAC is not a group of individuals speaking for themselves, nor a group of religious leaders interpreting a text. It is not the authoritative moral voice of America. Rather, it is a committee of people dedicated to offering advice on how to develop public policy that is ethically defensible. This means that the ethics of the policies as well the ethics of the underlying acts are at issue. For this reason, the NBAC considered its job to be to integrate arguments about the ethics of cloning with an understanding of American political and legal culture.

Newsweek ran a piece a number of years ago, before the end of the cold war, that recited a little ditty attempting to explain differences in national political cultures. It went something like this: in the United States, everything is allowed unless it is specifically prohibited; in East Germany, everything is prohibited unless it is specifically allowed; in the Soviet Union, everything is prohibited especially if it is allowed; and in Italy, everything is allowed especially if it is prohibited. While casual and perhaps too cute, this ditty nonetheless captures some fundamental approaches to governance. The NBAC took this advice to heart.

▲

The Prospect of Domestic Bioterrorism

JESSICA STERN

Terrorism is a word that has become part of our national vocabulary since 9/11, as has weapons of mass destruction. Today, the threat of terroristic use of biological agents is real, and a good deal of planning has been done to deal with this scenario. The following article was written before 9/11, even before the concerns of Y2K, but it raises a point about bioterrorism that has received relatively little attention—the threat from groups within the United States. Its conclusions may seem dated by the knowledge now available, but its analysis is worth reading.

▲

Would domestic terrorists use biological weapons? The conventional wisdom among experts has been that terrorists "want a lot of people watching, not a lot of people dead" and are unlikely to turn to weapons of mass destruction. A new school of thought proposes that improved technology has made biological attacks resulting in hundreds of thousands or millions of deaths all but inevitable. While terrorists are increasingly interested in weapons of mass destruction, proponents of the latter view exaggerate the threat. Using biological weapons to create mass casualties would require more than having biological agents in hand. The terrorists would need to disseminate the agent, which presents technical and organizational obstacles that few domestic groups could surmount. In addition, relatively few terrorists would want to kill millions of people, even if they could.

For most terrorists, the costs of escalation to biological weapons would seem to outweigh the benefits. Most modern terrorists have had substantively rational goals, such as attaining national autonomy or establishing a government purportedly more representative of the people's will. Escalating to such frightening weapons would result in a massive government crackdown and could

alienate the group's supporters. Biological weapons are also dangerous to produce. A number of Aum Shinrikyo members reportedly damaged their own health while working on biological agents. Additionally, some terrorists may perceive moral constraints.

Candidates for successful use of biological weapons represent the intersection of three sets: groups that want to use these weapons despite formidable political risks; groups that can acquire the agent and a dissemination device (however crude); and groups whose organizational structure enables them to deliver or disseminate the agent covertly. The intersection of these sets is small but growing, especially for low-technology attacks such as contaminating food or disseminating biological agents in an enclosed space. Major attacks are also becoming more likely. In the sections that follow, we consider eroding motivational, technical, and organizational constraints.

Motivational Factors

Getting Attention

Some terrorists may turn to biological weapons because they believe it would attract more attention

Stern, J. The prospect of domestic bioterrorism. Emerg Infect Dis [serial on the Internet]. 1999 Jul–Aug. Available from http://www.cdc.gov/ncidod/EID/vol5no4/stern.htm

to their cause than conventional attacks. Studies of perceived risk show an inexact correlation between scientists' assessment of risk and the level of fear invoked by risky technologies and activities. Biological weapons are mysterious, unfamiliar, indiscriminate, uncontrollable, inequitable, and invisible, all characteristics associated with heightened fear.

Economic Terrorism

Unlike conventional weapons, radiologic, chemical, and biological agents could be used to destroy crops, poison foods, or contaminate pharmaceutical products. They could also be used to kill livestock. (Conventional weapons could be used for the same purposes, albeit less efficiently.) Terrorists might use these agents to attack corporations perceived to be icons of the target country, for example, by contaminating batches of Coca-Cola, Stolichnaya vodka, or Guinness stout. Terrorists could attempt to disseminate anthrax with the explicit goal of imposing expensive clean-up costs on a target government.

Millenarianism

The millenarian idea is that the present age is corrupt and that a new age will dawn after a cleansing apocalypse. Only a lucky few (usually selected on the basis of adherence to doctrine or ritual) will survive the end of time and experience paradise. Some millenarians believe that the saved will have to endure the 7 years of violence and struggle of the apocalypse, and they want to be prepared. Shoko Asahara, leader of the doomsday cult that released sarin gas in the Tokyo subway in 1995, killing 12, told his followers that in the coming conflict between good and evil they would have to fight with every available weapon. A similar belief system explains the attraction to survivalism by Identity Christians, white supremacists who believe in an imminent Armageddon.

Premillennial Tension

Slight tension connected with the millennium presumably affects most people. Many are concerned about the Y2K problem, the prospect that computer systems will malfunction or fail at the end of 1999. Some fear the breakdown of air-traffic control systems and are planning to avoid traveling around January 1, 2000. Others fear an accidental launch of Russian nuclear missiles due to malfunctioning computers. Many are stockpiling food and medicine or will have extra cash on hand in case automated banking systems fail. Some feel vague religious fears. Members of antigovernment groups and religious cults are often vulnerable psychologically and appear to be especially affected by premillennial tension. Larry Wayne Harris, a white supremacist and born-again Christian, predicts that the Y2K bug will cause a civil war in the United States and that after January 1, 2000, the government will be unable to deliver welfare checks and food stamps for at least 3 years. He predicts that biological attacks could be carried out by domestic groups fighting for their heritage, traditions, and communities, causing devastating plagues like those described in the Bible's Book of Revelation. He urges all U.S. citizens to prepare. For some domestic groups, preparation involves stockpiling weapons and training to use them.

Exacting Revenge or Creating Chaos

Politically motivated terrorists who desire to change societies rather than destroy them might avoid killing very large numbers of people because the political costs would exceed the benefits. Some terrorists, however, want to annihilate their enemies or demolish the societal order. William Pierce, leader of the neo-Nazi organization National Alliance, aims to initiate a worldwide race war and establish an Aryan state. "We are in a war for the survival of our race," he explains, "that ultimately we cannot win . . . except by killing our enemies. . . . It's a case of either we destroy them or they will destroy us, with no chance for compromise or armistice." Creating social chaos is thus a worthwhile objective in Pierce's view. Ramzi Yousef, organizer of the World Trade Center bombing, claimed he was exacting revenge against the United States. Osama bin Laden seems to have similar motives.

Mimicking God

Terrorists hoping to create an aura of divine retribution might be attracted to biological agents. The fifth plague used by God to punish the Pharaoh in the Bible's Book of Exodus was murrain, a group of cattle diseases that includes anthrax. In the fifth chapter of Samuel I, God turned against the Philistines and "smote them with **emerods.**" Medical historians consider these emerods a symptom of bubonic plague. Some terrorists may believe they are emulating God by employing these agents.

The Aura of Science

Terrorists may want to impress their target audience with high technology or with weapons that appear more sophisticated than conventional ones. Terrorists may find technology appealing for various reasons. William Pierce, who studied physics at California Institute of Technology, is interested in high-technology weapons. In his novel The Turner Diaries, right-wing extremists use nuclear, chemical, biological, and radiologic weapons to take over the world. Pierce believes he can attract more intelligent recruits to his organization over the Internet than through radio or leaflets.

The Copycat Phenomenon

Domestic extremists have shown greater interest in chemical and biological weapons in the last 5 years. For example, in 1998, members of the Republic of Texas were convicted of threatening to assassinate with biological agents President Clinton, Attorney General Janet Reno, and other officials. In May 1995, 6 weeks after the Aum Shinrikyo incident on the Tokyo subway, Larry Wayne Harris bought three vials of *Yersinia pestis,*

the bacterium that causes bubonic plague. No law prohibited Harris or any other U.S. citizen from acquiring the agent. The law has been tightened up since, although many fear it is still not restrictive enough. The Federal Bureau of Investigation (FBI) Director Louis Freeh reports that "a growing number while still small of 'lone offender' and extremist splinter elements of right wing groups have been identified as possessing or attempting to develop or use" weapons of mass destruction.

In February 1998, Harris boasted to an informant that he had enough military-grade anthrax to wipe out all of Las Vegas. Eight bags marked "biological" had been found in the back of a car he and his accomplice were driving. Several days later, federal authorities learned that the anthrax Harris had brought to Las Vegas was a vaccine strain not harmful to human health. Nevertheless, the incident frightened many people and sparked a proliferation of anthrax hoaxes and threats in the second half of 1998 continuing into 1999 by groups including Identity Christians and other antigovernment groups, extortionists, antiabortion activists, and presumed prochoice groups. In many cases, the perpetrator's motives were unknown, but some incidents appear to have been student pranks, demonstrating the extent to which the threat of anthrax has entered U.S. consciousness.

Technical Factors

With the end of the cold war and the breakup of the Soviet Union, weapons of mass destruction and their components have become easier to acquire. Underpaid former Soviet weapons experts may be providing biological weapons and expertise to Iran. South African biological weapons scientists have offered their expertise to Libya. State-sponsored groups are most capable of overcoming technical barriers to mass-casualty attacks, but the sponsor would presumably weigh the risk for retaliation before supporting this type of terrorist attack.

College-trained chemists and biologists could presumably produce biological agents, although they might have trouble disseminating them as aerosols. Microorganisms can be disseminated by air in two forms: as liquid **slurries** or as dry powders. While producing liquid slurries is relatively easy, disseminating them as respirable infectious aerosols over large open areas is not. Although dry powders can be disseminated far more easily, high-quality powders require substantial development, involving skilled personnel and sophisticated equipment. Milling biological agents would require a level of sophistication unlikely to be found among many domestic terrorist groups. Far more likely are low-technology incidents such as contaminating foods, poisoning livestock, or disseminating industrial poisons in an enclosed space. Such attacks could still be lethal. Major attacks cannot be ruled out; however, governments need to prepare.

Organizational Factors

In the mid-1980s, a little-known survivalist group called The Covenant, the Sword, and the Arm of the Lord (CSA) acquired a large drum of cyanide with the intention of poisoning water supplies in major U.S. cities. At the time, CSA was unusual among terrorist groups in that its sole objective was large-scale murder rather than influencing government policies. CSA overcame two of three large obstacles to successful employment of a chemical agent. It had the motivation to use a chemical agent to kill large numbers and no political or moral constraints. The group had acquired a chemical agent, although not in sufficient quantity to contaminate city water supplies. The group's leaders had not recruited technically trained personnel and chose an unworkable dissemination technique. Moreover, the group lacked discipline and was easily penetrated by FBI. It is unlikely that CSA would make such mistakes if it were operating today, when antigovernment groups are so much more aware of the potential of poison weapons for inflicting mass casualties.

CSA was run as a relatively open compound. Some members wrote articles in local papers espousing antigovernment beliefs, and some worked in neighboring towns. Several former CSA members became informants, often because they hoped to get their sentences reduced for other, unrelated, crimes. In recent years, however, antigovernment groups have become more aware of the danger of penetration by law-enforcement authorities and have devised a new way of organizing themselves called "leaderless resistance." Members are encouraged to act on their own, minimizing their communication with the leadership of the movement. Timothy McVeigh operated according to this model. His bombing of the Oklahoma City Federal Building was originally conceived of by CSA, although it is not clear that McVeigh knew of CSA's earlier plot. If future terrorists with chemical or biological agents act on their own or in small, secretive groups, FBI may have difficulty apprehending them.

One of CSA's objectives was to establish a computerized, nationwide system linking right-wing groups. This goal has been achieved, although CSA is not exclusively or even principally responsible for this achievement. The nationwide linking of right-wing groups has implications that have not been adequately appreciated by the law enforcement community. The Internet makes terrorist acts easier to carry out. It facilitates leaderless resistance by allowing leaders of the movement to communicate with sympathizers worldwide without having to meet face-to-face with their followers.

The Likeliest Perpetrators

A small but growing number of domestic terrorists could attempt to use biological weapons in the belief that doing so would advance their goals. The most likely are religious and extreme right-wing groups and groups seeking revenge who view secular rulers and the law they uphold as illegitimate. They are unconstrained by fear of government or public backlash, since their actions are carried out to please God and themselves, not to impress a secular constituency. Frequently, they do not claim credit for their attacks since their ultimate objective is to create so much fear and chaos that the government's legitimacy is destroyed. Their victims are often viewed as subhuman since they are outside the group's religion or race.

Religiously motivated groups are increasing. Of 11 international terrorist groups identified by the Rand Corporation in 1968, none were classified as religiously motivated. By 1994, a third of the 49 international groups recorded in the Rand-St. Andrews Chronology were classified as religious. Religious groups are not only becoming more common; they are also more violent than secular groups. In 1995, religious groups committed only 25% of the international incidents but caused 58% of the deaths.

Identity Christians believe that the Book of Revelation is to be taken literally as a description of future events. Many evangelical Protestants believe in a doctrine of rapture: that the saved will be lifted off the earth to escape the apocalypse that will precede the Second Coming of Christ. Followers of Christian Identity (and some other millenarian sects), however, expect to be present during the apocalypse. Because of this belief, some followers of Christian Identity believe they need to be prepared with every available weapon to ensure their survival.

Organizational pressures could induce some groups to commit extreme acts of violence. Followers tend to be more interested in violence for its own sake than in the group's purported goals, making them less inhibited by moral or political constraints than the leaders. Leaders may have difficulty designing command and control procedures that work. Offshoots of established groups may be particularly dangerous. Groups may also become most violent when the state is closing in on them, potentially posing difficulties for those fighting terrorism. Another factor is the nature of the leader. Charismatic leaders who isolate their followers from the rest of society often instill extreme paranoia among their followers. Such

groups can be susceptible to extreme acts of violence.

Asked who he thought the most likely domestic perpetrators of biological terrorism were, John Trochman, a leader of the Montana Militia, said that extremist offshoots of Identity Christian groups are possible candidates, as are disaffected military officers. Some antigovernment groups are attempting to recruit inside the U.S. military. William Pierce also foresees the use of biological weapons by antigovernment groups. "People disaffected by the government include not only the kind of people capable of making pipe bombs. Bioweapons are more accessible than are nuclear weapons."

Conclusions

Terrorism with biological weapons is likely to remain rare. This is especially the case for attacks intended to create mass casualties, which require a level of technologic sophistication likely to be possessed by few domestic groups. While state-sponsored groups are most likely to be capable of massive biological weapons attacks, the state sponsor would presumably have to weigh the risk for retaliation. As in the case of other low-probability high-cost risks, however, governments cannot ignore this danger; the potential damage is unacceptably high. Because the magnitude of the threat is so difficult to calculate, however, it makes sense to focus on dual-use remedies: pursuing medical countermeasures that will improve public health in general, regardless of whether major biological attacks ever occur. This would include strengthening the international system of monitoring disease outbreaks in humans, animals, and plants and developing better pharmaceutical drugs.

The risk for overreaction must be considered. If authorities are not prepared in advance, they will be more susceptible to taking actions they will later regret, such as revoking civil liberties. Attacks employing biological agents are also more likely and will be far more destructive if governments are caught unprepared.

⋏

In Search of a Good Death: Observations of Patients, Families, and Providers

Karen E. Steinhauser, PhD; Elizabeth C. Clipp, PhD, MS, RN; Maya McNeilly, PhD; Nicholas A. Christakis, MD, PhD, MPH; Lauren M. McIntyre, PhD; and James A. Tulsky, MD

As populations in the developed countries age, new interest has been generated about such matters as the study of aging and the many questions involved in end-of-life issues. Increasingly, in the United States and Europe, dying patients are electing to spend their last days at home, usually under the care of hospice programs. Research on the important components of a "good death" reveals that patients and caregivers alike have definite ideas about what is necessary to give comfort and meaning to the final stage of life.

⋏

Professional organizations and the public have recently made care of the dying a national priority. Despite this, however, we remain confused about what constitutes a good death. Some patients with terminal illnesses choose to leave the conventional medical setting and receive hospice care in their home, surrounded by family. Others seek experimental chemotherapy in an intensive care unit. In each of these vastly different scenarios, the perception of the quality of death is constructed by family, friends, and health care providers, not solely by the dying person. However, little empirical evidence exists to document these varied perspectives.

We conducted this study to describe the attributes of a good death, as understood by various participants in end-of-life care. To evaluate the relative importance of these attributes, we compared the perspectives of different groups of persons who had experienced death in their personal or professional lives.

. . . We used focus groups and in-depth interviews to identify the attributes of a good death. . . . We asked focus group participants to discuss their experiences with the deaths of family members, friends, or patients and to reflect on what made those deaths good or bad. . . .

Focus group participants ranged in age from 26 to 77 years (mean age, 47 years). Sixty-four percent were women, 70% were white, and 28% were African American. Most of the sample was Protestant (61%), 18% was Roman Catholic, and 8% identified themselves as Jewish. Six themes emerged: pain and symptom management, clear decision making, preparation for death, completion, contributing to others, and affirmation of the whole person.

Pain and Symptom Management

Many focus group participants feared dying in pain. Portrayals of bad deaths usually mentioned inadequate **analgesia** during cure-directed therapies that were perceived as too aggressive. . . .

Participants were concerned with both current pain control and control of future symptoms. Intrusive thoughts of breakthrough pain or extreme

Reprinted by permission of the American College of Physicians, from K. E. Steinhauser, "In Search of a Good Death: Observations of Patients, Families, and Providers," *Annals of Internal Medicine* 132, no. 10 (2000): 825–30.

shortness of breath produced anxiety that could be relieved with appropriate reassurance. One man with AIDS said, "I don't want to be in pain, and I've discussed it with my doctor. He said, 'Oh, don't worry about pain. We'll put you on a morphine drip.' That sort of eased my mind."

Clear Decision Making

Participants stated that fear of pain and inadequate symptom management could be reduced through communication and clear decision making with physicians. Patients felt empowered by participating in treatment decisions. . . .

Alternately, descriptions of bad deaths frequently included scenarios in which treatment preferences were unclear. Patients felt disregarded, family members felt perplexed and concerned about suffering, and providers felt out of control and feared that they were not providing good care. Decisions that had not previously been discussed usually had to be made during a crisis, when emotional reserves were already low. . . .

Preparation for Death

Participants voiced a need for greater preparation for the end of life. Patients usually wanted to know what they could expect during the course of their illness and wanted to plan for the events that would follow their deaths. One patient said, "I have my will written out, who I want invited to the funeral. I have my obituary. That gives me a sense of completion that I don't have to put that burden on someone else. It's to prepare myself for it."

Family members felt a need to learn about the physical and psychosocial changes that would occur as death approached. Participants spoke of scenarios in which a lack of preparation adversely affected patient care. . . .

Finally, the most experienced nonphysician providers spoke about the importance of exploring one's own feelings about death and the ways in which these feelings influence the ability to care for terminally ill patients. . . .

Most of the personal preparation described by health care providers had occurred individually, outside the context of their formal training. Only one physician in our study had received residency training in **palliative** medicine.

Completion

Participants confirmed the deep importance of spirituality or meaningfulness at the end of life. Completion includes not only faith issues but also life review, resolving conflicts, spending time with family and friends, and saying good-bye. . . .

In western culture, completion may primarily be a process of individual life review that is subsequently shared with family and friends. For patients from other cultures, completion may be more explicitly communal and may involve rituals that are important to the family during the dying process and after death. . . .

Issues of faith were often mentioned as integral to overall healing at the end of life and frequently became more important as the patient declined physically. However, we also heard that such issues are highly individualistic and that cues about their particular expression must be taken from the patient.

Contributing to Others

Several focus groups mentioned the importance of allowing terminally ill persons to contribute to the well-being of others. . . .

Contributions can take the form of gifts, time, or knowledge. As death approaches, many patients reflect on their successes and failures and discover that personal relationships outweigh professional or monetary gains. They are anxious to share that understanding with others. One family member said, "I guess it was really poignant for me when a nurse or new resident came into his room, and the first thing he'd say would be, 'Take care of your wife' or 'Take care of your husband. Spend time with your children.' He wanted to make sure he imparted that there's a purpose for life."

Affirmation of the Whole Person

Participants repeatedly declared the importance of affirming the patient as a unique and whole person. Patients appreciated **empathic** health care providers. One patient said of his caretakers, "There's no question that they make me feel I can't ask." Family members were comforted by and spoke with great respect about those who did not treat their loved ones as a "disease" but understood them in the context of their lives, values, and preferences. . . .

Health care providers' descriptions of good deaths also focused on their personal relationships with patients and families. They were touched by the fact that these relationships were present even in the most dire medical crises. . . .

Distinctions in Perspectives of a Good Death

These six themes reflect the common ground shared by participants. However, we also saw differences between groups. Social and professional roles substantially shaped the views of our discussants. In fact, professional role distinctions were more pronounced than sex or ethnic differences. For example, all social workers spoke from a case management perspective and were highly attuned to the needs of the family as the unit of care. Chaplains eloquently discussed ethical issues and were the only group to relay the tension between individual and community rights. Family members spoke from the unique role of both patient advocate and recipient of care. All six themes were present in patient, family, and nonphysician health care provider focus groups. In contrast, physicians' discussions were uniformly more medical in nature, and no physicians spoke of "con-

tributing to others." One physician made a brief comment about completion, but other members of the group did not expand on it.

Discussion

Although death is a rite of passage in which we will all participate—as family member, provider, or, eventually, patient—we understand little of what is valued at the end of life. Our study confirmed the importance of four themes found in the palliative care literature: pain and symptom management, clear decision making, preparation for death, and completion. Two new themes, contributing to others and affirmation of the whole person, were unexpected and add to our understanding.

Every provider group offered regret-filled stories of patients who died in pain. Such findings are concordant with studies showing that 40% to 70% of Americans have substantial pain in the last days of their lives. Concern about undertreatment of pain is consistent across surveys of physicians, nurses, and recently bereaved family members. Our study also revealed a new dimension to this theme: anticipatory fears about pain and symptom control. Many dying persons are terrified of waking in the middle of the night with intense pain or air hunger. For them, a good death includes providers who anticipate these fears.

Providers and families in our study also identified the need for improved communication and clear decision making and feared entering a medical crisis without knowledge of patient preferences. Despite the recent attention devoted to advance care planning, this remains a source of great consternation. Medicine will never remove all uncertainty from the decision-making process. However, if values and preferences are clarified, tolerance for that uncertainty may increase.

Focus group members were concerned about our society's tendency to deny death and demanded greater preparation for dying. We heard many examples in which providers avoided end-of-life discussions because they did not want to remove hope. However, patients and families feared bad dying more than death. Bad dying was characterized by lack of opportunity to plan ahead, arrange personal affairs, decrease family burden, or say good-bye. For dying patients and their families, preparation does not preclude hope; it merely frames it. After a new diagnosis, patients usually hope for a cure. However, they also hope for lack of pain, lucidity, good quality of life, and a physician who is committed to being with them throughout the care process.

We heard extensive discussion of the need for "completion," a process involving meaningful time with family and close friends and attention to religious or spiritual beliefs. Terminally ill patients are often able to view their current experience as part of a broader life course trajectory. This may explain why they often rate their quality of life higher than observers, who often do not give appropriate weight to patients' emotional and spiritual development during the dying process. Traditional measures used to assess end-of-life quality do not usually account for this growth potential.

Our study introduced two novel components of a good death. First, a surprising number of participants spoke of the importance of terminally ill patients' contributions to the well-being of others. We fully expected to find that dying patients needed care, but we did not consider the extent to which they also needed to reciprocate. Social psychologists describe this need for "generativity" as one of the great emotional tasks of human development, particularly during later life. Dying patients need to participate in the same human interactions that are important throughout all of life. Second, focus group participants continually discussed the need to appreciate patients as unique and "whole persons," not only as "diseases" or cases. We were struck by the very personal language of this theme and by participants' desire to simply be known.

These six themes add to our understanding of what constitutes a good death and also generate hypotheses that have implications for both medical education and clinical practice. The culture of death changed dramatically during the 20th century. When people died primarily at home, family, community, and clergy assumed responsibility. As the location of death shifted to the hospital, physicians became the gatekeepers. As a result, death is now viewed through the lens of biomedical explanation and is primarily defined as a physiologic event. Most medical education and training reinforces this framework.

However, a strictly biomedical perspective is incomplete. For most persons involved with care at the end of life, death is infused with broader meaning and is considered a natural part of life, not a failure of technology. All focus groups, except physicians, spoke extensively about the need for life review and subsequent completion. This is not to suggest that these themes are unimportant to physicians; rather, they are not a usual focus of treatment. It may be useful to recognize that for most patients and families who are confronting death and dying, psychosocial and spiritual issues are as important as physiologic concerns. Patients and families want relationships with health care providers that affirm this more encompassing view.

In an economic environment that substantially limits physicians' time, developing such relationships may seem unrealistic. However, in a previous study, we noted that the median time for advanced directive discussions is less than 10 minutes, with no apparent correlation between length of discussion and discussion quality. Furthermore, an initial investment of time may improve the patient–physician relationship and save time in future conversations. Time may also be used more efficiently if providers have an a priori list of themes to touch on, such as the six discussed here.

There is no single formula for a good death. Many participants cautioned health care providers against implying, "You're not dying the right way because you're not dying the way we think you should." As one author has written, people die "in character." Professional providers who meet a dying patient for the first time are at a disadvantage because they catch only a cross-sectional glimpse of the lifetime of experiences that are shaping the dying process. Our data suggest that the quality of dying is related to acknowledgment of that lifetime context.

We heard many stories of health care providers' discomfort with death and dying. Whether such discomfort is caused by feelings of failure, a desire for professional distance, or inexperience, it can adversely affect care. Delivering bad news or discussing other end-of-life issues is a skill that is rarely natural; like other procedures, it must be learned. Furthermore, providers must be able to acknowledge and process the feelings that arise when caring for dying patients. Programs designed to facilitate this process are now common in police departments and crisis intervention programs, two occupational settings in which trauma and death are always present. However, such programs have not yet become a usual part of medical training or practice.

Physicians should also be reminded that they are not alone when caring for dying patients; many other health care providers (nurses, social workers, and chaplains) are available for comprehensive care. For example, physicians may ask a screening question (such as "What role does faith or spirituality play in your life?") that displays awareness of these important aspects. Physicians can then ask whether the patient would like to speak in greater depth with a chaplain. Although physicians may not be responsible for resolving the psychosocial and spiritual needs of patients, acknowledging the presence and complexity of these needs is a way of actively affirming the whole person.

Our study has several limitations. Most patients were recruited from a Veterans Affairs medical center, and therefore our findings may not be generalizable to other groups. Although our patients were mostly men, they represented a broad range of ages, educational levels, and socioeconomic backgrounds. Many also received care in the private sector, and their comments reflected experiences in many settings. Family focus group members were also recruited from the Veterans Affairs system. However, we collected extensive discussions of family perspectives during discussions with the hospice volunteer group and follow-up interviews with patients. Discussions were limited to deaths from chronic illness and did not include deaths caused by accident or trauma. However, participants described deaths that had occurred in hospices, hospitals, and at home. Good and bad deaths occurred in all settings.

Our study has implications for clinicians, educators, and researchers. Although there is no "right" way to die, the six themes identified here provide an initial framework for addressing topics that are important to patients and families. In addition, biomedical aspects of end-of-life care are crucial but merely provide a point of departure toward a good death. When physical symptoms are properly palliated, patients and families may have the opportunity to address the critical psychosocial and spiritual issues they face at the end of life. . . .

▲

Breakout

The Evolving Threat of Drug-Resistant Disease

Marc Lappé

As the world's population continues to expand into steadily shrinking ecosystems in a search for farmable land, forest and mineral resources, and space, the epidemiological impact will continue to grow. Particularly in the tropics, where this expansion is occurring the fastest, new diseases are emerging as humans come into contact with previously untouched species, from mammals to mosquitoes. Some of these creatures have lived for long times in ecological balance with parasites, viruses, and other vectors, but when confronted with new animals, including humans, new diseases emerge. Thus, the preservation or destruction of habitats can have a real effect on world health. We need only look at diseases such as AIDS; Ebola, Marburg, and Lassa fevers; malaria; and other emerging viral diseases to see the terrific potential dangers to public health.

Not all cases of emergent diseases occur in the tropics, as this article points out. The discovery and spread of Lyme disease in the United States is a direct result of increased human contact with deer and mice populations and the ticks they carry. Junin fever appeared in temperate climate areas of Argentina. Whether or not the Black Death was bubonic plague, the microbes existed in a stable relationship with rodents in Central Asia until human populations began to invade their habitat.

The appearance of new diseases is not simply the revenge of Mother Nature. Rather, as this author points out, it is the product of the evolution of viruses, bacteria, insects, and their hosts. Humans have just introduced a new species into the evolutionary equation.

▲

Ecosystem Disruption and Disease

All human illnesses have their roots in the forces that shaped evolution. . . . The emergence of new infectious diseases is a function of the extent to which pathogens can cross species lines to infect new hosts and the evolutionary resistance of those hosts to infection. . . .

Initially, no organism "wants" to cause disease. Provoking illness and death is generally an unfavorable way for a pathogen to remain alive. Hosts have evolved highly coordinated defenses against disease-causing organisms that make it difficult if not impossible for even the most wily invader to simply "set up shop" in a new body. . . . When the organism has a long-standing relationship with the host population, immunity is often set up in childhood, making adult reinfection difficult. But some parasites, viruses, and bacteria, such as the malarial or influenza organisms and the TB bacillus, have "learned" through aeons of coexistence with humans how to slip past these

defenses and survive, sometimes within the cells of the immune system themselves.

Paradoxically, other organisms have been successful precisely *because* they evoke immunological defences. Many produce an immune response that turns on the host, creating conditions that lead to autoimmune diseases. . . . And some organisms are pathogenic . . . because the by-products of an aroused immune system include mediators of inflammation and fever that generally make a person feel crummy. Parasites generally produce disease when their metabolic needs deprive their human hosts of needed resources. (A malarial infection "costs" the body more than 5,000 calories a day, some two to three times the normal intake in tropical climes.) Finally, there are the rare microorganisms that use up their own valuable genetic resources to make noxious chemicals (toxins) that poison their host. . . .

. . . When pathogens enter human populations for the first time, they often produce transient, highly fatal illnesses that may or may not take hold. Only infrequently does a "new" pathogen last long

---

From ***Breakout: The Evolving Threat of Drug-Resistant Disease***, by Marc Lappé. Copyright © 1995 by Marc Lappé. Reprinted by permission of Sierra Club Books.

enough in a human population and become transmitted well enough to become endemic, or to become a chronically recurring disease. It is an evolutionary maxim that to be successful . . . , a disease-causing organism must somehow become integrated into the ecosystem from which it initially emerged. Even when it has become fully integrated, disturbances of that ecosystem can spring a pathogen loose, placing any at-risk interloper in harm's way. In recent history, many of the human incursions into new ecosystems have been the precursors to the emergence of new diseases. . . .

A case in point is the first occurrence of a disease known as oropouche in Belém, Brazil. This disease, which causes a flu-like illness with severe muscle pain and high fever, ultimately affected more than 11,000 residents. The first reported cases occurred in 1961, just a few years after the completion of the highway through the Amazon that connected Belém with Brasilia. Indeed, just a year earlier, in 1960, the viral agent that eventually was found to be associated with oropouche was isolated from the corpse of a sloth found dead along the new highway. It took 19 more years to put together the ecological puzzle that linked this forest virus with human activity: When settlers cleared the forest for cacao plantations, they disturbed the habitat of a resident species of midge that harbored the suspect virus in its gut. Discarded cacao shells provided a new breeding ground for more of these insects. The resulting population explosion of these flies and their proximity to human habitation created the opportunity for the spread of the virus from midge bites.

. . . Why tropical areas have served as the epicenters for so many diseases is in part a result of their unique evolutionary history. The density and richness of species' interactions is hundreds of times greater in the tropics than in temperate zones. A single hectare of tropical rain forest may have more insect species than does the entire New England region of the United States or all of Great Britain. When new habitats are abruptly opened through extensive forest-clearing activities . . . , extinction of some narrowly confined species and invasion by many others may occur. In particular, as we saw

with the Brazilian midges, "opportunistic" species, including many insects and pathogens, may exploit the new environment. Sudden population expansions also afford expanded evolutionary opportunities. . . .

. . . In 1992, a subcommittee of the prestigious Institute of Medicine of the National Academy of Science concluded that human-made environmental disturbances were likely to account for most of the newly emergent diseases seen in contemporary human populations. And population movements often provide new routes for "microbial traffic."

We know such traffic has had devastating consequences in the past. The plague of the Black Death of the Middle Ages followed caravan trade routes from Asia to Europe. The major, near-genocidal destruction of indigenous peoples in the New World, the Hawaiian Islands, and Polynesia can be traced to the introduction of novel pathogens (intentionally or inadvertently) by conquering peoples. Clearly, policies that consider the potential of microorganisms to colonize and depopulate new hosts following ecological or political disturbances and new contacts are desperately needed in an era of global movement and rapid ecological dislocations.

. . . Among those most adept at surviving environmental disturbances are those species that are able to capitalize rapidly on new circumstances. Often these are species of rodents or arthropods, which, like the ixodid tick involved with Lyme disease, can serve as vectors of human disease. Humans may simply displace the previous "alpha" carnivore or kingpin species in an area or now actively exploit the local species for food. When they do so, the human form may become a new host for a parasitic or infectious disease that previously, for example, had been limited to monkeys or other primates in the area. This process of displacement and acquisition of new parasites has undoubtedly happened more than once in human history, with malaria and possibly AIDS being the most likely candidates for contemporary legacies of primate-centered environmental disruption.

New parasitic infections and mass epidemics accompanied the large-scale disruptions caused by the practice of agriculture in both the New and the Old World. The ecological disruption caused by the irrigation, dam building, and deforestation of the increasingly large-scale agricultural practices in the Yucatán Peninsula and central valley of Mexico may have contributed to the abrupt decline of Mayan civilization after A.D. 1000. Certainly this proved true in the Fertile Crescent and possibly in northern Africa, where agricultural practices brought together previously separated hosts and parasites and increased the likelihood of major new diseases such as leishmaniasis, river blindness, and schistosomiasis taking hold in the human population.

Indeed, the earliest forays into virgin forest at the dawn of the agrarian revolution may have been responsible for the most significant new disease of all—malaria. . . .

In fact, many of the most important diseases that have afflicted humankind had their origins in protected enclaves, tiny pockets of ecosystems where they originally had little or no impact on the life forms around them. A classic example is tick-borne Bitterroot fever, which was once confined to the specialized ticks and their rodent hosts in a tiny valley in Wyoming. It only became a human disease with the in-migration of the first human settlers. Then it spread with the ebb and flow of migrants elsewhere in the U.S. West.

. . . A more contemporary example is the emergence of Argentine hemorrhagic fever, a devastating disease associated with fever, muscle pains, rashes, internal bleeding, and central nervous system involvement leading to tremors or convulsions. Up to 20 percent of affected persons die. The cause of the disease is an organism known as the Junin virus. Prior to the expansion of corn farming in northern Argentina, this virus was a simple commensal in the wild mouse population. With the cultivation and storage of corn in the 1930s and 1940s, people came into contact with these and other rodents, leading to the appearance of this new and expanding disease entity. Argentine hemorrhagic fever now strikes some four to six hundred people each year.

The African cousin to the Argentine form of this disease, African hemorrhagic fever, is a much more lethal . . . and prevalent . . . viral disease. Like AIDS, it is suspected that the causative organism (the Ebola virus) probably arose first in monkeys and then was transmitted to the humans who invaded their habitat. The first victim was a trader who arrived at a mission hospital in northern Zaire in August 1976, bleeding internally, vomiting, and raging with fever. He died a few days later, but not before infecting half the nurses at the hospital and a large number of patients who carried the virus back with them to their native villages. By the time this short-lived epidemic waned, five hundred people had died. Fortunately, as would be predicted from an evolutionary perspective, this new agent was too virulent to establish a focus of further infectivity. Without the ability to survive outside its victim, any parasite that kills its host quickly diminishes its own chances of propagation.

Even though the first Ebola epidemic quickly subsided, it does not mean that the virus is gone. A related virus was inadvertently imported with a group of Philippine monkeys brought to a Reston, Virginia research laboratory in 1989, leading to belated but urgent curbs on the importation of monkeys. . . .

Less well known is the so-called Kyasanur Forest disease, a classic example of human disruption of a wildlife environment causing an outbreak of epidemic disease. The illness first appeared in 1957 in Karnataka, India, caused by a virus that previously had reproduced in game animals and in the ixodid tick. Human incursions into the wildlife refuges and the destruction of habitat led to contact between the tick and people, with the outbreak of a severe epizootic infection.

Even these few examples illustrate why it is so often true that we cannot disrupt natural relationships without imperiling our own welfare. This axiom is as old as human disease. The environmental disruptions caused by farming, logging, and, of course, war, have had more profound effects on the occurrence of disease than previously acknowledged. Major epidemics of pestilence and illness have been documented following every major human migration, war, or revolution. Coupled with new waves of exploration and commerce, local epidemics became pandemics, sweeping the globe in the thirteenth and fourteenth centuries as the Black Death, and today in the form of epidemics of influenza and cholera.

. . . One of the truisms of evolutionary theory is that most organisms that have evolved together exist in a state of dynamic equilibrium. When this equilibrium is disturbed, one or more of the involved species may undergo a dramatic shift in population.

Much of the farmland of New England, once forests, has been allowed to lie fallow, to return to the previous wooded state. In fact, more of New England is now forested than it has been since the colonial era. But the new forest lacks its previous checks and balances. And, most importantly of all, many more humans now live in close proximity to the new woodlands.

In the transitional stages between cleared farmland and forest, a number of species have expanded and contracted as their habitats changed. Rapidly expanding areas of weedy grasses and shrubs provide new habitats for rodent species in particular. Without the predator species such as wolves, bears, or mountain lions to control deer populations, these populations also expand. . . . And with that expansion, the arthropod parasites carried by deer and related hosts grow. Populations of ticks, in turn, carry an abundance of diseases. With a plethora of intermediate hosts in the form of various rodent species, including mice that carry nymph and larval forms as well as adult ticks, potentially infectious ticks can come in contact with humans or their pets, carrying previously rare diseases to nearby inhabitants. In some of these disturbed habitats, the *Borrelia* organism . . . has found new species of ticks to infect. Many of the ticks have also expanded their range by infecting new rodent intermediate hosts. This circumstance is so reminiscent of the conditions that preceded the outbreak of other major disease . . . that we might well have expected epidemiologists

to have sounded a warning about the need for environmental monitoring for pathogens that might transmit tick-borne diseases to humans. The unfortunate result of the lack of surveillance is the current epidemic of Lyme disease. . . .

Plague in Vietnam: A Case Study

Wars are a graphic example of massive ecological disruption. Like other major conflagrations, the Vietnam War compounded the misery of the citizenry by increasing the spread of deadly diseases such as cholera and dysentery. But ecosystem disruption in Vietnam occurred on a exceptionally large scale, creating the very conditions we hypothesized would lead to the emergence of new diseases. During the Vietnam War, some 30 million tons of herbicides were broadcast over the countryside to deny cover to enemy troops and, less publicized, to destroy civilian food crops. Coupled with napalm attacks, these herbicides (including the notorious Agent Orange, but also highly toxic Agents Purple and White) denuded the countryside and devastated previously forested regions, particularly along mangrove swamps in the south and hardwood forests in the highland areas of the west.

As in the Middle Ages and seventeenth century England, this large-scale disruption forced different rodent species into contact with the plague bacillus. The creation of large "dead zones" drove indigenous and Norway rats into new habitats and expanded their territories. Fleas went with them, moving the plague bacillus from rat species to bandicoots and other rodentlike species that had previously been free of plague. One of the first clues that plague had become integrated into the ecosystem in these areas was the discovery of plague in scout and tracker dogs that picked up ticks and fleas during their forays into the countryside near Pleiku and other outposts in the hill region of Vietnam.

While all eyes were on the dramatic physical events of the war in Vietnam, a more insidious horror was occurring within the environment.

A search of the literature reveals that studies had charted new outbreaks of plague in the disturbed areas as early as 1962–1963. Although certain areas of Vietnam, notably the highlands in the western region, were historic endemic areas for plague, virtually no cases of plague had been reported since the French occupation in the early part of the century. Then, in 1964, the first major outbreaks occurred in isolated areas inhabited by the Montagnard peoples. The outbreak spread in 1965 through 1966. But only in 1968 was the U.S. medical community alerted to the problem. By 1970, a major epidemic of plague was raging throughout South Vietnam. Military censorship prevented public dissemination of the extent of this outbreak until 2 more years had elapsed. By the end of the war, plague had spread widely through the provinces of South Vietnam.

Cultural traditions (for example, biting the flea to kill it) inadvertently spread the plague bacillus (*Yersinia pestis*) in its pneumonic or airborne form by allowing the germs to get into the respiratory passages. As in the classic Black Death of the Middle Ages, pneumonic plague was often more virulent than the bubonic form, particularly among Vietnamese children. In Quang Ngai Province, plague was a major source of death and morbidity for children under the age of 16. Often, only heroic treatment by U.S. medics saved infected children from being killed by this secondary effect of the war.

Before the war was over, plague had spread to new rodent species and had spread to other Southeast Asia regions. More critically, the bacillus itself had evolved to a form that could be carried in the pharyngeal tissues of the throat without causing symptoms, thereby bypassing the intermediate host (the flea) and permitting human-to-human transfer. By the end of the war, a new, atypical plague bacillus was being isolated from rodents, fleas, and humans in Vietnam. The disruption of the war thus expanded the plague bacillus' host range and habitat in Southeast Asia, and selection pressures led to the emergence of a new plague variant. . . .

Dengue Fever as a Model

A disease much like Lyme disease in terms of the rapidity of its spread and dispersion is commonly known as **dengue fever,** a mosquito-borne viral disease with deep historic roots in the subtropical areas of the world. Dengue exemplifies how ecological disruption can create novel opportunities for the rapid spread and dispersion of a disease vector. Also known as hemorrhagic fever because of the bleeding it produces in its victims, dengue was a long-standing disease in tropical Asia, but it was believed to be quiescent in the early part of [the twentieth] century. However, since the 1950s, dengue hemorrhagic fever has undergone a resurgence, becoming a major cause of death and hospitalization among Southeast Asian children.

Epidemics were first seen in Manila and Bangkok in 1954, largely as a result of flooding and resultant expansion of the mosquito population. Its victims are characteristically young children. Today, in the Philippines, Thailand, Burma, Cambodia, and Vietnam, dengue affects a broad cross section of the population and is responsible for some 600,000 victims per year in Southeast Asia. The rapid spread of dengue to North and South America beg[an] in the late 1970s.

Such explosive spread was not always the case. Since the turn of the century, public health authorities had assumed that this ancient scourge had all but disappeared from the Asian subcontinent. When dengue reemerged in 1954, it staged what one National Institutes of Health writer has described as a "spectacular comeback." In the first of three waves of epidemics in Southeast Asia, dengue struck the impoverished areas of this region with a vengeance, carrying a mortality rate of up to 40 percent. As a result of ecological disturbances and poor flood control that have produced expanded habitats for mosquitoes, we are now facing the prospect of its gaining a toehold in the United States.

Dengue's first foray to our continent occurred in 1981. In that year, dengue struck more than 300,000 Cubans, leading to 116,000 hospitalizations. And in 1985, the Asian tiger mosquito

Aedes aegypti, which carries the dengue virus, was imported into Florida in water carried in shipments of used tires from Southeast Asia. This insect carrier or vector is now widely distributed throughout the southernmost region of the country, threatening to carry dengue to a large population. That it has not yet done so is largely the result of Americans' penchant for avoiding mosquitos. In 1992, dengue's reach extended to the Australian continent, sending 616 people to the hospital.

Duane Gabler, currently the acting director of the Centers for Disease Control's division of Vector-Borne Viral Diseases, is alarmed about the prospect of dengue gaining a real foothold here. He has noted how readily dengue has made inroads in the Caribbean and South America. Only Bermuda, the Cayman Islands, Costa Rica, Uruguay, and Chile have escaped colonization by the mosquito.

According to Dr. Gabler, "We have a very real crisis on our hands." Pesticide spraying of *A. aegypti* mosquitos with malathion has had predictable effects—incomplete control (largely because of surviving indoor populations) and emergence of resistant strains. Until we recognize that the major source of the disease is the uncontrolled growth and dispersion of populations of this mosquito into new habitats, no feasible control is likely.

Past eradication efforts aimed at *A. aegypti* mosquitos were successful because their goal was restoring the ecological balance of natural predators and eliminating the standing water that is the mosquito's traditional breeding ground. In 1901, William Gorgas, then the sanitary engineer of Havana, successfully used such techniques to eradicate *Aedes* (also the carrier of yellow fever) in Cuba within 6 months. However, U.S. federal agencies see their only recourses as being the wholesale mobilization of citizens to take individual action to minimize contact with the mosquito and the development of a vaccine. But these avenues of protection fall far short of the revolutionary steps taken by Gorgas to limit the vec-

tor's access to populations through conversion of mosquito-breeding habitats and the introduction of natural predators (recently, the mosquito fish). Unfortunately, as both Lyme disease and dengue show, once ecological disturbance has occurred, the spread of a dangerous pathogen through a burgeoning vector population is extremely difficult to constrain.

How well we succeed in controlling this disease will determine in part our success in future efforts. We will not lack for new threats. A case in point is another mosquito-borne illness that also lurks just offshore of Florida. Eastern equine encephalitis (EEE) virus, the cause of a neurologically disabling illness among horses, has recently been found in another aedes strain (*A. albopictus*) in Florida, expanding its previous territory from southern Texas and Hawaii. Previously limited to Asia, as is its dengue-carrying counterpart, this species was probably also brought to the United States from Southeast Asian countries.

The Centers for Disease Control has now isolated sixteen different strains of newly recognized viruses of the arbovirus group (arthropod-borne viruses) from this mosquito. The EEE virus was among this group. Although this is presently the rarest mosquito-borne disease among humans in the United States, it is a potentially fatal illness, killing up to 30 percent of its victims. To their consternation, even as inspectors first discovered the mosquito among used tire shipments, they found that the EEE virus was already establishing itself in some bird species. . . .

Environmental disturbances are almost certainly at work today in shaping new patterns of disease and disability around the globe. Malaria has taken a startling upturn in Rwanda, a phenomenon linked to the global-warming-enhanced proliferation of its mosquito vectors. Seals fall ill in unprecedented numbers in Lake Baikal; dolphins succumb to a new bacterial illness that causes their skin to become as thin and weak as cellophane and their immune systems to fail; coral reefs die; sea urchins succumb to a new, temperature-dependent disease organism; and riverine fish develop tumors in epidemic proportion. These apparently "new" illnesses and epizootic infections all have the imprimateur of human activities that have radically disrupted the global environment. Inevitably, such massive die-offs are by their nature natural selective events. And whether their human counterparts in the form of our epidemics of AIDS, asthma, and tuberculosis will leave the next generation better prepared to resist these diseases than is the present one—or if we will need to depend solely on medical therapeutic interventions—remains to be seen. . . .

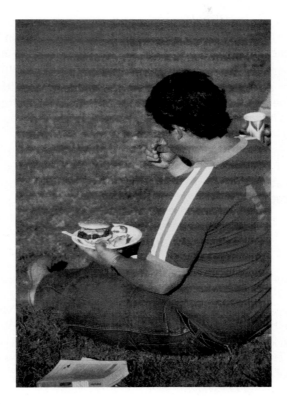

FIGURE 14–1 Obesity

One of the potentially serious public health concerns currently facing the American people is obesity. Because of changing lifestyles and workplace routines, the National Institutes of Health estimates that two-thirds of American adults are overweight and one-third are clinically obese—about 130 million people. Of even greater concern is the rapidly rising incidence of children and adolescents who are overweight—nearly 15 percent of all individuals aged 6 to 19 years.

KEY TERMS

Analgesia, 328 • Deontological, 320 • Dengue fever, 337 • Emerods, 325 • Empathic, 330 • Palliative, 329 • Sarin, 317 • Slurries, 326 • Tort, 322

QUESTIONS TO CONSIDER

1. What is your position on such controversial topics as cloning? Do any aspects of cloning research, such as stem cell research, have merit? If you were involved in a scholarly debate on cloning, what facts and evidence would you use to support your view? Be specific.

2. One of the concerns about the U.S. government's new regulations to combat terrorism has been the potential for infringement on privacy and personal freedoms. If a biowarfare incident occurred in a major city, what measures would you expect to see enforced? Would they limit personal freedom? If so, would the situation be yet another example of the public health maxim "The welfare of the many outweighs the freedom of the few," or would it be a special instance of the need for government control?

3. If you were alive in the year 2100, what would you list as the greatest accomplishments in medicine and related fields in the twenty-first century? Where do you think medicine is headed in the twenty-first century? What do you see as the most important obstacles that must be overcome?

4. What evidence do you see in Figure 14–1 that would explain the child's excess weight? What health problems would you expect to be future risk factors for him? Is obesity simply a matter of personal choice, or is it a problem with social, economic, and political ramifications?

RECOMMENDED READINGS

Barnett, Tony, and Alan Whiteside. *AIDS in the 21st Century: Disease and Globalization.* 2nd ed. New York: Palgrave Macmillan, 2003.

Beauchamp, Tom L. *Contemporary Issues in Bioethics.* Belmont, CA: Wadsworth, 2002.

Close, William T. *Ebola Through the Eyes of the People.* Big Piney, WY: Meadowlark Springs Production, 2001.

Cole, Leonard. *The Eleventh Plague: The Politics of Biological and Chemical Warfare.* New York: Freeman, 1997.

Donaldson, Robert M. *Yale Guide to Careers in Medicine and the Health Professions: Pathways to Medicine in the 21st Century.* Cambridge, MA: Yale University Press, 2003.

Farmer, Paul. *Infections and Inequalities: The Modern Plagues.* Berkeley: University of California Press, 2001.

Hunter, Susan. *Black Death: AIDS in Africa.* New York: Palgrave Macmillan, 2003.

Ludmerer, Kenneth M. *Time to Heal: American Medical Education from the Turn of the Century to the Era of Managed Care.* Oxford, UK: Oxford University Press, 1999.

Mangold, Tom, and Jeff Goldberg. *Plague Wars—The Terrifying Reality of Biological Warfare.* London: St. Martin's Press, 2001.

Peters, C. J. *The Virus Hunters: Thirty Years of Battling Hot Viruses Around the World.* New York: Anchor Books, 1998.

Rhodes, Richard. *Deadly Feasts: Tracking the Secrets of a Terrifying New Plague.* New York: Simon & Schuster, 1997.

Wilmut, Ian. *The Second Generation: Dolly and the Age of Biological Control.* Cambridge, MA: Harvard University Press, 2001.

Glossary

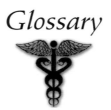

Acupuncture: Originally the Chinese practice of piercing specific points on the body to cure disease or relieve pain by restoring the flow of energy (*chi*)

Aflatoxin: Poison in molds that can cause liver cancer; endemic in developing countries

African sleeping sickness: Human and mammalian disease caused by *Trypanosoma brucei;* causes fatigue, coma, and eventual death

Agonal: Relating to the process of dying

Amaranth: New World herb cultivated as a food crop

Analgesia: Insensitivity to pain, even when fully conscious

Anamnesis: Patient history

Antiscorbutic: Remedy for scurvy

Apoplexy: Stroke; brain hemorrhage

A priori: Presupposed by evidence; presumptive

Arbovirus: Virus carried by arthropod vectors and transmitted through their saliva (e.g., yellow fever)

Ashipu: Babylonian exorcists who treated disease by driving out evil spirits

Astanga Hrdaya: One of the three major works composing Ayurvedic medicine, written about 500 B.C.E.; summary and clarification of Sushruta and Charaka samhitas, plus additional information

Atrabilious: Pertaining to black bile, the most dangerous of the four humors

Auscultation: Procedure for listening to sounds within the body

Avascular necrosis: Death of tissue due to lack of blood supply

Awelum: Upper class in ancient Babylon

Axilla: Underarm area

Ayurvedic, Ayurveda: Traditional system of Indian medicine, based on two texts written in the first through fourth centuries B.C.E.; emphasizes prevention, herbal cures, physiotherapy, and diet; still taught today

Azu: Physician-priests in ancient Babylon

Babesiosis: Rare but severe human illness caused by the protozoan *Babesia microti*

Baru: Ancient Babylonian diviners who interpreted omens and predicted the course and outcome of disease

Bilious, biliousness: In reference to the stomach —lack of appetite, constipation, headache; also, archaic term meaning *quick tempered*

Bluetongue: Viral infection of sheep, causing respiratory and gastrointestinal symptoms and a characteristic blue tongue

Bulbar: Pertaining to the medulla oblongata region of the brain stem that regulates respiration and cardiac function

Calculus: Solid substance, or "stone," which forms in the urinary tract

Capitation: Fixed amount of money paid to a hospital, clinic, or doctor for each person served; common method used by modern medical insurance companies to contain costs

Cerebral palsy: Brain disorder affecting motor skills, appearing before age 3 years

Chakras: Sanskrit term for several points of spiritual or physical energy in the human body

Charaka, Caraka: Indian author of the first of the great texts (samhitas); described hundreds of drugs and their uses for specific diseases; emphasized three forms of medicine: religious acts, diet and drugs, and psychic therapy

Chiropractic: System of diagnosis and healing based on the idea that health is related to the nervous system and can be treated by manipulation of the joints and spine

Chlorosis: Also known as *green disease;* a nineteenth-century diagnosis of a wasting disease of young women, characterized by pallor, weakness, palpitations, and anemia

Cineritial: Ashen

Colliers: Ships carrying coal

Confucian ethics: Branch of Confucius's philosophy emphasizing beneficence, humaneness, and nonmaleficence

Confucius (K'ung-Fu-tzu): Famous Chinese scholar and philosopher who emphasized benevolence, character, and virtue; had a strong influence on Chinese ethics

Conglutinations: Something glued together

Consumption: Nineteenth-century term for pulmonary tuberculosis

Coprolites: Fossilized feces; valuable evidence of the prehistoric diet

Couching: Ancient cataract surgery that displaced the lens out of the field of vision

Cranioplasties: Plastic surgery performed on the skull, often to correct a skull defect

Crush syndrome: Trauma to soft tissue due to a severe crushing injury, resulting in an obstructed blood supply; can cause a severe kidney reaction

Cyanobacteria: Blue-green algae

Defluxion: Fluid discharge, commonly from the nose

Dengue fever: Viral tropical disease transmitted by mosquitoes and preventable by immunization; in its hemorrhagic form, it is often fatal

Deontological: Pertaining to medical ethics

Depuration: Purification; removal of waste products

Diachronic: Occurring at several points in time

Diagenesis: Created in more than one place

Diagnostic Related Groups (DRGs): Classification of patients by diagnosis or surgical procedure for the purpose of determining payment of charges

Diathesis: Condition making a person unusually susceptible to a particular disease such as tuberculosis

Dinoflagellates: Aquatic photosynthetic organisms often found in marine plankton

Diploë: Soft, spongy substance between the plates of the skull

Doshas: Ayurvedic term for the three humors (vata, pitta, and kapha)

Dropsical: Having abnormal fluid retention, secondary to organ failure such as that of the kidneys or heart

Dyspepsia: Gastrointestinal distress, particularly after a large meal

Dyspnea: Shortness of breath; difficulty in breathing

Ecthyma: Large, inflamed skin pustules or pimples

Efflorescence: Blossoming

Elephantiasis: Skin disease causing thickening and roughening of the skin and swelling of the limbs

Emerods: Hemorrhoids

Empathic: Relating to a person's objective awareness of feelings and behaviors of others

Emunctory: Any organ that carries away waste material

Endemic: Agent of disease commonly present in a given population

Endogenous: Developing inside an organism

Enterovirus: Any virus that flourishes in the intestinal tract

Epidemics: Sudden outbreaks of disease, usually infectious, with excessive mortality and morbidity rates

Epistaxis: Nosebleed

Ergotism: Poisoning due to ingestion of rye or wheat infected with the fungus *Claviceps purpurea;* causes hallucinations, spasms, and dry gangrene; also known as *St. Anthony's Fire*

Erysipelatous: Having an acute disease involving fever and intense, local inflammation and swelling of the skin and subcutaneous tissues; caused by hemolytic streptococcus

Evisceration: Removal of the bowels

Exogenous: Developing outside an organism

Filial piety: One of the key concepts of Confucianism; requires reverence of elders and ancestors

Five Elements, Five Phases: In Chinese medical theory, fire, earth, metal, water, and wood; linked in cycles of creation and destruction (e.g., earth is the source of metal; water puts out fire)

Five viscera: In traditional Chinese medicine, the five solid organs (heart, lungs, liver, spleen, and kidneys), which are connected with other five-based elements such as climate, flavors, and spiritual resources in the basic concept of systematic correspondence

Flux: Dysentery; bloody diarrhea

Fornon: Forenoon; morning

Fuliginous and mordicant: Murky and acrid

Gallabu: Babylonian barbers who did slave brandings and dental and surgical procedures

Glanders: Contagious disease of horses and mules; can be transmitted to sheep, dogs, and humans

Hansen's disease: Modern name for a disease historically known as *leprosy*

Harris lines: Lines parallel to growth plates in long bones; indicate slowing or stoppage of growth

Hemiplegia: Paralysis of one side of the body

Hemostasis: Stopping active bleeding, either through constriction and coagulation or surgically

Hepatoscopy: Ancient method of forecasting the future based on examination of entrails—especially the liver—of sacrificial animals

Homeostasis: Stable condition in a normal body

Humors: Four fluids (blood, phlegm, yellow bile, and black bile) postulated by Hippocrates (and later) to make up the body in ancient times, the balance of which determines health and temperament; imbalance of any one of the humors was thought to cause disease

Hyperandrogenism: Excessive production of the male hormone androgen in women

Hyperplasia: Abnormal increase in the number of normal cells in tissue

Iatrochemistry: Medical school of thought that explains disease and health on the basis of the chemical properties of the body

Ichorous: Thin, watery discharge from a wound or tumor

Igneity: Fiery

Intercostals: Spaces between the ribs

Intermittent fever: Nineteenth-century diagnostic term for a fever that recurs after a period of normal temperature (e.g., malaria)

Kapha: "Phlegm"; term in Indian medicine for a substance that provides a fluid that makes the body hold together; one of the three doshas

Leishmaniasis: Also known as *kala-azar;* parasitic disease involving the skin, mucous membranes, and organs

Mandible: Jawbone

Mandragora: Mandrake plant; its root is used as an aid to contraception or as a treatment for insomnia

Marmas: Vital body points in Indian medicine where muscles, blood vessels, and joints come together

Materia medica: General term for all substances used as curative agents

Metastatic: Spread of a disease from one organ or tissue to another part of the body

Motor cortex: Area of the frontal lobe of the brain responsible for primary motor control

Moxibustion: Chinese treatment based on the use of cups or cones placed on the skin, in which certain herbs are burned, at key acupuncture points

Mushkenum: Middle class; freemen in ancient Babylon

Mycotoxins: Poisonous substances produced by mold

Myeloma: Malignant tumor composed of bone marrow cells

Myocardial infarction: Heart attack with irreversible injury to heart muscle

Nei Ching: Also known as *The Yellow Emperor's Classic of Internal Medicine;* a key Chinese text fundamental to all Chinese medical practices; written as a dialogue between Emperor Huang Ti and his minister of health and healing, Ch'i Po; explains the whole Chinese medical philosophy, including the concepts of yin and yang, pulse theory, and acupuncture

Neoplasms: New and abnormal tissue growths, either benign or malignant

Neuroblastoma: Malignancy of childhood that attacks spinal nerves

Non-naturals: Galen's term for health factors that a patient can control, such as food and drink, rest, exercise, and so forth

Nosocomial: Acquired in a hospital; nosocomial infections are more common in patients but can also affect staff

Nosologic, nosology: Classification of diseases

Oliguria: Diminished urine production

Ossification: Formation of bone or bony substance, or conversion of cartilage to bone

Osteitis: Inflammation of the bone

Osteoporosis: Reduced bone mass leading to fragile and brittle bones easily damaged by only minor trauma

Oxymel: Mixture of honey, water, vinegar, and spices

Paleopathology: Study of ancient disease and trauma through examination of fossilized remains

Palliative: Affording relief but not cure

Palsied: A condition marked by uncontrollable tremor of the body, or of a body part.

Pandemics: Epidemics affecting a wide geographic area

Parietal craniectomies: Neurosurgical procedures in which parts of the parietal bone are removed for access to the brain but are not replaced

Patent medicine: More properly a proprietary medicine; over-the-counter preparation

Peripubertal: Near puberty

Phagedenic: Ulcerative

Phrenitis: Inflammation of the brain, accompanied by high fever and delirium

Phthysis: Archaic term for tuberculosis

Pica: Appetite for abnormal substances (e.g., earth, coal, chalk)

Pitta: "Bile"; term in Indian medicine for the humor responsible for all metabolic functions; one of the three doshas

Pledgets: Compresses or pads

Pleurisy: Inflammation of the membrane lining the lungs

Polypharmacological: Involving a prescription composed of many, often excessive, ingredients

Postpolio sequelae: Also called *postpolio syndrome;* new symptoms appearing years after the initial polio attack, causing further loss of muscle function, joint pain, and fatigue

Pránahara: "Seats of Life"; network of vital points in the body (marmas), which, according to Sushruta, will cause pain, illness, or death if injured

Prodrome: Early symptom of disease

Prolapse: Fallen; displaced

Puerperal: Pertaining to childbirth

Puerperal fever: Also known as *childbed fever;* postpartum sepsis; often fatal

The Pulse Classic: Famous Chinese text by Wand Shu he, which set forth the basic principles of pulse theory essential to traditional Chinese medicine

Quinsy: Inflammation of the throat with fever and difficulty swallowing; can cause suffocation

Ramayana: One of two great epic poems of India, composed in Sanskrit about 300 B.C.E.

Remittent fever: Nineteenth-century term for a fever that varies during a twenty-four-hour period; most fevers are remittent

Rheumatic fever: Disease involving joint inflammation and damage to the heart following streptococcal infection

Rhinoplasty: Plastic surgery of the nose to correct a deformity or replace lost tissue

Rigveda: Collection of hymns forming a part of the Indian sacred literature called *Vedas*

Roentgenography: Radiography; making film images of internal structures by using x-rays or gamma rays

Salmonelloses: Bacterial diseases caused by ingestion of contaminated food, characterized by severe gastrointestinal symptoms; sometimes called *food poisoning*

Samhita: One of three texts that compose the fundamentals of Ayurvedic medicine; written by semilegendary authors

Sanitaria, sanitarium: Institutions, usually private, for recovery of specific diseases or conditions such as tuberculosis or alcholism

Sarin: Extremely toxic gaseous chemical-warfare agent

Schistosomiasis: Also known as *bilharzia,* or *snail fever;* spread by worms carried by water snails; endemic in parts of Africa and South America

Shang oracle bones: Animal bones used in Bronze Age China to communicate with the dead in order to predict the future

Slurries: Watery mixtures of insoluble materials such as mud

Solarium: Glass-enclosed room or porch used for therapeutic exposure to the sun

Solipsism: Philosophy that the self is the only thing that truly exists

Spina bifida: Congenital spinal defect in which the spinal cord may protrude

Subdural hematomas: Blood clots on the surface of the brain underneath the dural membrane, usually the result of head trauma

Surra: Protozoan disease of horses, mules, dogs, and cattle; found in Africa, Asia, and the Americas; spread by bloodsucking flies

Sushruta: Ayurvedic surgeon-author; his text (samhita) is the most recent of the three samhitas, dealing with surgical procedures such as couching, rhinoplasty, lithotomy, and amputations

Sutures (of the skull): Lines where the bones of the skull unite

Tachycardia: Rapid heartbeat

Tachypnea: Rapid, shallow breathing

Taoism, Taoist: Daoism; Chinese philosophy centered on nature and following the way (Dao) that it demonstrates, found through meditation and observation

Taphonomic, taphonomy: Study of processes affecting plant and animal remains as they fossilize

Theriacs: Ancient compound remedies using dozens, even hundreds, of substances

Thoracic: Related to the chest

Tonic-clonic: Type of seizure that causes loss of consciousness, muscle contractions, and tongue biting; also known as *grand mal*

Torpor: Inactivity; sluggishness

Tort: Wrongful act for which damages may be awarded

Travil: Travail; in active labor

Treatment modalities: Methods of treatment

Trephining: Removing a circular portion of the skull; also called *trepanation*

Trichothecenes: Chemicals produced by fungus and some plants that can contaminate food and cause vomiting, bleeding in the lungs and brain, and damage to bone marrow

Turbid: Cloudy; full of sediment

Uremic: Pertaining to the kidneys or the urinary system

Valetudinarium: Hospital

Vata: "Wind"; term in Indian medicine for the humor responsible for all motor activity; one of the three doshas

Váyu: "Air"; another word for *vata*

Vedas, Vedic: Ancient oral epics and sacred hymns and verses in India; date from 1500 B.C.E. to 500 B.C.E.

Venesection: Bloodletting; phlebotomy; opening a vein to allow blood to flow

Vesical: Pertaining to the bladder

Virilization: Becoming more masculine

Wardum: Male and female slaves in Babylon

Yin and yang: In Eastern philosophy, two complementary forces or principles that make up all aspects of life (e.g., hot-cold, male-female)

Photo Credits

p. ii *Frontispiece:* Courtesy of the Library of Congress; p. 58 *Figure 3–1:* Art Resource/ Reunion des Musees Nationaux; p. 138 *Figure 7–1:* Bildarchiv Preussischer Kulterbesitz/Art Resource, New York; p. 164 *Figure 8–1:* Library of Congress; p. 164 *Figure 8–2:* The Granger Collection, New York; p. 165 *Figure 8–3:* National Library of Medicine; p. 165 *Figure 8–4:* The Granger Collection, New York; p. 166 *Figure 8–5:* National Library of Medicine; p. 166 *Figure 8–6:* The Granger Collection, New York; p. 167 *Figure 8–7:* National Library of Medicine; p. 167 *Figure 8–8:* The heart and the circulation, facsimile of the Windsor book (pen and ink on paper), Vinci, Leonardo da (1452–1519) (after)/Bibliotheque des Arts Decoratifs, Paris, France, Archives Charmet/Bridgeman Art Library International; p. 210 *Figure 10–1:* Army Military History Institute; p. 219 *Figure 10–2:* Corbis/Bettmann; p. 253 *Figure 11–1:* Courtesy of the Library of Congress; p. 300 *Figure 13–1:* © Bettmann/Corbis; p. 313 *Figure 13–2:* Ellen McCurley—The Pendulum Project; p. 339 *Figure 14–1:* Robert E. Daemmrich/Getty Images Inc.—Stone Allstock.